W0105737

Ataxia-Telangiectasia

NATO ASI Series

Advanced Science Institutes Series

A series presenting the results of activities sponsored by the NATO Science Committee, which aims at the dissemination of advanced scientific and technological knowledge, with a view to strengthening links between scientific communities.

The Series is published by an international board of publishers in conjunction with the NATO Scientific Affairs Division

A Life Sciences	Plenum Publishing Corporation
B Physics	London and New York
C Mathematical and Physical Sciences	Kluwer Academic Publishers Dordrecht, Boston and London
D Behavioural and Social Sciences	
E Applied Sciences	
F Computer and Systems Sciences	Springer-Verlag Berlin Heidelberg New York
G Ecological Sciences	London Paris Tokyo Hong Kong
H Cell Biology	Barcelona Budapest
I Global Environmental Change	

NATO-PCO DATABASE

The electronic index to the NATO ASI Series provides full bibliographical references (with keywords and/or abstracts) to more than 30 000 contributions from international scientists published in all sections of the NATO ASI Series. Access to the NATO-PCO DATABASE compiled by the NATO Publication Coordination Office is possible in two ways:

- via online FILE 128 (NATO-PCO DATABASE) hosted by ESRIN, Via Galileo Galilei, I-00044 Frascati, Italy.

- via CD-ROM "NATO Science & Technology Disk" with user-friendly retrieval software in English, French and German (© WTV GmbH and DATAWARE Technologies Inc. 1992).

The CD-ROM can be ordered through any member of the Board of Publishers or through NATO-PCO, Overijse, Belgium.

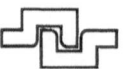

Series H: Cell Biology, Vol. 77

Ataxia-Telangiectasia

Edited by

Richard A. Gatti

Department of Pathology
University of California Los Angeles
School of Medicine
Los Angeles, CA 90024-6975, USA

Robert B. Painter

Laboratory of Radiobiology and Environmental Health
University of California San Francisco
San Francisco, CA 94143-0750, USA

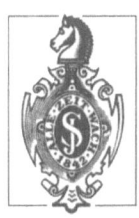

Springer-Verlag
Berlin Heidelberg New York London Paris Tokyo
Hong Kong Barcelona Budapest
Published in cooperation with NATO Scientific Affairs Division

Proceedings of the NATO Advanced Research Workshop on Ataxia-Telangiectasia, held at Newport Beach, CA, USA, May 17–20, 1992

ISBN 978-3-642-78280-0   ISBN 978-3-642-78278-7 (eBook)
DOI 10.1007/978-3-642-78278-7

Library of Congress Cataloging-in-Publication Data.
Ataxia-telangiectasia / edited by Richard A. Gatti, Robert B. Painter. p. cm. – (NATO ASI series. Series H. Cell biology; vol. 77)
"Proceedings of the NATO Advanced Research Workshop on Ataxia-Telangiectasia, held at Newport Beach, CA, USA, May 17-20, 1992" – T.p. verso. "Published in cooperation with the NATO Scientific Affairs Division." Includes bibliographical references and index.

1. Ataxia telangiectasia–Congresses. I. Gatti, Richard A. II. Painter, Robert B. III. North Atlantic Treaty Organization. Scientific Affairs Division. IV. NATO Advanced Research Workshop on Ataxia-Telangiectasia (1992: Newport Beach, Calif.) V. Series. [DNLM: 1. Ataxia Telangiectasia–congresses. WL 320 A8618 1992] RC607.A83A84 1993 618.92'683–dc20 DNLM/DLC for Library of Congress 93-20625

This work is subject to copyright. All rights are reserved, whether the whole or part of the material is concerned, specifically the rights of translation, reprinting, reuse of illustrations, recitation, broadcasting, reproduction on microfilm or in any other way, and storage in data banks. Duplication of this publication or parts thereof is permitted only under the provisions of the German Copyright Law of September 9, 1965, in its current version, and permission for use must always be obtained from Springer-Verlag. Violations are liable for prosecution under the German Copyright Law.

© Springer-Verlag Berlin Heidelberg 1993
Softcover reprint of the hardcover 1st edition 1993

Typesetting: Camera ready by authors
31/3145 - 5 4 3 2 1 0 - Printed on acid-free paper

DEDICATION

To Debby

DEDICATION

CONTENTS

CONTRIBUTORS

PREFACE
   Richard A. Gatti and Robert B. Painter

PART I. INTRODUCTION

ATW5 PARTICIPANTS (Photo)

BRIEF HISTORICAL OVERVIEW
   Robert P. Sedgwick 1

PART II. ISOLATION OF A-T GENE(S)

**Cloning and characterization of a candidate gene for A-T
complementation Group D**
Leon N. Kapp and John P. Murnane 7

**Precise localization of a gene responsible for ataxia-
telangiectasia on chromosome 11q**
*F. Cornelis, Michael James, D. Cherif, Takashi Tokino, J.
Davies, D. Girault, C. Bernard, M.F. Croquette, D. Theau, H.
Avet-Loiseau, Michael Litt, R. Berger, Yusuke Nakamura, Mark
Lathrop and Cecille Julier* 23

How many A-T genes?
*Ethan Lange, Richard A. Gatti, Eric Sobel, Patrick Concannon
and Kenneth Lange* 37

**Isolation of human cDNAs that complement the ataxia-
telangiectasia phenotype in cultured fibroblasts**
*M. Stephen Meyn, Jennifer M. Lu-Kuo and Laura B.K.
Herzing* 55

Complementation of the cellular A-T phenotype by gene transfer
*Yael Ziv, Tsafi Danieli, Galit Rotman, Adam Sartiel, Anat Bar-
Shira, Nicholas G.J. Jaspers, Richard Swirski, Robert T.
Schimke, Roger L. Eddy, Thomas B. Shows and Yosef
Shiloh* 65

**Use of microcell hybrids for analysis of the 11q23 region and
improved localization of the A-T Group A/C genes**
Yusuke Ejima, Mitsuo Oshimura and Masao S. Sasaki 75

**AT-like radiosensitive rodent cell mutants: an alternative
approach to the isolation of the A-T gene(s)**
*Margaret Z. Zdzienicka, Gerald W C T Verhaegh, Wim Jongmans,
Nicholas G.J. Jaspers, Mitsuo Oshimura, Michael R. James and
Paul H.M. Lohman* 87

PART III. A-T HETEROZYGOTES AND COMPLEMENTATION

Identification of A-T heterozygotes
David Scott, Lucy A Jones, Sean A G Elyan, Ann Spreadborough,
Richard Cowan and Gerald Ribiero 101

Correction of post-gamma ray DNA repair deficiency in ataxia-telangiectasia complementation group A fibroblasts by cocultivation with normal fibroblasts
Malcolm C. Paterson and Razmik Mirzayans 117

The A-T gene does not make a major contribution to familial breast cancer
Richard Wooster, Douglas F. Easton, Deborah Ford, Jonathan
Mangion, Bruce A.J. Ponder, Julian Peto and Michael
Stratton 127

Mammography screening for A-T heterozygotes
Amos Norman and Rodney Withers 137

PART IV. DEFINING THE A-T DEFECT

Lymphoid V(D)J recombination: accessibility and reaction fidelity in normal and ataxia-telangiectasia cells
Chih-Lin Hsieh and Michael R. Lieber 143

Murine scid cells and human ataxia-telangiectasia cells complement each other's radiosensitivity
Kenshi Komatsu 155

Ataxia-telangiectasia: defective in a p53-dependent signal transduction pathway
Michael B. Kastan 163

DNA recombination in the transgenic mouse brain
Linda Kingsbury and Itoshi Sakano 175

PART V. A-T VARIANTS

Clinical variants of ataxia-telangiectasia
Ozden Sanal, A. Izzet Berkel, Fugen Ersoy, Ilhan Tezcan and
Haluk Topaloglu 183

Epidemiology of ataxia-telangiectasia in Italy
Luciana Chessa and Massimo Fiorilli 191

Epidemiology of ataxia-telangiectasia in Costa Rica
Oscar Porras, Olga Arguendas, Margarita Arata, Max Barrantes,
Luis Gonzalez and Elizabeth Saenz 199

Clinical and cellular heterogeneity in ataxia-telangiectasia
A. Malcolm R. Taylor, Carmel M. McConville and C. Geoffrey
Woods, Phillip J. Byrd and Diana Hernandez 209

PART VI.   OVERVIEWS

Biochemical defects in ataxia-telangiectasia
Martin F. Lavin *235*

Radiobiology of ataxia-telangiectasia
Robert B. Painter *257*

Treatment of ataxia-telangiectasia
Susan L. Perlman *269*

INDEX *279*

CONTRIBUTORS

Margarita Arata, Departments of Immunology and Oncology, National Children's Hospital, Apartado 1654 1000 San Jose, Costa Rica

Olga Arguendas, Departments of Immunology and Oncology, National Children's Hospital, Apartado 1654 1000 San Jose, Costa Rica

H. Avet-Loiseau, Unite d'Hematologie Pediatrique, CHR, Nantes, France

Anat Bar-Shira, Department of Human Genetics, Sackler School of Medicine, Tel Aviv University, Ramat Aviv 69978, Israel

Max Barrantes, Departments of Immunology and Oncology, National Children's Hospital, Apartado 1654 1000 San Jose, Costa Rica

R Berger, INSERM U301, 27 rue Juliette Dodu, Paris 75010, France

A. Izzet Berkel, Division of Pediatric Immunology, Hacettepe University Medical School, Ankara, Turkey

C Bernard, Department of Medical Genetics, Oregon Health Sciences University, Portland, Oregon, USA

Phillip J. Byrd, CRC Department of Cancer Studies, The Medical School, University of Birmingham, Edgbaston, Birmingham B15 2TT, UK

D. Cherif, INSERM U301, 27 rue Juliette Dodu, Paris 75010, France

Luciana Chessa, Dipartimento di Medicina Sperimentale, University "La Sapienza", Viale Regina Elena 324, 00161 Roma, Italy

Patrick Concannon, Virginia Mason Research Center, Seattle, WA 98101, USA

F Cornelis, Centre d'Etude du Polymorphism Humain, 27 rue Juliette Dodu, Paris 75010, France

Richard Cowan, Department of Clinical Oncology, Christie Hospital NHS Trust, Manchester M20 9BX, UK

M.F. Croquette, Hopital Saint-Antoine, Lille, France

Tsafi Danieli, Department of Human Genetics, Sackler School of Medicine, Tel Aviv University, Ramat Aviv 69978, Israel

J Davies, Centre d'Etude du Polymorphism Humain, 27 rue Juliette Dodu, Paris 75010, France

Douglas F. Easton, Section of Epidemiology, Institute of Cancer Research, 15 Cotswold Road, Sutton, Surrey, SM2 5NG, UK

Roger L. Eddy, Department of Human Genetics, Roswell Park Cancer Institute, Buffalo, NY 14263, USA

Yusuke Ejima, Radiation Biology Center, Kyoto University, Yoshida-konoecho, Sakyo-Ku, Kyoto 606 Japan

Sean AG Elyan, CRC Department of Experimental Radiation Oncology, Paterson Institute for Cancer Research, Manchester M20 9BX, UK

Fugen Ersoy, Division of Pediatric Immunology, Hacettepe University Medical School, Ankara, Turkey

Massimo Fiorilli, Istituto di Clinica Medica III, University "La Sapienza", Viale Regina Elena 324, 00161 Roma, Italy

Deborah Ford, Section of Epidemiology, Institute of Cancer Research, 15 Cotswold Road, Sutton, Surrey, SM2 5NG, UK

Richard A. Gatti, Department of Pathology, UCLA School of Medicine, Los Angeles, CA 90024-6975, USA

D Girault, Service d'Immunologie Pediatrique, Hopital Necker, Paris, France

Luis Gonzalez, Departments of Immunology and Oncology, National Children's Hospital, Apartado 1654 1000 San Jose, Costa Rica

Diana Hernandez, CRC Department of Cancer Studies, The Medical School, University of Birmingham, Edgbaston, Birmingham B15 2TT, UK

Laura B.K. Herzing, Department of Pediatrics, Yale University School of Medicine, 333 Cedar Street, New Haven, CT 06510, USA

Chih-Lin Hsieh, Laboratory of Experimental Oncology, Department of Pathology, Stanford University School of Medicine, Stanford, CA 94305-5324 USA

Michael R. James, Centre d'Etude du Polymorphism Humain, 27 rue Juliette Dodu, Paris 75010, France

Nicholas G.J. Jaspers, Department of Cell Biology and Genetics, Erasmus University, 3000 DR Rotterdam, Netherlands

Lucy A Jones, CRC Department of Cancer Genetics, Paterson Institute for Cancer Research, Manchester M20 9BX, UK

Wim Jongmans, MGC Department of Radiation Genetics and Chemical Mutagenesis, State University of Leiden and J.A. Cohen Institute, Interuniversity Research institute for Radiopathology and Radiation Protection, Wassenaarseweg 72 2333 AL Leiden, The Netherlands

Cecille Julier, Centre d'Etude du Polymorphism Humain, 27 rue Juliette Dodu, Paris 75010, France

Leon N. Kapp, Laboratory of Radiobiology and Environmental Health, Box 0750, University of California, San Francisco, San Francisco, CA 94143, USA

Michael B. Kastan, Department of Oncology, Johns Hopkins University School of Medicine, 600 N. Wolfe Street, Baltimore, MD 21287, USA

Linda Kingsbury, Division of Immunology, Department of Molecular and Cell Biology, University of California, Berkeley, California 94720, USA

Kenshi Komatsu, Radiation Biophysics, Atomic Disease Institute, Nagasaki University School of Medicine, Sakamoto-machi, Nagasaki 852, Japan

Ethan Lange, Departments of Pathology and Mathematics, UCLA School of Medicine, Los Angeles, CA 90024-6975, USA

Kenneth Lange, Department of Biomathematics, UCLA School of Medicine, Los Angeles, CA 90024-6975, USA

Mark Lathrop, Centre d'Etude du Polymorphism Humain, 27 rue Juliette Dodu, Paris 75010, France

Martin F. Lavin, Queensland Cancer Fund Research Unit, Queensland Institute of Medical Research, The Bancroft Centre, 300 Berston Road, Brisbane QLD 4029, Australia

Michael R. Lieber, Laboratory of Experimental Oncology, Department of Pathology, Stanford University School of Medicine, Stanford, CA 94305-5324 USA

Michael Litt, Department of Medical Genetics, Oregon Health Sciences University, Portland, Oregon, USA

Paul H.M. Lohman, MGC Department of Radiation Genetics and Chemical Mutagenesis, State University of Leiden and J.A. Cohen Institute, Interuniversity Research institute for Radiopathology and Radiation Protection, Wassenaarseweg 72 2333 AL Leiden, The Netherlands

Jennifer M. Lu-Kuo, Department of Pediatrics, Yale University School of Medicine, 333 Cedar Street, New Haven, CT 06510, USA

Jonathan Mangion, Section of Molecular Carcinogenesis, Institute of Cancer Research, 15 Cotswold Road, Sutton, Surrey SM2 5NG, UK

Carmel M. McConville, CRC Department of Cancer Studies, The Medical School, University of Birmingham, Edgbaston, Birmingham B15 2TT, UK

M. Stephen Meyn, Department of Genetics, Yale University School of Medicine, 333 Cedar Street, New Haven, CT 06510, USA

Razmik Mirzayans, Molecular Oncology Program, Department of Medicine, Cross Cancer Institute, 11560 University Avenue, Edmonton, Alberta T6G 1Z2, Canada

John P. Murnane, Laboratory of Radiobiology and Environmental Health, Box 0750, University of California, San Francisco, San Francisco, CA 94143, USA

Yusuke Nakamura, Department of Biochemistry, Cancer Institute, Kami-Ikebukuro, Tokyo, Japan

Amos Norman, Department of Radiation Oncology, UCLA School of Medicine, Los Angeles, CA 90024-6975, USA

Mitsuo Oshimura, Department of Molecular and Cell Genetics, School of Life Sciences, Tottori University, Nishimachi 86, Yonago 683, Japan

Robert B. Painter, Laboratory of Radiobiology and Environmental Health, Box 0750, University of California, San Francisco, San Francisco, CA 94143, USA

Malcolm C. Paterson, Molecular Oncology Program, Department of Medicine, Cross Cancer Institute, 11560 University Avenue, Edmonton, Alberta T6G 1Z2, Canada

Susan L.Perlman, Department of Neurology, UCLA School of Medicine, Los Angeles, CA 90024-6975, USA

Julian Peto, Section of Epidemiology, Institute of Cancer Research, 15 Cotswold Road, Sutton, Surrey, SM2 5NG, UK

Bruce AJ Ponder, CRC Human Cancer Genetics Research Group, University of Cambridge, Tennis Court Road, Cambridge, CB2 1QP, UK

Oscar Porras, Departments of Immunology and Oncology, National Children's Hospital, Apartado 1654 1000 San Jose, Costa Rica

Gerald Ribiero, Department of Clinical Oncology, Christie Hospital NHS Trust, Manchester M20 9BX, UK

Galit Rotman, Department of Human Genetics, Sackler School of Medicine, Tel Aviv University, Ramat Aviv 69978, Israel

Elizabeth Saenz, Departments of Immunology and Oncology, National Children's Hospital, Apartado 1654 1000 San Jose, Costa Rica

Hitoshi Sakano, Division of Immunology, Department of Molecular and Cell Biology, University of California, Berkeley, California 94720, USA

Ozden Sanal, Division of Pediatric Immunology, Hacettepe University Medical School, Ankara, Turkey

Adam Sartiel, Department of Human Genetics, Sackler School of Medicine, Tel Aviv University, Ramat Aviv 69978, Israel

Masao S. Sasaki, Radiation Biology Center, Kyoto University, Yoshida-konoecho, Sakyo-Ku, Kyoto 606 Japan

Robert T. Schimke, Department of Biological Sciences, Stadford University, Stanford, CA 94305-5020, USA

David Scott, CRC Department of Cancer Genetics, Paterson Institute for Cancer Research, Manchester M20 9BX, UK

Robert P. Sedgwick, 1136 West Sixth Street, #711, Los Angeles, CA 90025, USA

Yosef Shiloh, Department of Human Genetics, Sackler School of Medicine, Tel Aviv University, Ramat Aviv 69978, Israel

Thomas B. Shows, Department of Human Genetics, Roswell Park Cancer Institute, Buffalo, NY 14263, USA

Eric Sobel, Department of Biomathematics, UCLA School of Medicine, Los Angeles, CA 90024-6975, USA

Ann Spreadborough, CRC Department of Cancer Genetics, Paterson Institute for Cancer Research, Manchester M20 9BX, UK

Michael Stratton, Section of Molecular Carcinogenesis, Institute of Cancer Research, 15 Cotswold Road, Sutton, Surrey SM2 5NG, UK

Richard Swirski, Department of Biological Sciences, Stanford University, Stanford, CA 94305-5020, USA

A. Malcolm R. Taylor, CRC Department of Cancer Studies, The Medical School, University of Birmingham, Edgbaston, Birmingham B15 2TT, UK

Ilhan Tezcan, Division of Pediatric Immunology, Hacettepe University Medical School, Ankara, Turkey

D. Theau, 18, rue d'Aiguillon, Brest, France

Takashi Tokino, Department of Biochemistry, Cancer Institute, Kami-Ikebukuro, Tokyo, Japan

Haluk Topaloglu, Division of Neurology, Hacettepe University Medical School, Ankara, Turkey

Gerald WCT Verhaegh, MGC Department of Radiation Genetics and Chemical Mutagenesis, State University of Leiden and J.A. Cohen Institute, Interuniversity Research institute for Radiopathology and Radiation Protection, Wassenaarseweg 72 2333 AL Leiden, The Netherlands

Rodney Withers, Department of Radiation Oncology, UCLA School of Medicine, Los Angeles, CA 90024-6975, USA

C. Geoffrey Woods, Department of Clinical Genetics, Churchill Hospital, Headington, Oxford OX3 7LJ, UK

Richard Wooster, Section of Molecular Carcinogenesis, Institute of Cancer Research, 15 Cotswold Road, Sutton, Surrey SM2 5NG, UK

Margaret Z. Zdzienicka, MGC Department of Radiation Genetics and Chemical Mutagenesis, State University of Leiden and J.A. Cohen Institute, Interuniversity Research institute for Radiopathology and Radiation Protection, Wassenaarseweg 72 2333 AL Leiden, The Netherlands

Yael Ziv, Department of Human Genetics, Sackler School of Medicine, Tel Aviv University, Ramat Aviv 69978, Israel

PREFACE

The chapters included in this volume were based on the material presented at the Fifth International Workshop (ATW5), which took place in Newport Beach, California, May 17-20, 1992. However, these are not the *proceedings*. The participants were not asked to arrive at the workshop with manuscripts in hand, in which case the chapters would only reflect what was known about A-T before May 1992. Nor were individual reimbursements withheld until manuscripts were submitted, an interesting ploy sometimes used by organizers of workshops to encourage cooperation in meeting book deadlines. Instead, on the last day of the workshop, some participants were invited to write either a "position paper" or an overview on the area of A-T research that they knew best. While a deadline of two months was suggested, and adhered to by many, other chapters arrived much later, some even after the new year began. But since each senior author was selected to serve a unique function in escorting the curious reader through the complexity of the A-T phenotype, as of early 1993, it was important to wait for the very "last but not least".

The waiting period provided an opportunity for each investigator to mull over what transpired at ATW5 and shortly thereafter. It also allowed certain key experiments to be confirmed or extended. Kapp and coworkers were able to supply further insight into the nature of their ATDC gene. Lange *et al* reanalyzed the linkage evidence for genetic heterogeneity; this analysis was unfortunately not ready at the time of ATW5. Kastan's work on cell cycle responses of irradiated A-T cells was not presented at ATW5 but was included in this volume because of its potential importance in further defining the A-T defect. The five chapters describing and discussing A-T variants (Lange *et al*, Sanal *et al*, Chessa and Fiorilli, Porras *et al*, and Taylor *et al*) reflect a certain optimism that it will soon be possible to begin correlating specific genetic mutations with clinical variations.

This volume cannot bring the reader up to date on the fine mapping and positional cloning of the A-T gene(s). That work is moving faster than the publication process. It is also highly technical, filled with now irrelevant false starts and failed experiments, and is somewhat proprietary.

The cloned A-T gene(s) will be a sort of biological "rosetta stone". The A-T gene promises to translate into a single common denominator for such otherwise unrelated phenomena as the cell cycle defects, failure of the thymus to develop, specific chromosomal translocation breakpoints, cancer susceptibility, radiosensitivity, and cerebellar degeneration. It will provide insight into DNA repair/processing, mechanisms of somatic gene rearrangement, and mitotic recombination (there is still no evidence for increased *meiotic* recombination). The issue of whether A-T mutations can lead to breast cancer will be resolved. Cancer patients who experience side-reactions to conventional doses of radiation therapy can be tested for A-T mutations. The A-T families will be rewarded for their moral and financial support of A-T research over the past ten years if an effective treatment, or cure, can be found for the progressive ataxia that so debilitates A-T sufferers. Finally, through understanding the function of the A-T protein, it may be possible to develop a radioprotective agent that could be used to shield normal tissues during radiotherapy -- or perhaps even to shield a city or countryside (animals included) from the radiation threat of a nuclear accident, such as Chernobyl?

The volume ends with three overviews: biochemical defects in A-T (Lavin), the radiobiology of A-T (Painter), and supportive treatment for A-T patients (in the absence of a specific treatment!)(Perlman). These overviews are intended to invite the uninitiated reader to take a fresh look at the evidence and perhaps develop some new insights for unravelling, or effectively treating, this challenging disease entity.

14 March 1993   **Editors**

I. Introduction

Participants of the Fifth International Workshop on Ataxia-Telangiectasia, May 17-20, 1992, Newport Beach, CA, USA

Albertini, Richard (Burlington, USA)
Arlett, Colin (Brighton, UK)
Bedilion, Tod (UCLA-Molecular Biology)
Bick, Miriam (UCLA-Pathology)
Boder, Elena (Los Angeles, USA)
Byrd, Phillip (Birmingham, UK)
Charmley, Patrick (Seattle, USA)
Chen, Philip (Brisbane, Australia)
Chen, Xiaoguang (UCLA-Pathology)
Chessa, Luciana (Rome, Italy)
Chiang, Chi-shiun (UCLA-Radiation Oncology)
Chiplunkar, Sujata (UCLA-Pathology)
Concannon, Patrick (Seattle, USA)
Cook, Robert (UCLA-Biomedical Physics)
Croce, Carlo (Philadelphia, USA)
Ejima, Yosuke (Kyoto, Japan)
Gatti, Richard (UCLA - Pathology)
Grody, Wayne (UCLA-Pathology)
Haile, Robert (UCLA- Public Health)
Hernandez, Diana (Birmingham, UK)
Herzing, Laura (New Haven, USA)
Hong, Ji-Hong (UCLA-Radiation Oncology)
Hsieh, Chih-Lin (Stanford, USA)
Huo, Yong (UCLA-Pathology)
James, Michael (Paris, France)
Jaspers, Nicholas (Rotterdam, Netherlands)
Kaleita, Thomas (UCLA-Pediatric Neurology)
Kapp, Leon (San Francisco, USA)
Kingsbury, Linda (Berkeley, USA)
Komatsu, Kenshi (Nagasaki, Japan)
Lange, Ethan (UCLA-Pathology
Lange, Kenneth (UCLA-Biomathematics)
Lavin, Martin (Brisbane, Australia)
Lewensohn, Rolf (Stockholm, Sweden)
Li, Fred (Boston, USA)
Lieber, Michael (Stanford, USA)
Lynn, William (Galveston, USA)
McBride, William (UCLA-Radiation Oncology)
McConville, Carmel (Birmingham, UK)
McCurdy, Deborah (Irvine, USA)
McElligott, David (San Diego, USA)
Meyn, Stephen (New Haven, USA)
Murnane, John (San Francisco, USA)
Painter, Robert (San Francisco, USA)
Paterson, Malcolm (Edmonton, Canada)
Perlman, Susan (UCLA-Neurology)
Peterson, Raymond (Mobile, USA)
Porras, Oscar (San Jose, Costa Rica)
Puckett, Carmie (Pasadena, USA)
Salser, Winston (UCLA-Molecular Biology)
Sanal, Ozden (Ankara, Turkey)

Sawicki, Mark (UCLA-Surgery)
Scott, David (Manchester, UK)
Sedgwick, Robert (Los Angeles, USA)
Sherrington, Paul (Cambridge, UK)
Shilling, Paul (San Diego, USA)
Shiloh, Yosef (Tel Aviv, Israel)
Skog, Sven (Stockholm, Sweden)
Sobel, Eric (UCLA-Biomathematics)
Sparkes, Robert (UCLA-Medicine/Pediatrics)
Stoppa-Lyonnet, Domenique (Paris, France)
Swift, Michael (North Carolina, USA)
Taylor, Malcolm (Birmingham, UK)
Teraoka, Sharon (UCLA-Molecular Biology)
Thick, Jane (Birmingham, UK)
Tolun, Asli (Istanbul, Turkey)
Uhrhammer, Nancy (UCLA-Pathology)
Wagner, Margaret (Guest)
Weemaes, Corrie (Nijmegen, Netherlands)
Withers, Rodney (UCLA-Radiation Oncology)
Woods, Christopher Geoffrey (Oxford, UK)
Wooster, Richard (Sutton, UK)
Wright, Jocyndra (Seattle, USA)
Yang, Huanming (UCLA-Pathology)
Zdzienicki, Margaret (Leiden, Netherlands)

Some of the participants at ATW5 (from top left):

1. Robert Sedgwick, GUEST SPEAKER
2. Sedgwick, Gatti, Painter
3. Taylor, McConville

4. Byrd, McConville, Woods
5. Lois Rosen (HOST), Shiloh
6. Kapp, Murnane

7. Concannon, Charmley, Wright
8. Herzing, Meyn
9. Arlett, Kingsbury

10. Arlett, Barbara and Richard Albertini
11. Chiplunkar, Uhrhammer, Yang
12. Peterson, Boder, Pam Smith (HOST)

13. Wooster
14. Tolun, Sanal
15. Swift, Salser
16. Paterson

17. Scott, Stoppa-Lyonnet
18. Weemaes, Jaspers
19. Murnane, Zdzienicki

20. George Smith (HOST), Gatti
21. Chessa, Chen, Lavin, James
22. Komatsu, Ejima

Tana Gatti, PHOTOGRAPHER.

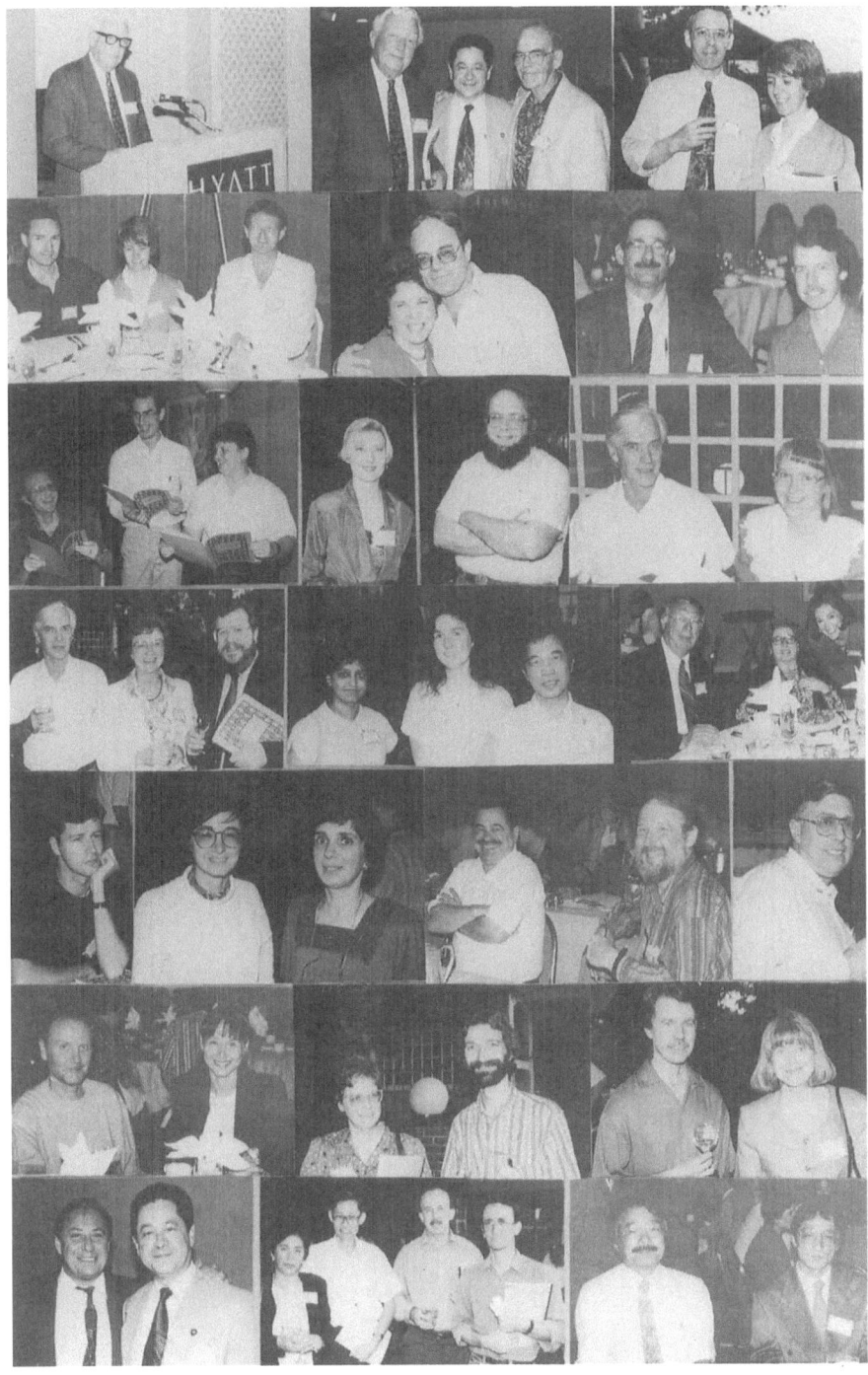

ATAXIA-TELANGIECTASIA: A BRIEF HISTORICAL OVERVIEW

Robert P. Sedgwick, M. D.
1136 West Sixth Street, #711
Los Angeles, California 90025
USA

Despite two early case reports[1][2] the clinical-pathological
delineation of ataxia-telangiectasia (A-T) as a disease entity
occurred over the years 1957-1963.[3][4][5][6] By 1963 it was
possible to publish a review of 101 cases world-wide illustrat-
ing the stereotyped nature of the disorder: progressive cerebellar ataxia in childhood, autosomal recessive heredity, oculocutaneous telangiectasia, frequency of sinopulmonary infection,
peculiarity of eye movements, frequency of lymphoreticular malignancy and pathological demonstration of cortical cerebellar
atrophy and dystrophic thymus.[6] Publications in 1963, 1964
and 1966[7][8][9] confirmed inconstant hypogammaglobulinemia
(particularly IgA) and described immunological defect as shown
by deficient response to a variety of antigenic stimuli and delayed and impaired skin homograft rejection. It was postulated
that the fundamental immunological defect was a consequence of
the thymic deficiency and suggestion was made that A-T patients
may be critical keys to the study of complex host factors involved in immunogenesis and malignancy. In 1968 the peculiar
generalized nucleocytomegaly was recognized confirming the fact
that A-T is a multisystem disorder.[10] The elevation of alpha-
fetoprotein as an important laboratory marker was reported in
1972.[11] Epidemiologic studies over the period 1976 to 1990
have confirmed the increased risk of diabetes mellitus and malignancy in heterozygotes.[12]

Clinical radiosensitivity in A-T patients was first reported
in 1967[13] and abnormal lymphocyte chromosomal aberrations when
exposed to radiation in 1973.[14] In 1975 it was demonstrated
that A-T fibroblasts were abnormally susceptible to ionizing radiation (but not to the ultra-violet).[15] Numerous studies
have confirmed these findings and led to the study of A-T on the

the cellular and molecular level.[15][16][17][18][19]

There have by now been five international A-T workshops permitting exchange of new research information. The main thrust of present research is in molecular genetics. Five complementation groups have been described. A gene locus at   11q22-23 now seems certain.   This progress has been recently summarized.[21] In this short review it has been possible to mention only a few high points in the A-T story. The disease has stimulated a vast literature and been the subject of study and reports by a multitude of investigators throughout the world. Clearly the isolation of the responsible A-T gene and its metabolic consequences will provide the "golden key" for genetic counseling and (hopefully) for specific therapy.

REFERENCES

Aguilar MM, Kamoshita S, Landing GH, Boder E, Sedgwick RP (1968)
    Pathological observations in ataxia-telangiectasia. A report
    on 5 cases. J Neuropathol exp Neurol 27:659-676
Arlett CF, Harcourt SA (1980) Survey of radiosensitivity in a
    variety of human cell strains. Cancer Res 117:40:926-932
Biemond A (1957) A palaeocerebellar atrophy with extrapyramidal
    manifestations in association with bronchiectasis and telan-
    giectasis of the conjunctiva bulbi as a familial syndrome. In
    L van Bogaert and J Radermecker (eds) Proc 1st Intern Congr
    of Neurological Sciences Brussels July 1957 London Pergamon
    Press 4:206
Boder E, Sedgwick RP (1957) Ataxia-telangiectasia. A familial
    syndrome of progressive cerebellar ataxia, oculocutaneous tel-
    angiectasia and frequent pulmonary infection. A preliminary
    report on 7 children, an autopsy and a case history. Univ Sth
    Calif Med Bull 9:15-28
Boder E, Sedgwick RP (1963a) Ataxia-telangiectasia. A review of
    101 cases. In G Walsh (ed) Little Club Clinics in Develop Med
    London, Heinemann Medical Books 8:110-118
Cox R, Hosking GP, Wilson J (1978) Ataxia telangiectasia. Evalu-
    ation of radiosensitivity in cultured skin fibroblasts as a
    diagnostic test. Arch Dis Child 53:5:386-390
Fireman P, Boesman M, Gitlin D (1964) Ataxia telangiectasia. A
    dysgammaglobulinemia with deficient gamma IA (B2A)-globulin.
    Lancet 1:1193-1195
Gatti RA (1991) Molecular genetics of ataxia-telangiectasia.
    Handbook of Clinical Neurology 16:60:425-431
Gotoff SP, Amirmokri E, Liebner EJ (1967) Ataxia-telangiectasia
    Neoplasia, untoward response to X-irradiation, and tuberous
    sclerosis. Am J Dis Child 114:617-625

Hanawalt P, Painter R (1985) On the nature of a 'DNA-processing' defect in ataxia-telangiectasia. In: RA Gatti and M Swift (eds) Ataxia-Telangiectasia. New York, Alan R Liss Inc. Kroc Found Ser 19:67-71

Hecht F, Hecht BK (1985) Ataxia-Telangiectasia breakpoints in chromosome rearrangements reflect genes important to T and B lymphocytes. In: RA Gatti and M Swift (eds) Ataxia-Telangiectasia. New York, Alan R Liss Inc. Krock Found Ser 19:189-195

Hecht F, MCCaw BK, Koler R (1973) Ataxia-Telangiectasia-clonal growth of translocation lymphocytes. N Engl J Med 289:6:286-291

Lehmann AR, James MR, Stevens SS (1982) Miscellaneous observations on DNS repair in ataxia-telangiectasia. In BA Bridges and DG Harnden (eds) Ataxia-Telangiectasia, New York, Wiley 347-353.

Louis-Bar D (1941) Sur un syndrome progressif comprenant des télangiectasies capillaires cutanées et conjonctivales symétriques, à disposition naevode et de troubles cérébelleux. Confin neurol (Basel) 4:32-42

Pascual-Pascual SI, Pascual-Castroviejo I, Fontan G, Lopez-Martin V (1981) Ataxia-Telangiectasia (A-T). Contribution with eighteen personal cases. Brain Dev 3:3:289-296

Paterson MC, Anderson AK, Smith BP, Smith PJ (1979) Enhanced radiosensitivity of cultured fibroblasts from ataxia-telangiectasia heterozygotes manifested by defective colony-forming ability and reduced DNS repair replication after hypoxic gamma-irradiation. Cancer Res 39:9:3725-3734

Peterson RDA, Kelly WD, Good RA (1964) Ataxia-telangiectasia: Its association with a defective thymus, immunological-deficiency disease, and malignancy. Lancet 1:1189-1193

Strich S (1966) Pathological findings in 3 cases of ataxia-tellangiectasia. J Neurol, Neurosurg, Psychiatry 29:489-499

Swift M (1990) Genetics Aspects of Ataxia-Telangiectasia. Immunodefic Rev 2:67-81

Syllaba L, Henner K (1926) Contribution à l'indépendance de l'athétose double idiopathique at congénitale. Atteinte familiale, syndrome dystrophique, signe du réseau vasculaire conjonctival, intégrité psychique. Rev neurol 1:541-562

Taylor AM, Harnden DG, Arlett CF, Harcourt SA, Lehmann AR, Stevens S, Bridges BA (1975) Ataxia-Telangiectasia: a human mutation with abnormal radiation sensitivity. Nature 4: 258 (5534) 427-429

Waldmann TA, McIntire KR (1972 Serum-alpha-fetoprotein levels in patients with Ataxia-Telangiectasia Lancet 25; 2 (787) 1112-1115

Wells CE, Shy GM (1957) Progressive familial choreoathetosis with cutaneous telangiectasia. J Neurol Neurosurg Psychiat 20: 98-104

Young RR, Austen KF, Moser HW (1964a) Abnormalities of serum gamma 1A globulin and ataxia telangiectasia. Medicine 43:423-433

II. Isolation of A–T Gene(s)

Cloning and Characterization of a Candidate Gene for A-T Complementation Group D

Leon N. Kapp and John P. Murnane
Laboratory of Radiobiology and Environmental Health
Box 0750
University of California, San Francisco
San Francisco, CA 94143

INTRODUCTION

Ataxia-telangiectasia (A-T) has been of interest to radiobiologists because A-T cells have two important responses to X-radiation: hypersensitivity to the killing effects of radiation (Taylor et al.1975), and DNA synthesis that is not inhibited by exposure to ionizing radiation (i.e., radioresistant DNA synthesis) (Painter and Young, 1980). The exact defect in A-T cells is unknown; cloning of an A-T gene should lead to a new understanding of both human radiosensitivity and the regulation of DNA synthesis after radiation-induced DNA damage. One obvious method for cloning an A-T gene would be to introduce random normal human DNA segments into A-T cells in culture and then to screen these cells to find cell clones that had become at least partially radioresistant when compared with the original A-T cell line. This approach was begun in this Laboratory in 1983 and resulted in the isolation of a candidate A-T gene at the end of 1990. Currently, work is in progress to characterize this candidate gene and to determine whether it is the gene for A-T complementation group D.

NATO ASI Series, Vol. H 77
Ataxia-Telangiectasia
Edited by R. A. Gatti and R. B. Painter
© Springer-Verlag Berlin Heidelberg 1993

MATERIALS AND METHODS

All methods used in these studies are reported in detail in Kapp and Painter (1989) and Kapp et al. (1992). The methods are briefly described here.

Cell culture and growth
An SV40-transformed A-T cell line (AT5BIVA) was used. Cells were maintained in minimal essential medium with 12% fetal calf serum. Synchronization was obtained with the thymidine double-block method (Bootsma et al., 1964; Kapp and Painter, 1989).

Transfection
A human genomic library in cosmid pCV108k was used (Lau and Kan, 1983). Transfection was performed with the calcium phosphate precipitation method (Wigler et al., 1978), with the precipitate remaining in contact with the cells for 18 h. After removal of the precipitate, the cells were incubated in medium for 24 h and G418 (400 mg/ml) was added.

Irradiation
Cells were irradiated in plastic Falcon flasks with either a ^{60}Co source at the Lawrence Berkeley Laboratory or a Philips RT250 therapeutic unit.

Cosmid library construction
A cosmid library from 1B3 was constructed as described by Sambrook et al.(1989). Genomic 1B3 DNA was partially digested with MboI, and fragments of 30-50 kb were ligated to BamHI-digested pWE16 cosmid DNA. Clones containing the *neo* gene were selected by infecting NM554 bacteria and growing them on agar plates with kanamycin.

Cosmid and cDNA library screening
A commercially available HeLa cell cDNA library (Stratagene) was screened (Murnane, 1986) with a probe made from cosmid fragments that did not contain repetitive sequences. A chromosome 11-specific cosmid library obtained from L. Deaven (Los Alamos National Laboratory) was screened (Sambrook et al., 1989) with the 3.0-kb cDNA obtained from the HeLa library.

Southern and RNA blot analysis
High molecular weight cellular DNA was isolated and Southern blot analysis was performed as described previously (Murnane, 1986). mRNA was isolated with a kit from Invitrogen. RNA gel electrophoresis and blot analysis were performed as described previously (Sambrook et al., 1989).

Functional complementation
DNA from the cosmid K-1 and cDNA were transfected into AT5BIVA cells with the calcium phosphate precipitate method (Kapp et al., 1992). Clones of interest were selected by growth in G418 (400 mg/ml). Individual clones were then tested for X-ray survival characteristics (Kapp and Painter, 1989).

Radiation hybrid mapping
The chromosomal location of *ATDC* was determined by analysis of 100 radiation hybrids (Cox et al., 1990; Kapp et al., 1992) that contained defined regions of 11q23.

RESULTS AND DISCUSSION

Human DNA from normal cells was transfected into AT5BIVA cells by the calcium phosphate-DNA precipitate method (Kapp and Painter, 1989). The donor DNA was in a pCV108k cosmid library that contains a *neo* gene and 40-kb segments of normal human DNA. This approach presented a number of difficulties but was the most promising method available in 1983 when this work was begun.

Considering the size of the human genome (3×10^9 bp) and the size of the human DNA fragments in each cosmid, it would require 3.5×10^5 transfected cells to give a 99% probability that one of the transfectants would contain the complementing A-T gene (Clarke and Carbon, 1976). Since the task of generating a minimum of 3.5×10^5 clones with the starting A-T cell line was one of the largest obstacles, any significant improvement in transfection frequencies would greatly reduce the size of the necessary experiments.

The cell line used for these experiments was AT5BIVA, an SV40-transformed A-T fibroblast cell line that belongs to complementation group D (Jaspers et al., 1988). With the standard calcium phosphate-DNA transfection method, these cells had an average transfection frequency of approximately 5×10^{-4}. However, it was found that synchronized populations gave a 10-fold or higher transfection frequency of 5×10^{-3} to 1×10^{-2} (Kapp and Painter, 1989). The most efficient cell populations for transfection were obtained by mitotic selection, but these synchronous cell populations were relatively small. When we used a thymidine double-block synchrony method (Bootsma et al., 1964; Kapp and Painter ,1989), virtually the entire cell population could be synchronized, resulting in a very large recipient cell preparation with an average transfection frequency of approximately 5×10^{-3}.

Another problem was in what form to introduce the normal genomic DNA and selection marker into the cells. Co-transfection with high molecular weight human genomic DNA, along with a plasmid or cosmid vector containing a selective marker such as the *neo* gene, has been used to generate cell clones that contain large stretches of normal genomic DNA (Lehmann et al., 1986). Growth in selective medium containing G418 would select for these transfected cells. However, we chose a human cosmid library for this purpose. The human library's advantage was that a candidate A-T gene (if found) would be within 40 kb of the selective marker, making it easier to retrieve the transfected DNA from the hybrid A-T cell line. In contrast, with co-transfection, a larger amount of DNA might be integrated into an A-T cell, but the integrated human gene that complements A-T might be too far from the selective gene to allow cloning and rescue.

Another consideration was the source of the genomic DNA, which could have been either human or rodent. The advantage of using rodent DNA was that it would be easier to recover from the complemented A-T cells because of the presence of rodent-specific repetitive sequences; however, a drawback would be that the complementing DNA might not be closely homologous to the human A-T gene. In contrast, the use of human donor DNA would increase the probability that any cloned A-T cDNA would be the correct gene, but it might be harder to identify and clone the transfected human DNA from A-T cells.

Finally, the nature of the selection with ionizing radiation was also critical, because the difference in radiosensitivity between A-T and normal cells is not large enough that a single dose of radiation would kill the A-T cells but not the complemented A-T cells. For this reason, a series of three sequential and increasing doses were used to select for complemented A-T cells. In addition, after each irradiation the colonies were allowed to grow to more than 300 cells so that trypsinization, replating (with a 20% plating efficiency), and irradiation would not cause the loss of potentially important clones. That is, the protocols used were aimed at preserving cells from each of the original transfectants through the selection process to help maximize the likelihood that a complemented A-T cell would survive the selection, radiation, and cloning procedures (Kapp and Painter, 1989)

On the basis of the above considerations, the following conditions were chosen: a human genomic library in the pCV108k cosmid (Lau and Kan, 1983) containing the *neo* gene for selection was transfected into a population of AT5BIVA cells synchronized by thymidine double block (Kapp and Painter, 1989). Approximately 24 h after transfection, G418 was added to the medium to ensure that all the surviving cells had incorporated normal human genomic DNA, and G418 remained in the cell culture medium from this point on. These cells were then exposed to 1.2 Gy of X-radiation. After 3 weeks of culture, which permitted the growth of large colonies, the cells were trypsinized, dispersed, replated, and exposed to 6 Gy of X-radiation. After another 3 weeks, the resulting colonies were again dispersed and were exposed to 10 Gy of X-radiation. All colonies appearing after this third irradiation were isolated with cloning cylinders and expanded into cell lines.

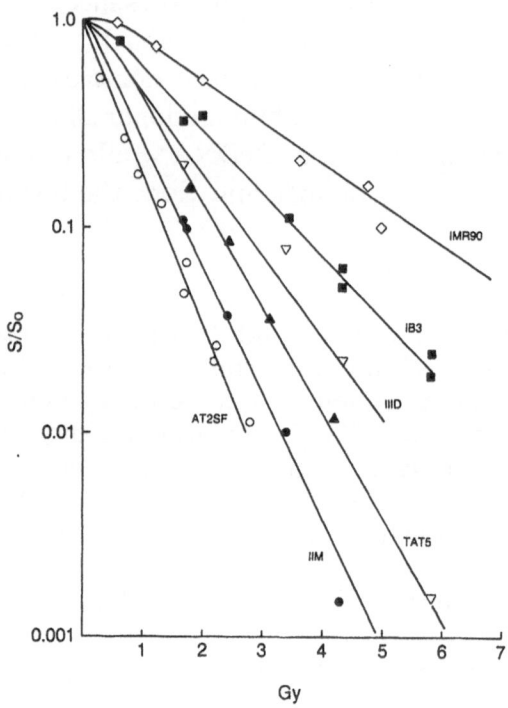

Fig. 1   Survival as a function of X-ray dose for AT5BIVA cells (TAT5), untransformed A-T cells (AT2SF), normal IMR90 cells, and cell lines selected after transfection of AT5BIVA cells with the pCV108k cosmid library (IIm, IIId, 1B3). Reproduced from Kapp and Painter (1989) with permission of Taylor & Francis.

The transfection process generated 450,000 to 500,000 clones (Kapp and Painter, 1989). After selection with radiation, 29 clones were produced, each of which was examined with the use of radiation survival curves (Fig. 1). The survival curves for these clones showed D_0 values between those of the parental AT5BIVA cells and control human IMR90 cells, and approximately 15 of the clones showed radioresistance above that of the parental AT5BIVA cells. However, repeated testing of these clones by means of survival curves indicated that many of them were not stably radioresistant, although all of them remained G418 resistant. A single clone (1B3) was stably radioresistant, with D_0 values in the lower range of the values for normal cells.

Southern blots in which the *neo* gene was used as a probe indicated that 1B3 cells contained three or four integrated cosmids. Presumably, one of these cosmids was associated with the partial radioresistance seen in these cells. Several other cell clones isolated in this same experiment had identical bands, demonstrating that they were all derived from the same original transfected cell. Interestingly, in cell line 1B3 the integrated cosmid sequences appeared to be amplified, providing a possible explanation for why 1B3 maintained its radioresistance, whereas radioresistance was gradually lost from the other related clones (Kapp and Painter, 1989). For additional confirmation that an integrated cosmid was associated with the radioresistance of 1B3, heavily irradiated (50 Gy) 1B3 cells were fused to parental AT5BIVA cells (Kapp and Painter, 1989). The fused cells were selected for G418 resistance, which resulted in the isolation of 24 such clones. When tested by means of survival curves, the radiosensitivity of these clones fell into two groups (rather than into a spectrum, as with the original selection protocol): either A-T-like or 1B3-like, with about one quarter of the clones displaying 1B3-like radioresistance. These results strongly supported the association between the integrated cosmid sequences and the increased radioresistance in the 1B3 cell line.

To rescue the integrated cosmid sequences, we constructed a human genomic library from 1B3 genomic DNA by using the cosmid vector pWE16 (Kapp et al., 1992). The bacteria strain NM554 was then infected with this library and plated on agar plates with kanamycin. Since the pWE16 vector itself does not contain any genes conferring kanamycin resistance, the kanamycin resistance in colonies appearing on these plates must arise from the integrated *neo* genes in the 1B3 cell DNA. (Because the *neo* gene contains both a mammalian and a bacterial transcriptional promoter, it provides antibiotic resistance in both cell types.) Any colonies appearing under these conditions would thus contain the *neo* gene along with up to 40 kb of adjoining genomic DNA from 1B3 cells, much of which would be derived from the original pCV108k library. Fifty-five kanamycin-positive clones (K1-K55) were obtained by this method.

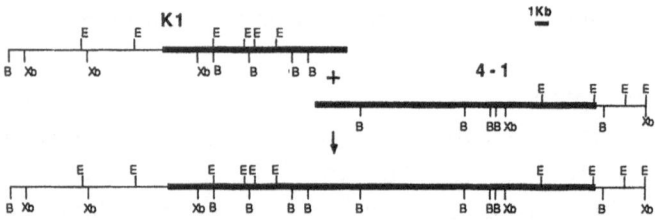

Fig. 2 Restriction map of cosmids K-1 and 4-1 and the composite 30-kb genomic region containing *ATDC*. B, BglII; E, EcoRI; Xb, XbaI.

The next step was to determine which of these clones contained DNA that complemented radiosensitivity in the A-T cell line (Kapp et al., 1992). Since the genes for AT had been localized to chromosome 11q23, any of the 55 clones that contained DNA from this region would be likely to contain a candidate gene for A-T complementation group D. By fluorescent *in situ* hybridization, two of these clones, K-1 and K-41, were found to hybridize exclusively to 11q23. Restriction maps showed that K-1 and K-41 overlapped almost completely, with K-41 being slightly larger. The rescue from the integration site in 1B3 of DNA that comes from 11q23 is strong evidence that a gene within the transfected DNA complements radiosensitivity in cells from A-T complementation group D, because the A-T genes from complementation groups A, C, and D have all been mapped to 11q23 (Gatti et al., 1991).

To determine whether the K-1or K-41 cosmid actually contained an expressed gene, four separate probes were made with EcoRI fragments of K-1, which contained no repetitive sequences (Kapp et al., 1992). A HeLa cell cDNA library was then screened, and a large number of positive cDNA clones were isolated. Restriction enzyme mapping and nucleotide sequence analysis showed that they were all related. Six of the largest clones (3.0 kb) appeared to be nearly full length, because they had poly-A on one end and a complete open reading frame with termination codons just 5´ to the first methionine codon. Nucleotide sequence analysis of the cDNA for this gene, which has been named *ATDC*, demonstrated no significant homology to any known genes. Comparison of the restriction maps of the cosmids and 3.0-kb cDNA, as well as Southern blot analysis of K-1 with probes made from the cDNA, indicated that nearly one half of the sequences contained in the cDNA were missing from the cosmid clones K-1 and K-41. The 3´ end of this gene, therefore, was missing from the integrated sequences contained in cell line 1B3. However, the SV40 bidirectional transcriptional termination sequences from the original pCV108k cosmid are located downstream from the truncated ATDC gene, forming a functional transcription unit. The presence of only part of this transfected gene could therefore explain the partial correction of the A-T characteristics in this cell line. Although this gene appears to be the likely candidate for the complementation of radiosensitivity in the 1B3 cell line, the K-1 cosmid is being screened for other genes that may be present.

To find the missing 3´ end of the *ATDC* gene, we used the 3.0-kb cDNA as a probe to screen a human genomic chromosome 11-specific library (Kapp et al., 1992). Two positive cosmid clones (4-1 and 3-1) were found in this library. Restriction maps of these clones demonstrated that they contained overlapping sequences, and one region in 4-1 was found to overlap with clones K-1 and K-41. Cosmid clone 4-1 therefore contains the 3′ end of the *ATDC* gene, which was missing from clones K-1 and K-41. A composite map of K-1 and 4-1, containing all of the genomic sequences for the 3.0-kb cDNA, is more than 30 kb in length (Fig. 2). Multiple copies of both 3-1 and 4-1 were identified within the chromosome 11-specific library; however, no clones containing the 5′ end of the *ATDC* gene were found, possibly owing to overamplification. The choice of this library was fortunate for this work but does indicate the importance of having a complete library for this type of screening.

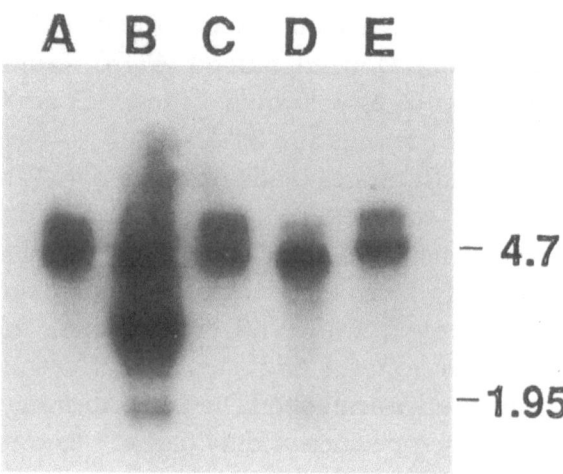

Fig. 3   RNA blot analysis of poly-A-selected mRNA from cell lines LM217 (lane A), HeLa (lane B), 1B3 (lane C), AT3BISV (lane D), and AT5BIVA (lane E), with the 3.0-kb cDNA as a probe. The positions of human and bacterial ribosomal RNA size markers (in kilobases) are shown. Reproduced from Kapp et al. (1992) with permission of The University of Chicago Press.

Southern blot analysis of human genomic DNA with the 3.0-kb cDNA as a probe gave results that were consistent with the structure seen by restriction mapping analysis of the cosmid clones (Kapp et al., 1992). *ATDC* therefore is a single-copy gene, because no unidentified bands were evident. Identical results were seen with DNA from several A-T cell lines, including the parental AT5BIVA, AT3BISV (group A), and AT2SF (group unknown), indicating that no major DNA rearrangements are present in this gene in these cells.

Although *ATDC* is a single-copy gene, RNA blot analysis from several cell lines (normal and A-T) showed the presence of five different mRNA transcripts of 1.8, 2.6, 3.0, 4.7, and 5.7 kb (Kapp et al., 1992) (Fig. 3). The most abundant transcript seen in HeLa cells was 3.0 kb, consistent with the cDNA clones isolated from the HeLa cell cDNA library. However, other normal (LM217) and AT (AT5BIVA and AT3BISV) cells predominantly had the larger transcripts. The complemented A-T line 1B3 appeared identical to the normal line (LM217) in its expression of the 4.7- and 5.7-kb transcripts. These results are consistent with alternative processing of this gene. Although this is an interesting feature of many mammalian genes, it also greatly complicates the analysis of *ATDC*..

CURRENT RESEARCH

Current research is directed at attempting to prove conclusively that mutations in the *ATDC* gene are responsible for A-T complemention group D. Three main approaches are being taken. First, we have mapped the location of the gene on chromosome 11q23 much more accurately. The second approach is to demonstrate that this gene can correct the radiosensitivity in the AT5BIVA cell line, and the third approach is to identify specific mutations within this gene in A-T cells from complementation group D.

Using radiation hybrids that contain mapped fragments of human chromosome 11, we determined that the *ATDC* gene is located just telomeric to the THY1 marker at 11q23 (Kapp et al., 1992) (Fig. 4). This is outside the linkage region for the A-T gene(s) for complementation groups A and C, which have been mapped to a more centromeric region between the markers STMY and D11S424 (Gatti et al., 1991). However, a second linkage region that has often been noted near THY1 could result from a small subset of A-T individuals, possibly group D (approximately 15% of A-T patients). Recent work has indicated that the gene for group D is more telomeric than the genes for groups A and C (Sobel et al., 1992); however, the statistical significance of these studies is weak (see Gatti et al , this volume).

To test the genomic sequences (K-1) and the 3.0-kb cDNA in an expression vector for their ability to confer radioresistance, these

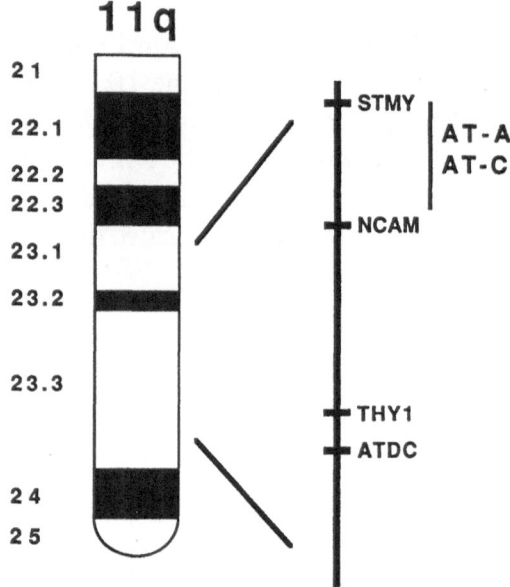

Fig. 4 A map of chromosome 11q23 showing the linkage regions for A-T complementation groups A and C and the location of *ATDC*.. The various markers used for linkage analysis are shown.

19

sequences were transfected in the parental AT5BIVA cell line (Kapp et al., 1992). After transfection, the cells were grown in G418, and the resulting G418 clonal lines were tested for radioresistance. A small degree of complementation was found with the cDNA (in 6 of 33 clones) and the truncated gene in K-1 (in 1 of 50 clones) (Fig. 5). This lack of full complementation could arise for several reasons. The large size of *ATDC* may make full complementation difficult because

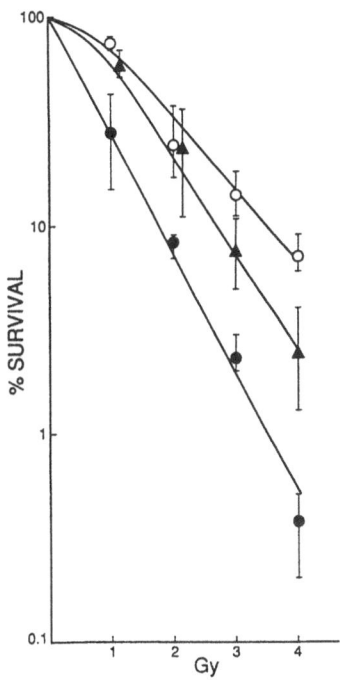

Fig. 5   Survival as a function of X-ray dose for AT5BIVA (solid circles), 1B3 (open circles), and C6 (triangles).   C6 was selected by transfecting the cosmid K-1 into parental AT5BIVA cells. Reproduced   from Kapp et al. (1992) with permission of The University of Chicago Press.

of problems associated with the integration of large intact DNA fragments into human cells. In addition, because the *ATDC* gene produces mRNAs larger than that coded for by the 3.0-kb cDNA, it is possible that K-1 may not contain all of the coding sequences originally transfected into 1B3.

AT5BIVA cell clones transfected with the cDNA in an expression vector also did not achieve full complementation. However, this approach is complicated because of the five different mRNA transcripts produced by this gene. Multiple transcripts can arise from the presence of multiple promoters, alternative splicing, and/or alternative poly-A addition sites. Furthermore, because the 3.0-kb mRNA is not always present in all cells, complete functional complementation may require a cDNA from one of the larger transcripts.

Because Southern blot analysis did not reveal a major DNA rearrangement in the *ATDC* gene in the AT5BIVA cell line, attempts to demonstrate a mutation in this gene have focused on identification of point mutations. Characterization of the 3.0-kb cDNA has demonstrated the presence of nine exons, and the polymerase chain reaction (PCR) is currently being used to analyze all of the known coding regions. PCR primers have been derived from the surrounding introns for the seven smaller exons, and two large exons have been broken up into multiple products. These PCR products are being analyzed by size, single-stranded conformation polymorphism, heteroduplex denaturation gel analysis, and nucleotide sequencing. To date, no specific mutations have been identified in DNA from AT5BIVA. This approach is complicated by the rarity of the positively identified group D cell lines available and the fact that many point mutations that lead to gene inactivation occur outside the coding region.

Additional studies are also in progress to learn more about the nature of the *ATDC* gene. The mRNA is being characterized to determine the various factors that influence the alternative processing and levels of transcription of the various mRNA transcripts. Finally, antibodies to the ATDC gene product are being produced to establish the intracellular location and tissue specificity of this protein.

REFERENCES

Bootsma D, Budke L, Vos O (1964) Studies on synchronous division of tissue culture cells initiated by excess thymidine. Exp Cell Res 33:301-309

Clarke L, Carbon J (1976) A colony bank containing synthetic Col E1 hybrid plasmids representative of the entire E. coli genome. Cell 9:91-99

Cox DR, Burmeister M, Price ER, Kim S, Myers RM (1990) Radiation hybrid mapping: a somatic cell genetic method for constructing high-resolution maps of mammalian chromosomes. Science 250:245-250

Gatti, RA, Boder E, Vinters HV, Sparkes RS, Norman A, Lange K (1991) Ataxia-telangiectasia: an interdisciplinary approach to pathogenesis. Medicine 70:99-117

Jaspers NG, Gatti RA, Baan C, Linssen PCML, Bootsma D (1988) Genetic complementation analysis of ataxia telangiectasia and Nijmegen breakage syndrome: a survey of 50 patients. Cytogenet Cell Genet 49:259-263

Kapp LN, Painter RB (1989) Stable radioresistance in ataxia-telangiectasia cells containing DNA from normal human cells. Int J Radiat Biol 56:667-675

Kapp LN, Painter RB, Yu LC, van Loon N, Richard CW 3d, James MR, Cox DR, Murnane JP (1992) Cloning of a candidate gene for ataxia-telangiectasia group D. Am J Hum Genet 51:45-54

Lau Y-F, Kan YW (1983) Versatile cosmid vectors for the isolation, expression, and rescue of gene sequences: Studies with the human a-globin gene cluster. Proc Natl Acad Sci, USA 80:5225-5229

Lehmann AR, Arlett CF, Burke JF, Green MHL, James MR, Lowe JE (1986) A derivative of an ataxia-telangiectasia (A-T) cell line with normal radiosensitivity but A-T-like inhibition of DNA synthesis. Int J Radiat Biol 49:639-643

Murnane JP (1986) Inducible gene expression by DNA rearrangements in human cells. Mol Cell Biol 6:549-558

Painter RB, Young BR (1980) Radiosensitivity in ataxia-telangiectasia: A new explanation. Proc Natl Acad Sci, USA 77:7315-7317

Sambrook J, Fritsch EF, Maniatis T (1989) Molecular cloning: a laboratory manual, 2d ed. Cold Spring Harbor Laboratory, Cold Spring Harbor, New York

Sobel E, Lange E, Jaspers NGJ, Chessa L, Sanal O, Shiloh Y, Taylor AMR, Weemaes CM, Lange K, Gatti RA (1992) Ataxia-telangiectasia: linkage evidence for genetic heterogeneity. Am J Hum Genet 50:1343-1348

Taylor AMR, Harnden DG, Arlett CF, Harcourt SA, Lehmann AR, Stevens S, Bridges BA (1975) Ataxia-telangiectasia: a human mutation with abnormal radiation sensitivity. Nature 258:427-429

Wigler M, Pellicer A, Silverstein S, Axel R (1978) Biochemical transfer of single-copy eucaryotic genes using total cellular DNA as donor. Cell 14:725-731

PRECISE LOCALIZATION OF A GENE RESPONSIBLE FOR ATAXIA-TELANGIECTASIA ON CHROMOSOME 11q.

F. Cornélis[1,2], M. James[1,2], D. Cherif[1,3], T. Tokino[4], J. Davies[1,2], D. Girault[5], C. Bernard[6], M. F. Croquette[7], D. Théau[8], H. Avet-Loiseau[9], M. Litt[10], R. Berger[3], Y. Nakamura[4], M. Lathrop[1,2] and C. Julier[1,2].

[1]Centre d'Etude du Polymorphism Humain and [2] INSERM U358, 27 rue Juliette Dodu, Paris 75010.*

INTRODUCTION

Ataxia-telangiectasia (A-T) is a recessive disorder of childhood characterized by progressive cerebellar ataxia, occulocutaneous telangiectasias, and a high incidence of cancer and infection. Other distinctive features of the disease include: hypersensitivity of fibroblasts and lymphocytes to ionizing radiation; cellular and humoral immunodeficiencies; chromosomal instability and non-random chromosomal rearrangements in lymphocytes; and elevated levels of alpha-fetoprotein (Boder, 1985). The molecular basis of A-T is thought to be an abnormality of DNA repair (Hanawalt and Painter, 1985). In culture, cells from A-T patients show an increased sensitivity to ionizing radiation when compared to normal cells. Four complementation groups (denoted A,C,D and E) have been described (Jaspers et al., 1988); although the disease is clinically indistinguishable in the four groups, radiation-sensitivity is rendered normal by fusion of cells deriving from A-T patients from different groups (whereas fusion of cells from patients from the same group has no effect).

The A-T heterozygote frequency is estimated at 0.68% to 7.7% in populations of European origin in North America (Swift et al., 1986). Although heterozygous carriers are generally healthy, epidemiological studies suggest that they may be predisposed to cancer, with a risk 2 to 3-fold greater than matched controls (Swift et al., 1991; Swift et al., 1987). In particular, women carrying the A-T gene have a relative risk for breast cancer estimated to be 6- to 7-fold greater compared to controls; thus, >5% of breast cancer patients may be

* [3]INSERM U301, 27 rue Juliette Dodu, Paris 75010.
[4]Department of Biochemistry, Cancer Institute, Kami-Ikebukuro, Tokyo.
[5]Service d'Immunologie Pediatrique, Hopital Necker, Paris.
[6]Service de Neurologie Infantile, CHR, Lille.
[7]Hôpital Saint-Antoine, Lille.
[8]18, rue d'Aiguillon, Brest.
[9]Unité dHématologie Pédiatrique, CHR, Nantes.
[10]Department of Medical Genetics, Oregon Health Sciences University, Portland, Oregon.

NATO ASI Series, Vol. H 77
Ataxia-Telangiectasia
Edited by R. A. Gatti and R. B. Painter
© Springer-Verlag Berlin Heidelberg 1993

carriers of the A-T gene (Borresen *et al.*, 1990; Pippard *et al.*, 1988; Swift *et al.*, 1991; Swift *et al.*, 1987). Cultured cells from A-T heterozygotes exhibit increased sensitivity to ionizing radiation, although the differences from control cells are not as striking as in homozygotes (Paterson *et al.*, 1985). These findings have led to the speculation that breast cancer patients who are carriers of the A-T gene may exhibit increased sensitivity to radiation therapy (Norman *et al.*, 1988).

Genetic linkage studies have led to the assignment of a gene responsible for A-T to chromosome 11q (Gatti *et al.*, 1988). Although the families included in the initial study were largely unassigned, or from complementation group A, no evidence of heterogeneity in the gene localizations has been found in subsequent studies (McConville *et al.*, 1990a; McConville *et al.*, 1990b). Recent studies have confirmed the assignment of the gene responsible for A-T group C to chromosome 11q (Ziv *et al.*, 1991). Further confirmation that A-T is caused by a gene, or genes on chromosome 11 has been provided by Komatsu et al. (Komatsu *et al.*, 1990) who showed that an A-T group D cell line shows radiation responses similar to control cells after transfer of human chromosome 11 from a somatic cell hybrid, whereas transfer of human chromosome 12 had no effect on the phenotype.

To provide a precise localization of the gene, or genes on chromosome 11q that may be responsible for A-T, we undertook genetic linkage studies of 20 families, with at least 2 affected members. These families were characterized with up to 20 polymorphic marker loci localized to the A-T region by a combination of linkage studies in CEPH reference pedigrees, and by high resolution fluorescent in situ hybridization.

MATERIALS AND METHODS

A-T and CEPH families

DNA from 59 reference families available from CEPH were used for linkage mapping chromosome 11q, as reported previously (Julier *et al.*, 1990).

A-T families characterized for all the markers described in this study consisted of 9 multiplex families from France (7 with 2 affected offspring, 1 with 3 affected offspring and 1 with 1 affected offspring), and 11 multiplex families from the United States (9 with 2 affected offspring, and 2 with 3 affected offspring) provided by Dr M. Swift (Department of Pediatrics, New York Medical College, Valhalla, NY.) An additional 18 nuclear families (3 with 3 affected offspring, 5 with 2 affected offspring, 8 with 1 affected offspring), and two extended pedigrees (1 containing 3 affected individuals, and the other 2 affected individuals) were characterized with 1-5 marker loci. In 9 families, one marriage was known to have occurred between related individuals. An additional family contained two cosanguinious marriages, one between 2nd cousins (parents of two children with A-T), and one between cousins (grandparents of the children).

DNA markers

The article by Julier et al. (Julier *et al.*, 1990) contains details of the polymorphisms and mapping of the following loci and probes: D11S389 (pCJ52.99M2), D1S388 (CJ52.4), D11S98 (ph9-11), D11S85 (ph6-3), D11S84 (p2-7-1D6), D11S385 (pCJ52.75M1), D11S35 (ph2-22), D11S384 (CJ52.193), D11S424 (pCJ52.77M1), D11S386 (CJ52.5T1), D11S351 (p1CJ52.208M2, 2CJ52.208M2), D11S144 (pMCT128.1), D11S29 (pL7), PBGD (pstpstPNE), D11S350 (pHHH172), D11S147 (pHBI18P2, HBI18P1), D11S34 (ph2-11) and D11S83 (ph2-25). Previously unpublished polymorphisms for some of these loci are shown in Table 1. Polymorphisms detected by probe lambdaHD2G1 (dopamine receptor gene, DRD2) are described by Grandy et al. (Grandy *et al.*, 1989). The probe cCI11-45, which detects a TaqI polymorphism is described in Tokino et al. (Tokino *et al.*,). Genotype data in the CEPH panel of reference families for cCI11-45 was produced at the Cancer Institute, Tokyo. Data on DRD2 was a gift from M. Leppert and R. White, Salt Lake City.

Locus	Probe	Enzyme	Alleles Sizes	Frequency	Other Poly- morphic Systems
D11S388	CJ52.4	MspI	5.4	0.29	3
			5.2	0.71	
D11S386	CJ52.5T2	TaqI	4.4	0.66	1
			3.5	0.34	
D11S351	CJ52.208	MspI	13.0	0.84	2
			5.6	0.05	
			2.0	0.11	

Table 1. New restriction fragment length polymorphisms detected by previously published probes. The size and frequency of the particular polymorphic fragments and the number of other published polymorphic systems for each locus are shown.

Genotyping for DNA markers

DNA was extracted from whole blood using standard methods (Sambrook *et al.*, 1989). The DNA was digested by TaqI, MspI or PstI, electrophoresed through a 0.8% agarose gel and alkaline tranferred to nylon membrane (Reed and Mann, 1985). The probes were labeled by random priming using [alpha-^{32}P]dCTP, to a specific activity of 10^9 cpm/μg (Feinberg and Vogelstein, 1984). Prehybridization and hybridization were at 65°C in a mixture composed of 7% PEG8000 / 10% SDS (Tokino *et al.*, 1991), and 100 µg/ml of denatured sonicated salmon sperm DNA (for probes free of repetitive sequences) or human DNA (for probes containing repetitive sequences). Probes containing repetitive sequences were preannealed in the hybridization mixture for 1h before hybridizing to the DNA blot. The final post hybridization wash was given in 0.1xSSC, 0.1%SDS at 65°C, and membranes were exposed to Cronex 7 films at -80°C, with intensifying screens.

In situ hybridization

Physical localizations were obtained for 9 of the markers in this study by fluorescent *in situ* hybridization on metaphase chromosomes with simultaneous R-banding (Cherif *et al.*, 1990). An additional marker, DRD2, was mapped by reference to a cosmid containing NCAM (gift from G. Evans) as explained in the text.

To obtain metaphase chromosome preparations, lymphocyte cultures of healthy males were synchronized by methotrexate and treated with BrdU (5-Bromodeoxyuridine) during the last S-phase. Colcemid was added for the last 15 minutes before harvesting according to the usual technique (hypotonic solution: 0.075M KCl; fixative: methanol/glacial acetic acid, 3/1). After spreading, the slides were kept in darkness at -20°C until use.

Cosmid probes were labeled by nick translation with bio-11dUTP according to the BRL (Bethesda Research Laboratories) protocol. Just before hybridization, the slides were immersed in 70% formamide/2xSSC, pH7 for 2 minutes at 70°C. Cosmid probes were preannealed with excess human DNA as a competitor for 3 hours prior to hybridization. The hybridization signal was revealed by avidin-FITC and amplified once with additional layers of biotinylated goat anti-avidin and avidin-FITC, as described in Pinkel *et al.*, 1986. R-bands were obtained after staining with Hoechst 33258, UV light exposure, and immersion in Earle solution (pH 6.5) at 87°C for 2 minutes. After banding, a second round of signal amplification was necessary for the detection of the hybridized probe on the banded chromosome.

Linkage analysis

Linkage analysis was performed with version 5.1 of the LINKAGE programs (Pinkel *et al.*, 1986) modified to allow efficient likelihood calculations for families containing recessive disease traits. Gene frequency estimates for the marker loci were obtained from parents in the reference pedigrees. Initially, we combined data from the CEPH and A-T families (with consanguinity relationships ignored) to obtain a high resolution linkage map of the marker loci, with the algorithm described in Lathrop et al. (Lathrop *et al.*, 1988). Briefly, a trial map order is obtained from pairwise recombination estimates. The likelihoods of this order, and alternatives based on permutations of loci, or tightly-linked groups of loci are

Locus (probe)	No sex difference	Constant ratio		Variable ratio	
		Male	Female	Male	Female
1. DS11S389 (pCJ52.99M2)	0.07	0.05	0.10	0.08	0.07
2. D11S388 (pCJ52.4)	0.01	0.00	0.01	0.00	0.01
3. D11S85 (ph6-3)	0.02	0.01	0.03	0.00	0.03
4. D11S98 (ph9-11)	0.00	0.00	0.00	0.00	0.00
5. D11S84 (p2-7-1D6)	0.08	0.06	0.11	0.03	0.13
6. D11S385 (pCJ52.75M1)	0.00	0.00	0.00	0.00	0.00
7. D11S35 (ph2-22)	0.04	0.03	0.05	0.02	0.01
8. D11S384 (CJ52.193)	0.03	0.03	0.05	0.04	0.07
9. D11S424 (pCJ52.77M1)	0.02	0.01	0.02	0.01	0.02
10. D11S444 (CI11-45)	0.03	0.02	0.04	0.03	0.04
11. DRD2 (lambdaHD2G1)	0.02	0.01	0.02	0.00	0.02
12. D11S386 (CJ52.5)	0.07	0.05	0.01	0.05	0.11
13. D11S351 (CJ52.208)	0.00	0.00	0.00	0.00	0.00
14. D11S144 (pMCT128.1)	0.01	0.1	0.02	0.02	0.01
15. D11S29 (pL7)	0.03	0.02	0.03	0.00	0.05
16. D11S350 (pHHH172)	0.00	0.00	0.00	0.00	0.00
17. PBGD (pstpstPNE)	0.03	0.02	0.05	0.02	0.03
18. D11S147 (HBI18)	0.07	0.04	0.08	0.03	0.11
19. D11S34 (ph2-11)	0.21	0.17	0.29	0.20	0.22
20. D11S83 (ph2-25)					

Table 2. Chromosome 11 marker loci in the region of the gene responsible for A-T. Loci are shown in the inferred gene order with recombination distances estimated under three different models of sex-specific recombination rates. Some systems were characterized by different probes (plasmid subclones or fragments derived from the same cosmid) in which case only the name of the cosmid is shown.

compared to find a new trial order with higher likelihood. The process is repeated until convergence.

All obligate and probable recombination events were identified after initial determination of the gene order, and the data were verified prior to re-analysis. Sex-specific recombination rates were evaluated under 3 different hypotheses (no sex-difference, uniform sex-difference, and variable sex-difference) as previously described (O'Connell *et al.*, 1987). Likelihoods for different localizations of the A-T gene were initially evaluated by the location score method (Lathrop *et al.*, 1984). The results were confirmed by re-estimation of the recombination rates with the A-T gene included in the map under selected gene orders. All linkage analyses assumed lack of interference. Genetic distances were calculated from Haldane's map function.

RESULTS

Genetic map of chromosome 11q in the region of A-T

Marker loci in the region of the gene responsible for A-T were selected for study based on linkage, or physical mapping data. Many of these markers are contained in the previous map based on genotypes on CEPH reference families (Julier *et al.*, 1990). Here, genotypes from the CEPH pedigrees and disease families were combined to improve the inference of the gene order, and obtain better estimates of the recombination distances between adjacent markers. The results of the order inference and recombination estimates under the different sex-specific recombination hypotheses are shown in Table 2.

The order of D11S85 (ph6-3) and D11S98 (ph9-11) cannot be resolved with respect to D11S388 (CJ52.4) and D11S84 (p2-7-1D6) from these data, as few recombination events were detected between these loci. Similarly, alternative placements of DRD2 with respect to CJ52.5 and CI11-45 cannot be excluded, based on the linkage results. Although linkage favours the order D11S44 (CI11-45)-DRD2- D11S386 (CJ52.5), the odds against the inversion of the last two loci are only 38:1. The odds against the placement of D11S444 (CI11-45) in the segment spanned by D11S384 (CJ52.193) and D11S424 (CJ52.77) are 2:1. Finally, the orientations of three other pairs of loci could not be determined, as no recombination events were observed: D11S385 (pCJ52.75M1)-D11S35 (ph2-22), D11S351 (p1CJ52.208M2, p2CJ52.208M2, p3CJ52.208)-D11S144 (pMCT128.1), and D11S350 (pHHH172)-PBGD. Other orders tested during the construction of the map could be rejected with odds >100:1. Figure 1 shows the genetic orders and distances for markers included in the study, showing the loci whose order could not be resolved for the linkage data, and the odds against the inversions of adjacent loci. Under a constant sex-difference model, the estimated female/male genetic distance ratio in the region was 2; the ratio differs significantly from 1 (X^2_1=48.2; p<0.00001). No evidence was found for a significant variation in the sex-specific distance ratio in different intervals (X^2_{15}=18.8; p>0.1).

29

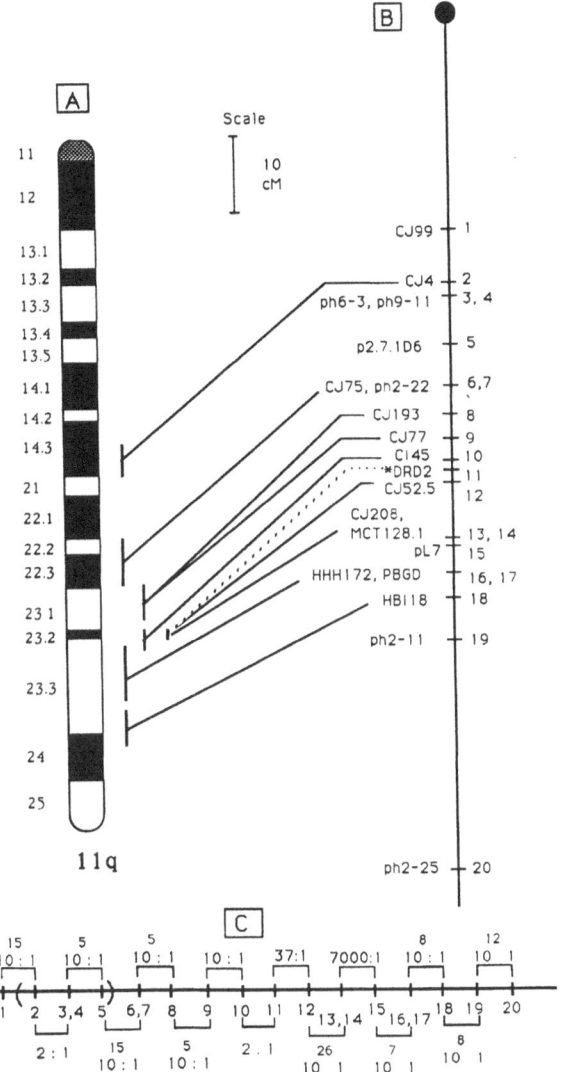

Figure 1. *In situ* and genetic maps of the A-T region of chromosome 11q. (A) Ideogram of chromosome 11q showing *in situ* localizations of nine cosmids. (B) Chromosome 11q markers under the inferred gene order. Distances between markers have been calculated from the sex-average recombination rates. Probe names have been abbreviated from Table 2. Cosmids localized by *in situ* are indictaed by solid lines to the ideogram. The physical localization for DRD2 was inferred indirectly by study of a cosmid that contains NCAM (see text), and is indicated by a dashed line. (C) The order of markers and the relative odds against the inversion of adjacent loci as determined from the linkage analysis. Loci numbers correspond to those given in Table 2. All other orders that were tested could be rejected with relative odds greater than 100:1, except for order involving certain permutations of the markers indicated in ().

In situ studies

Fluorescent *in situ* studies were undertaken with some of the cosmid clones to further refine the placement of marker loci in the region of the A-T locus. A partial physical map that contains 4 of the markers characterized here is given in Cherif et al. (Cherif *et al.*, 1990), and new data were collected for an additional 6 markers. The results of the physical mapping studies are shown in Figure 1. The placement of DRD2 was inferred from the study of a cosmid clone containing NCAM, since NCAM and DRD2 have been shown to hybridize to a single pulse-field gel electrophoresis fragment (Cherif *et al.*, 1990). The order of the markers inferred from the physical and linkage studies are compatible, although in several instances, loci could be ordered unambiguously from the linkage data. However, CI11-45 was mapped by *in situ* hybridization distal to CJ52.77, for which the linkage evidence was equivocal.

Linkage to A-T

The maximum lod score was 7.0 at $-\theta = 0.08$ (0.03-0.16 1-lod- unit confidence interval), obtained with D11S388 (CJ52.4). D11S384 (CJ52.193) gave a lod score of 5.9 at $-\theta=0.0$ (0.00-0.06 1-lod-unit confidence interval). Two other markers, D11S424 (CJ52.77) and D11S351 (CJ52.208), exhibited maximum lod scores of 6.1 and 5.6, respectively. Lod scores >3 were found with 3 other probes (Table 3).

Locus (probe)	0.00	0.01	0.02	0.03	0/04	0.05	0.10	0.20
1 D11S389 (CJ52.99)	-inf	1.9	2.4	2.6	2.7	2.7	2.7	1.9
2 D11S388 (CJ52.4)	-inf	3.4	5.2	6.0	6.5	6.8	6.9	5.2
3 D11S85 (ph6-3)	-inf	-3.2	-2.1	-1.5	-1.1	-0.8	-0.1	0.2
4 D11S98 (ph9-11)	-inf	-2.5	-0.9	-0.1	0.5	0.9	1.7	1.6
5 D11S84 (p2-7-1D6)	2.4	2.3	2.2	2.2	2.1	2.0	1.7	1.0
6 D11S385 (CJ52.75)	-inf	1.3	1.8	2.0	2.2	2.2	2.2	1.5
7 D11S35 (ph2-22)	-inf	2.5	2.9	3.0	3.1	3.1	2.9	2.0
8 D11S384 (CJ52.193)	5.9	5.7	5.6	5.4	5.3	5.1	4.3	2.9
9 D11S424 (CJ52.77)	-inf	5.4	5.9	6.1	6.1	6.1	5.4	3.5
10 D11S444 (CI11-45)	-inf	2.2	2.9	3.2	3.4	3.5	3.4	2.5
11 DRD2 (HD2G1)	-inf	1.8	2.3	2.5	2.6	2.7	2.6	1.9
12 D11S386 (CJ52.5)	-inf	-0.3	0.7	1.3	1.7	2.0	2.6	2.0
13 D11S351 (CJ52.208)	-inf	3.0	4.3	5.0	5.4	5.6	5.6	3.8
14 D11S144 (MCT128.1)	-inf	-1.3	0.8	1.8	2.5	2.9	3.6	2.8
15 D11S29 (L7)	-inf	-3.8	-2.4	-1.7	-1.2	-0.8	0.1	0.4
16 D11S350 (HHH172)	-inf	-1.9	-0.8	-0.3	0.1	0.4	1.0	0.9
17 PBGD (pstpstPNE)	-inf	-9.2	-6.8	-5.4	-4.4	-3.7	-1.7	-0.4
18 D11S147 (HBI18)	-inf	-8.2	-4.5	-2.4	-1.0	0.0	2.4	2.8
19 D11S34 (ph2-11)	-inf	-11.4	-8.9	-7.5	-6.4	-5.6	-3.2	-1.4
20 D11S83 (ph2-25)	-inf	-15.4	-11.9	-9.9	-8.4	-7.4	-4.3	-1.7

Table 3. Lod scores between chromosome 11 markers and A-T.

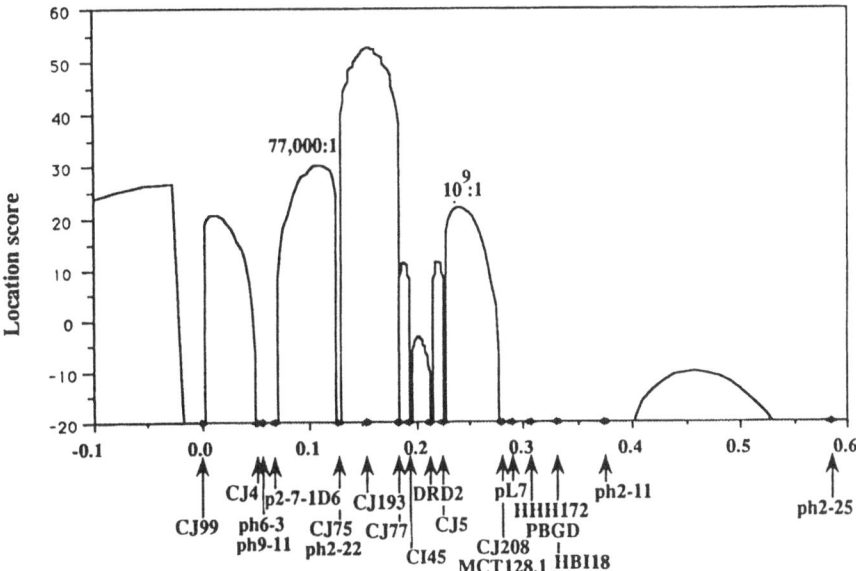

Figure 2. Location scores showing the location of the gene responsible for A-T with respect to the chromosome 11 markers studied here. The x-axis is in centiMorgans. Marker loci are indicated by an abbreviation of the probe names listed in Table 2. Distances have been calculated from male recombination rates obtained under the constant sex- difference model. The odds against several alternative locations are indicated.

Gene frequency estimates for the marker alleles were varied within a range of 20% to test the sensitivity of the lod scores, as the probability that marker alleles are identical by descent in consanguineous pedigrees depends on the assumed gene frequencies. Although the results did not change the conclusions for most, the maximum lod score for D11S384 (CJ52.193) ranged from 6.7 to 5.5 at $-\theta=0$. All signficant lod scores also remained >3 when consanguinity relationships where excluded from the analysis; in particular, the maximum lod score between A-T and D11S384 (CJ52.193) was 4.8 at $-\theta=0$ when consanguinity was ignored. Application of the test of homogeneity in recombination rates (Ott, 1983) showed no evidence of genetic heterogeneity amongst the A-T families (results not shown).

To further refine the placement of the gene responsible for A-T with respect to the markers studied here, we calculated location scores with respect to the fixed order of markers obtained from the combination of genetic and physical studies, with genetic distances given under the constant sex-difference model in Table 2. Initially, the consanguinity relationships were not taken into account and the two extended pedigrees were reduced to core nuclear families in order to increase the efficiency of the multilocus analysis. As shown in Figure 2, the results gave strong support for a location of the gene close to the locus D11S384 (CJ52.193), and flanked by the markers D11S385 (CJ52.75) - D11S35 (ph2-22) (proximal), and D11S424 (CJ52.77) (distal) on the chromosome. The possibility that the gene responsible for A-T resides in other intervals of our genetic map could be strongly rejected (odds >10^7:1). A 1-lod-unit confidence interval calculated from the location scores places the A-T gene within 2 cM of D11S348 (CJ52.193).

Re-estimatation of the recombination rates between loci in the map with different placements of the A-T gene did not significantly modify these results. We also verified that the assumption of different orders for the marker loci in the regions where this order could not be precisely determined from linkage data did not modify the conclusions (results not shown). In particular, the inversion of D11S424 (CJ52.77) and D11S444 (CI11-45), or DRD2 and D11S386 (CJ52.5) in the region flanking the probable location of the A-T locus had no effect on the odds against alternative placements for A-T. We also undertook investigations of the effect of including or excluding the consanguinity with up to 6 marker loci in different regions of the map. The inclusion of consanguinity increased the statistical evidence in favour of the localization of the A-T locus in the interval containing D11S384 (CJ52.193) (results not shown).

DISCUSSION

Initially, the gene responsible for A-T was mapped to chromosome 11 by linkage to two markers, D11S144 (MCT128.1) and Thy-1 (Gatti et al., 1988). Several recent studies have refined the localization of the A-T locus. Sanal et al. (Sanal et al., 1990) have published data on 31 A-T families supporting a localization of the gene to region of 16.8 cM spanned by STMY (Stromelysin) and D11S144 (MCT128.1). McConville et al. (McConville et al., 1990a) studied a smaller set of families, and provided evidence for a localization of A-T distal to D11S144 (MCT128.1), near Thy1 (i.e. outside of the interval STMY- D11S144). However, when they undertook a second study with additional families, they concluded that the A-T locus was situated within the interval defined by DRD2-STMY, and therefore, proximal to D11S144 (MCT128.1) (McConville et al., 1990b). The latter authors estimate a distance of approximately 10 cM for the interval between STMY and D11S144 (MCT128.1), a much smaller distance than that reported by Gatti et al. and Sanal et al. (Sanal et al., 1990). The most recent A-T consortium report gives D11S132/NCAM as the telomeric flanking marker (Foroud et al., 1991). Our results (Figures 1 and 2) and radiation-hybrid mapping data of Richard et al. (Richard III et al., 1992) show that D11S424 and CI11-45, the new markers flanking A-T on the telomeric side are centromeric to D11S132/NCAM/DRD2.

Finally, an investigation of a single complementation group C family has also shown significant linkage to markers in this region (Ziv *et al.*, 1991).

Further information on the location of the A-T locus is essential for efforts to isolate and characterize the gene responsible for the disease. Previously, we have constructed a primary genetic linkage map of chromosome 11q (Julier *et al.*, 1990), and this map provided a basis for the selection of markers to be characterized in the present study. The high resolution genetic and *in situ* maps of the A-T region presented here permit a precise localization of the disease locus. Several of the marker loci contained in the maps exhibited significant lod scores when characterized in families informative for linkage with A-T, and no evidence of genetic heterogeneity was found. The locus D11S384, detected with the probe CJ52.193 has a lod score of 5.9 with A-T, and exhibits no recombination with the disease in our families. Location score analysis places the gene responsible for A-T within 2 cM of this locus. Both D11S384 (CJ52.193) and the A-T locus are contained in an interval of approximately 7 cM spanned by D11S385 (CJ52.75)-D11S35 (ph2-22) and D11S424 (CJ52.77). The evidence against the localization of A-T to other intervals in the map was very strong (odds >10^7:1). These results are consistent with physical mapping and linkage data given in McConville et al. (McConville *et al.*, 1990b), who have shown that CJ52.75 and ph2-22, along with STMY, hybridize to a single pulse-field gel fragment. Their linkage data supports the placement of the A-T gene between this complex of loci and DRD2, in agreement with the localization given here. The data presented here and the radiation hybrid mapping of the same markers (Richard III *et al.*, 1992) clearly distinguishes the recently cloned candidate A-T group D gene (Kapp *et al.*, 1992) from the groups A and C genes.

ACKNOWLEDGEMENTS

We thank Dr Michael Swift (Department of Pediatrics, New York Medical College, Valhalla, NY.) for providing DNA of the 11 American families used in this study and Drs J. Aicardi, A. Aurias, M. Debray, A. Fisher, M. Landrieu, B. Pertuiset, M. Tardieu, M. Tourneux, L. Vallée, A. David, J.M. Mussini, G. Potel and Pr. Griscelli for help in the collection of the french A-T families. We thank J. Dèrrè for expert technical assistance. We are grateful to M. Leppert and R. White for providing genotype data on DRD2, and to G. Evans for a cosmid clone containing NCAM. Support was provided by grants from HFSP (M.L., C.J, M.J. and Y.N.), and INSERM and the French Minister of Recherche and Technology (M.L., R.B., D.C.).

REFERENCES

Boder, E. (1985). Ataxia-telangiectasia: An overview. In R. Gatti and M. Swift (ed.), Ataxia-telangiectasia: Genetics, Neuropathology, and Immunology of a Degenerative Disease of Childhood. Alan R. Liss, New York., pp. 1-63.

Borresen, A.-L., Anderson, T. I., Tretli, S., Heiberg, A., and Moller, P. (1990). Breast cancer and other cancers in Norwegian families with ataxia-telangiectasia. *Genes Chrom Cancer* **2**: 339-40.

Cherif, D., Julier, C., Delattre, O., Derre, J., Lathrop, G. M., and Berger, R. (1990). Simultaneous localization of cosmids and chromosome R-banding by fluorescence microscopy: application to regional mapping of human chromosome 11. *Proc Natl Acad Sci U S A* **87**: 6639-43.

Feinberg, A. P., and Vogelstein, B. (1984). Random priming method of labeling DNA *Anal Biochem* **132**: 6-13.

Foroud, T., Wei, S., Ziv, Y., Sobel, E., Lange, E., Chao, A., Gorodia, T., Huo, Y., Tolun, A., Chessa, L., Charmley, P., Sanal, O., Salman, N., Julier, C., Concannon, P., McConville, C., Taylor, A. M. R., Shiloh, Y., Lange, K., and Gatti, R. A. (1991). Localization of an ataxi-telangiectasia locus to a 3-cM interval on chromosome 11q23: Linkage analysis of 111 families by an international consortium *Am. J. Hum. Genet.* **49**: 1263-1279.

Gatti, R. A., Berkel, I., Boder, E., Braedt, G., Charmley, P., Concannon, P., Ersoy, F., Foroud, T., Jaspers, N. G., and Lange, K. (1988). Localization of an ataxia-telangiectasia gene to chromosome 11q22-23. *Nature* **336**: 577-80.

Grandy, D. K., Litt, M., Allen, L., Bunzow, J. R., Marchionni, M., Makam, H., Reed, L., Magenis, R. E., and Civelli, O. (1989). The human dopamine D2 receptor gene is located on chromosome 11 at q22-q23 and identifies a TaqI RFLP. *Am J Hum Genet* **45**: 778-85.

Hanawalt, P., and Painter, R. (1985). On the nature of a "DNA-processing defect in ataxia-telangiectasia. In R. Gatti and M. Swift (ed.), Ataxia-telangiectasia: Genetics, Neuropathology, and Immunology of a Degenerative Disease of Childhood. Alan R. Liss, New York., pp. 67-71.

Jaspers, N. G., Gatti, R. A., Baan, C., Linssen, P. C., and Bootsma, D. (1988). Genetic complementation analysis of ataxia telangiectasia and Nijmegen breakage syndrome: a survey of 50 patients. *Cytogenet Cell Genet* **49**: 259-63.

Julier, C., Nakamura, Y., Lathrop, M., O'Connell, P., Leppert, M., Litt, M., Mohandas, T., Lalouel, J. M., and White, R. (1990). A detailed genetic map of the long arm of chromosome 11. *Genomics* **7**: 335-45.

Kapp, L. N., Painter, R. B., Yu, L.-C., van Loon, N., Richard III, C. W., James, M. R., and Murnane, J. P. (1992). Cloning of a candidate gene for ataxia telangiectasia *Am. J. Hum. Genet.* **51**:45-54.

Komatsu, K., Kodama, S., Okumura, Y., Koi, M., and Oshimura, M. (1990). Restoration of radiation resistance in ataxia telangiectasia cells by the introduction of normal human chromosome 11. *Mutat Res* **235**: 59-63.

Lathrop, G. M., Lalouel, J. M., Julier, C., and Ott, J. (1984). Strategies for multilocus linkage analysis in humans. *Proc Natl Acad Sci USA* **81**: 3443-6.

Lathrop, G. M., Nakamura, Y., Cartwright, P., O'Connell, P., Leppert, M., Jones, C., Tateishi, H., Bragg, T., Lalouel, J. M., and White, R. (1988). A primary map of markers for human chromosome 10. *Genomics* **2**: 157-64.

McConville, C. M., Formstone, C. J., Hernandez, D., Thick, J., and Taylor, A. M. (1990a). Fine mapping of the chromosome 11q22-23 region using PFGE, linkage and haplotype analysis; localization of the gene for ataxia telangiectasia to a 5cM region flanked by NCAM/DRD2 and STMY/CJ52.75, phi 2.22. *Nucleic Acids Res* **18**: 4335-43.

McConville, C. M., Woods, C. G., Farrall, M., Metcalfe, J. A., and Taylor, A. M. (1990b). Analysis of 7 polymorphic markers at chromosome 11q22-23 in 35 ataxia telangiectasia families; further evidence of linkage. *Hum Genet* **85**: 215-20.

Norman, A., Fagan, R. A., and Chan, S. L. (1988). The importance of genetics for the optimization of radiation therapy. *Am J Clin Oncol* **11**: 84-8.

O'Connell, P., Lathrop, G. M., Law, M., Leppert, M., Nakamura, Y., Hoff, M., Kumlin, E., Thomas, W., Elsner, T., Ballard, L., Goodman, P., Azen, E., Sadler, J., Cai, G., Lalouel, J. M., and White, R. (1987). A primary genetic linkage map for human chromosome 12. *Genomics* **1**: 89-102.

Ott, J. (1983). Linkage analysis and family classification under heterogeneity. *Ann Hum Genet* **47**: 311-20.

Paterson, M. C., MacFarlane, S. J., Gentner, N. E., and Smith, B. (1985). Cellular hypersensitivity to chronic radiation in cultured fibrolasts from ataxia-telangiectasia heterozygotes. In R. Gatti and M. Swift (ed.), Ataxia-telangiectasia: Genetics, Neuropathology, and Immunology of a Degenerative Disease of Childhood. Alan R. Liss, New York., pp. 73-87.

Pinkel, D., Strume, T., and Gray, J. W. (1986). Cytogenetic analysis using quantitative, high sensitivity, fluorescence hybridization *Proc Natl Acad Sci USA* **83**: 2934-2938.

Pippard, E. C., Hall, A. J., Barker, D. J. P., and Bridges, B. B. (1988). Cancer in homozygotes and heterozygotes of ataxia-telangiectasia and xeroderma in Britain. *Cancer Res* **48**: 2929-32.

Reed, K., and Mann, D. (1985). Rapid transfer of DNA from agarose gels to nylon membranes. *Nucleic Acids Res* **13**: 7207-21.

Richard III, C. W., Cox, D. R., Kapp, L., Murnane, J., Cornelis, F., Julier, C., Lathrop, M., and James, M. R. (1992). A radiation hybrid map of human chromosome 11q22-q23 containing the ataxia-telangiectasia disease locus. *Submitted*

Sambrook, J., Fritsch, E., and Maniatis, T. (1989). Molecular Cloning: A Laboratory Manual

Sanal, O., Wei, S., Foroud, T., Malhotra, U., Concannon, P., Charmley, P., Salser, W., Lange, K., and Gatti, R. A. (1990). Further mapping of an ataxia-telangiectasia locus to the chromosome 11q23 region. *Am J Hum Genet* **47**: 860-6.

Swift, M., Morrell, D., Cromartie, E., Chamberlin, A. R., Skolnick, M. H., and Bishop, D. T. (1986). The incidence and gene frequency of ataxia-telangiectasia in the United States. *Am J Hum Genet* **39**: 573-83.

Swift, M., Morrell, D., Massey, R. B., and Chase, C. L. (1991). Incidence of cancer in 161 families affected by ataxia-telangiectasia. *New Eng J Med* **325**: 1831-36.

Swift, M., Reitnauer, P. J., Morrell, D., and Chase, C. L. (1987). Breast and other cancers in families with ataxia-telangiectasia. *New Eng J Med* **316**: 1289-94.

Tokino, T., Takahashi, E., Mori, M., Tanigami, A., Glaser, T., Park, J. W., Jones, C., Hori, T., and Nakamura, Y. (1991). Isolation and mapping of 62 new RFLP markers on human chromosome 11. *Am J Hum Genet* **48**: 258-68.

Ziv, Y., Rotman, G., Frydman, M., Dagan, J., Cohen, T., Foroud, T., Gatti, R. A., and Shiloh, Y. (1991). The ATC (ataxia-telangiectasia complementation group C) locus localizes to 11q22-q23. *Genomics* **9**: 373-5.

How Many Ataxia-Telangiectasia Genes?

Ethan Lange[1,2], Richard A. Gatti[1], Eric Sobel[3],
Patrick Concannon[4] and Kenneth Lange[3]

Department of Pathology[1]
Department of Biomathematics[3]
School of Medicine
Department of Mathematics[2]
University of California, Los Angeles
Los Angeles, CA 90024

The Virginia Mason Research Center[4]
Seattle, WA 98101

Introduction

In this chapter we review the evidence for genetic heterogeneity and clinical variability of A-T. Because of the existence of five complementation groups [Jasper et al. 1988], a homogeneity model is automatically suspect. There are also clinical variants of A-T, and those are discussed briefly.

On the basis of linkage analysis of group A pedigrees alone, there clearly is an ATA locus at 11q22-23 between the proximal cluster of marker loci STMY, D11S385 (CJ75), and D11S35 and the distal cluster of marker loci D11S424 (CJ77), D11S132, D11S386 (CJ5), NCAM, and DRD2 [Gatti et al. 1988a; McConville et al. 1990a, 1990b; Sanal et al. 1990; Foroud et al. 1991]. The region defined by these two clusters extends about 6-8 cM on a sex-averaged map and about 3-4 cM on a male-specific map (Figure 1). Group C pedigrees also map to the same region [Ziv et al. 1991]. At this writing it is unclear whether the ATA and ATC genes represent mutations at the same or different loci.

The relationship of these two genes to a putative ATD gene needs further analysis. Komatsu et al. [1990] corrected the radiosensitivity of group D fibroblasts via fusion with a normal chromosome 11q. In independent experiments, Kapp et al. [1989, 1992] isolated a candidate group D gene that maps by radiation hybrids to the region between THY1 and D11S83, about 30 cM distal to the ATA/ATC region. The status of this candidate gene is currently unclear since no mutations have been found in the three group D patients examined so far [Kapp et al. (this volume)].

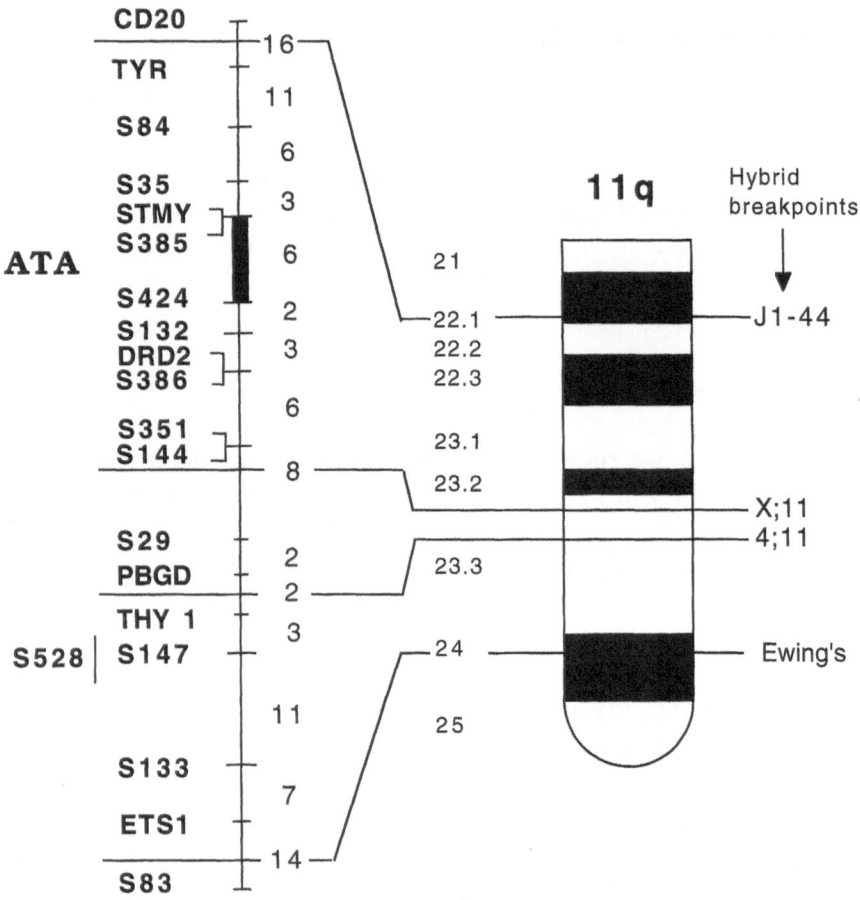

Figure 1. Linkage map (sex-averaged cM) of chromosome 11q showing localization of A-T gene(s). Hybrid cell breakpoints anchor the linkage map to a cytogenetic map.

A Brief History of A-T Mapping

To the advantage of everyone involved in mapping A-T, the A-T disease phenotype is well defined, in most cases easily diagnosed, completely penetrant, and of early onset. In addition, the radiosensitivity of A-T cells can be corrected *in vitro* by DNA transfection, thus permitting candidate genes to be screened *in vitro*. To everyone's disadvantage, affected families were initially hard to locate and are generally small, making it difficult to generate significant LOD scores by linkage analysis. Because we feared that the five defined complementation groups might represent five genes mapping to different genomic regions, it seemed to us several years ago that linkage analysis could only be successful if we could assign each family to a definite complementation group or if we could focus our mapping efforts on a single, large inbred pedigree that was genetically homogeneous.

We eventually found a large, 61-member Amish pedigree that was subsequently assigned to group A. After screening 171 genetic markers, we detected no recombinants and a LOD score of 1.8 to the biallelic marker THY1 on chromosome 11q23 [Gatti et al. 1988a, 1988b]. Follow-up studies with additional group A families confirmed linkage of the ATA locus to THY1. A second nearby biallelic marker, D11S144, also showed linkage, with no recombinants and a LOD score of 1.7 in the Amish pedigree. A certain amount of good fortune was involved in these initial discoveries because THY1 is approximately 25 cM distal to the most likely ATA location; D11S144 lies about 12 cM proximal to THY1 and correspondingly closer to the ATA locus. Both markers were uninformative in branches of the Amish pedigree that were later shown to contain recombinants distal to ATA. Several recombinants proximal to ATA would have masked linkage from that direction as well (Figure 2).

Subsequent progress in mapping the A-T gene or genes has been slow, but steady. Several labs acted on the necessity of developing a detailed marker map of the 11q22-23 region [Maslen et al. 1988; Charmley et al. 1990; Julier et al. 1990; McConville et al. 1990b; Wei et al. 1990]. Many more A-T families were collected. The work involved in these tasks has been substantial.

Parallel to these laboratory studies, we exploited advances in computer hardware and in database management software. We also developed a Monte Carlo method for computing location scores [Lange and Matthysse 1989; Lange and Sobel 1991]. Location scores are the multipoint analogs of conventional LOD scores. Location scores summarize available linkage information in a more powerful manner than LOD scores do. In this report we use location scores to assess the evidence for genetic heterogeneity in the A-T consortium families. Because of the expense and delay in doing further complementation assignments, there is little chance for a more definitive statistical analysis of genetic heterogeneity until the A-T gene or genes are cloned and sequenced.

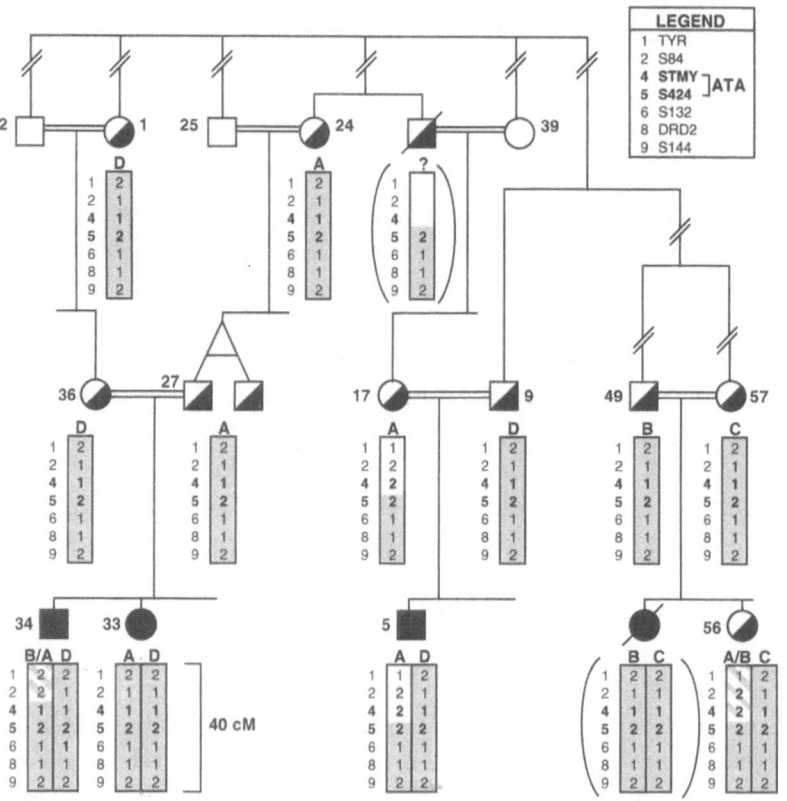

Figure 2. Haplotypes of Amish pedigree. Affected haplotypes are shaded. Cross-hatching represents recombination in that generation.

Location Scores Applied to A-T

Two distinct types of computational problems arise in creating linkage maps of the human genome. If the task is to map a common genetic marker, then the preselected pedigrees of the Centre d'Etude du Polymorphisme Humain (CEPH) can be used to good advantage [Dausset et al. 1990]. The simple and consistent structure and the nearly complete typing of these pedigrees allow straightforward linkage calculations. Although computational bottlenecks appear for more than 10 markers, with special mathematical techniques [Lathrop et al. 1986; Lander and Green 1987; Lange and Weeks 1989; Goradia et al. 1992] one can analyze marker gene flow at 20 or more loci using CEPH pedigrees.

On the other hand, if the task is to map a disease trait, particularly a rare recessive disease, the pedigrees that segregate the trait will often include a significant amount of missing data and graphical complications such as consanguinity. With such pedigrees, standard multipoint linkage calculations can seriously degrade with as few as one or two markers. Usually such calculations are performed as part of the method of location scores [Lathrop et al. 1984]. Here the marker locations are considered fixed either by previous linkage evidence or by physical mapping results [Lathrop et al. 1984; Charmley et al. 1990; Wei et al. 1990], and an attempt is made to position the trait locus relative to the markers by computing the joint probability of the trait and marker phenotypes. The more markers one is able to include, the more complete a picture of the recombination events one is able to reconstruct. These scores are plotted across the region of interest, and the trait location with the largest likelihood is noted.

Lange and Sobel [1991] recently developed a Monte Carlo method for computing location scores that allows simultaneous analysis of the trait and large numbers of marker loci. Current software is limited to biallelic markers, but theoretical advances should soon permit the lifting of this restriction. Briefly, the Monte Carlo method involves simulating the ordered genotypes for all marker loci conditioned on the observed marker phenotypes. One then samples several realizations from this simulation. Because marker genotypes and phases are known for each realization, one can compute by standard deterministic methods the joint likelihood of the trait and marker loci at each possible position of the trait loci. Averaging these joint likelihoods over the sampled realizations provides an approximate location score curve.

Lange and Sobel [1991] showed that this Monte Carlo algorithm gives good numerical agreement on two simple data sets for which exact likelihoods can be computed. Simultaneously, Foroud et al. [1991] used the Monte Carlo method on A-T data to good effect. These data, slightly updated and corrected here, consist of 94 A-T pedigrees typed at 14 biallelic markers in the 11q22-23 region. Of the 94 pedigrees, 22 are consanguineous, 12 belong to complementation group A, four belong to group C, and one belongs to group V1. The remaining pedigrees are unassigned, but otherwise typical A-T pedigrees. Roughly a third of all marker information is missing in the 94 pedigrees. Of the 14 original markers described by Foroud et al. [1991], the locus APO has been dropped from the current data, and the locus D11S424 (CJ52.77) has been added.

The location score curve for the revised data is shown in Figure 3. This figure clearly implies that the 6 cM interval from STMY to D11S424 is the most likely interval for an A-T locus. The next most likely interval extends from D11S84 to STMY and is less likely by a factor of at least 10^{-5}. Dropping three $\log_{10}$ units below the maximum likelihood provides a conservative 4 cM support interval for an A-T locus. This support interval is centered between STMY and D11S424 and agrees well with the 4 cM interval around D11S384 (CJ193) suggested by Cornelis et al. [this volume].

Dissection of Heterogeneity by Location Scores

As a follow-up to Foroud et al. [1991], Sobel et al. [1992] employed the same 94 A-T pedigrees to address the question of heterogeneity. In particular, Sobel et al. [1992] noted the presence of a secondary mode in the A-T location score curve in the vicinity of Kapp's candidate ATD locus. Equally intriguing, this mode was slightly more pronounced when the 16 known group A and C families were omitted from the analysis and was absent when only the A and C families were included. These pedigree observations seemed to bolster the case for a separate D locus, but it must be stressed that no formal statistical tests were performed at that writing to assess the importance of the secondary mode. Here we evaluate the location score curve evidence more rigorously.

Our strategy compares two models. Model 1 assumes one location

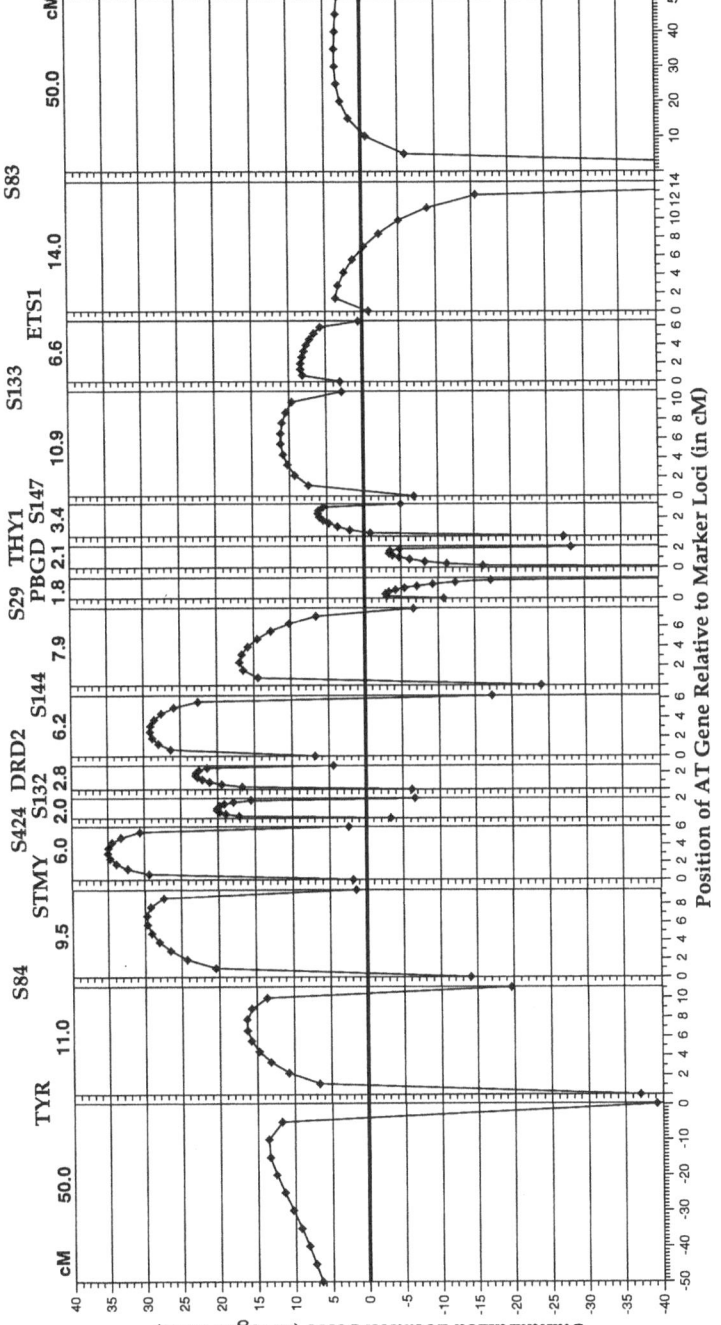

Figure 3: Location scores using all pedigrees.

s for the A-T gene along the chromosome, and model 2 assumes two locations s and t. In model 2 we further postulate a prior probability α of an unassigned pedigree segregating an A-T mutation at location s; the pedigree then segregates an A-T mutation at location t with the complementary probability $1 - \alpha$. Under model 1 the likelihood of the data is

$$L_1(s) \;=\; \prod_i \mathrm{Pr}_s(ped_i),$$

where i ranges over all pedigrees, and where $\mathrm{Pr}_s(ped_i)$ denotes the likelihood of the observed phenotypes on the ith pedigree when the A-T gene is located at s. Under model 2 the likelihood of the data is

$$L_2(\alpha, s, t) \;=\; \prod_i [\alpha \mathrm{Pr}_s(ped_i) + (1 - \alpha)\mathrm{Pr}_t(ped_i)].$$

The maximum likelihood procedure in comparing two models is to maximize each corresponding likelihood with respect to its parameters. In the present context, we must be careful since the location score curve appears multimodal. Typically each marker interval for the A-T gene shows a single mode of the curve and a plunge of the curve toward $-\infty$ as the A-T gene approaches either end of the interval. Thus, we are really faced with a sequence of optimization problems – one for each interval or pair of intervals. Since our Monte Carlo program evaluates a likelihood $\mathrm{Pr}_s(ped_i)$ within each interval at only a finite number of points s, these optimization problems are discrete in s and t, but continuous in α. The discrete part of the optimization is handled by exhaustive consideration of each s or pair s and t subject to the constraint that s and t are confined to the few relevant points on their relevant intervals. The continuous part of the optimization is easily done by the bisection algorithm on α for each fixed pair s and t.

Once $L_1(s)$ and $L_2(\alpha, s, t)$ are maximized, we can compare the models by likelihood ratios evaluated at the optimal points. For model 2 we can also compute the posterior probability that a particular pedigree i segregates form 1 of the disease. Assuming that the optimal values of the parameters are true, Bayes' theorem indicates that this posterior probability is given by the expression

$$\frac{\alpha \mathrm{Pr}_s(ped_i)}{\alpha \mathrm{Pr}_s(ped_i) + (1 - \alpha)\mathrm{Pr}_t(ped_i)}$$

evaluated at the optimal points. Posterior probabilities can be used as a diagnostic in understanding the implications of model 2 [Ott 1991] on a pedigree-by-pedigree basis.

In the A-T data there are 15 intervals for the location of the single A-T locus of model 1 and $\frac{15 \times 14}{2} = 105$ pairs of intervals for the location of the two different A-T loci of model 2. As already noted, STMY – D11S424 is the best interval under model 1. The two best intervals under model 2 are STMY – D11S424 and D11S144 – D11S29. These two best intervals are barely distinguishable from the second best pair STMY – D11S424 and DRD2 – D11S144. In the model 2 calculations, the prior probability that a family is assigned to the proximal interval of a pair of intervals was taken as 1 rather than α for those 16 families assigned to groups A or C. The single V1 family was treated as unassigned. The ratio of maximum likelihoods for model 2 versus model 1 is 41.4, not a convincing argument for choosing model 2 over the more parsimonious model 1.

The advantage of model 2 over model 1 is even less striking if we compare the single best interval STMY – D11S424 to the pair of intervals STMY – D11S424 and D11S147 – D11S133. Recall that D11S147 – D11S133 is the location of the putative ATD locus. In this comparison the ratio of maximum likelihoods is 29.8 for model 2 versus model 1. As outlined above, we computed posterior probabilities for the various unassigned pedigrees segregating an STMY – D11S424 A-T gene rather than an D11S147 – D11S133 A-T gene. These calculations are based on an estimated prior probability α of .86. This estimate of α does agree well with the frequency of non-group D patients. Naturally the posterior probability for each of the 16 families already assigned to complementation groups A and C must be 1.

Among the 78 unassigned pedigrees, only three estimated posterior probabilities fell below .5. The highest of these three was .45. The second highest, .24, belonged to a pedigree that appears not to link to 11q22-23. The single affected in this pedigree suggests the possibility of a spontaneous mutation. The lowest posterior probability, .02, belonged to a consanguineous pedigree that is heterozygous on the interval STMY – D11S424 and homozygous on the interval D11S147 – D11S133. Although there are no obvious crossovers within STMY – D11S424, heterozygosity is inconsistent with the plausible hypothesis of a single ancestral gene meeting in the inbred affecteds. Since typing with other markers close to

D11S147 – D11S133, such as D11S29, THY1 and D11S528, does reveal heterozygosity in the patients, the evidence for assigning this pedigree to the interval D11S147 – D11S133 is ambiguous. Perhaps in this pedigree, the A-T genes found in the affecteds originate from more than one ancestor. These two anomalous pedigrees could also belong to the rare complementation group E.

Because the location score analysis is based on a subset of the markers and on biallelic systems only, there is some loss of information. Construction of haplotypes for each of the 94 families reinforces the case for genetic homogeneity. We have typed CA repeats at the loci D11S35, DRD2, and D11S528 and additional biallelic probes on the loci D11S385, NCAM, D11S386, and D11S351. With the exception of the two pedigrees identified above with the lowest posterior probabilities, all pedigrees seem consistent with the hypothesis of a single A-T gene on the interval STMY – D11S424.

The one remaining puzzle is the appearance of the secondary mode of the location score curve on the interval D11S147 – D11S133 [Sobel et al. 1992]. In reconsidering this mode, the three deep gaps between D11S29 and D11S147 seem as impressive as the secondary mode. This insight suggested to us that it might be useful to repeat the location score analyses omitting the intermediate marker PBGD. The results of recomputing location scores with this omission were striking (Figure 4). Clearly, the evidence for heterogeneity has disappeared. It is difficult to pinpoint the exact cause of this change. Most likely, the locus PBGD had hidden typing errors that obscured the true pattern of inheritance in its vicinity. It is noteworthy that the odds for placing the A-T gene at STMY – D11S424 increased when PBGD was omitted from the analysis.

Variants

Although early genetic studies emphasized the uniformity of the A-T syndrome, variants do exist [Hecht and McCaw 1977; Ying and Decoteau 1981; Weemaes et al. 1981; Fiorilli et al. 1983; Byrne et al. 1984; Seemanova et al. 1985; Conley et al. 1986; Taylor et al. 1987; Aicardi et al. 1988; Jaspers et al. 1988; Maserati et al. 1988; Wegner et al. 1988; Curry et al. 1989; Ziv et al. 1989; Ziv et al. 1992; Chessa and Fiorilli (this volume); Porras et al. (this volume); Sanal et al. (this volume); Taylor and Woods (this volume)]. It is unclear whether these

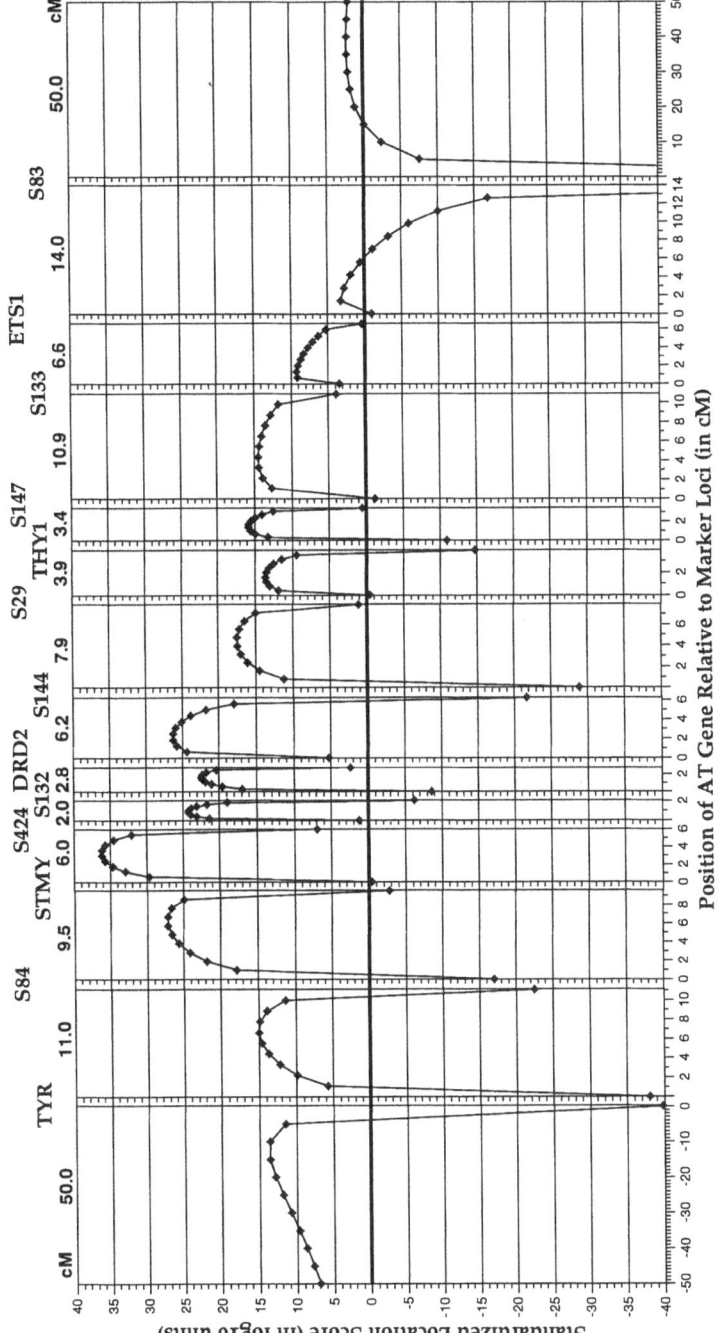

Figure 4: Location scores using all pedigrees but omitting marker PBGD.

variants represent unusual alleles at a single A-T locus, other rare A-T loci, or other disease entities. Most of the answers to such questions will come with the isolation of the A-T gene(s). Once the normal DNA sequence of the gene is known, it will be possible to look for mutations in the sequences of variant patients. No doubt a few variants will turn out to be compound heterozygotes.

Current A-T variants can be briefly categorized on both clinical and laboratory grounds. Some of the variable *clinical* features are listed in Table 1; variable *laboratory* features are listed in Table 2. Occasionally

Table 1. Clinical Variations of A-T

Age of onset of ataxia
Presence or absence of telangiectasia
Presence or absence of immunodeficiency
Severity of immunodeficiency
Associations with other disorders:
    diabetes
    cardiac anomalies
    endocrine defects
    gastric cancer
    epilepsy
    nystagmus
    clubbing

Table 2. Laboratory Variations of A-T

Serum alphafetoprotein – abnormal in > 95%
Radioresistant DNA synthesis – abnormal in > 95%
Chromosomal aberrations – abnormal in > 75%
Cell survival after *in vitro* irradiation
Cell survival after *in vitro* exposure to radiomimetic
    agents

A-T patients do not manifest well-defined telangiectasia [Ying and Decoteau 1981; Byrne et al. 1984; Aicardi et al. 1988; Maserati et al. 1988]. At least three families exist in which some members have classical A-T, while others have only severe telangiectasia with or without ataxia [Sanal et al. (this volume)].

The relationship between A-T and other DNA repair and chromosomal instability syndromes also needs to be clarified. Some patients have been described with classical clinical features of A-T but with little or no increased radiosensitivity, as measured by either radioresistant DNA synthesis (RDS) or colony survival [Chessa and Fiorilli (this volume)]. Unfortunately, a patient with normal radiosensitivity can never be assigned to a complementation group. Perhaps some of these 'experiments of nature' will also help us to recognize other A-T genes, forming a more extensive A-T family of genes.

It is important to keep in mind that variants account for only a small fraction of all A-T patients. At least 95 per cent of A-T families appear to link to the 11q22-23 region. We have some preliminary data suggesting linkage of the related, but more difficult to localize, Nijmegen Breakage Syndrome [Weemaes et al. 1981] to 11q22-23 region markers as well.

Table 3 attempts to summarize some of the issues concerning variants. We prefer to divide A-T patients and variants into four *generic* categories. Category A) includes classical A-T patients meeting the minimal criteria of consistency with: recessive inheritance; progressive, early-onset cerebellar ataxia; radiosensitivity; and ocular apraxia. Category B) includes those patients in complementation group V1 [Seemanova et al. 1985; Curry et al. 1989] as well as patients satisfying the minimal criteria of radiosensitivity and progressive cerebellar ataxia but lacking some of the other classical clinical indications of A-T. Unassigned patients in category B) are natural candidates for complementation studies. Category C) includes patients with ataxia who do not manifest radiosensitivity. Complementation tests are impossible for these patients, so they will have to be analyzed in other ways. Category D) includes patients with other radiosensitivity syndromes, but without ataxia or telangiectasia. Complementation studies for these individuals should prove revealing when feasible. DNA sequencing will also be useful in determining whether any of the category C) and D) patients are A-T mutants.

TABLE 3
ATAXIA-TELANGIECTASIA SYNDROMES

	A	T	radio sens	familial	chrom aberr	AFP	apraxia	CA	immune defect	MR	micro ceph
A – Classic AT											
Generic	+	(+)	+	+	(+)	(+)	(+)	(+)	(+)	-	-
B – "AT variants"											
Generic	(+)	(+)	+	+	+	(+)	(+)	(+)	(+)	+	+
Curry (V$_1$)[a] [1989]	+	+	+	+	+	+	+	-	-	+	+
Nijmegen (V$_1$) [1981]	-	-	+	+	+	-	-	-	+	+	+
Seemanova #7 (V$_1$) [1985]	-	-	+	+	+	?	-	-	-	-	+
Junker [b]	+	(+)	?	+	(-)	+	+	+	-	-	-
Byrne [1984]	+	-	?	+	(-)	-	+	+	+	+	?
Fiorilli #6 [1988]	+	-	?	-	+	+	+	?	-	+	?
C – "AT-Like" disorders											
Generic	+	(+)	-	+	-	-	(+)	-	-	(+)	-
D – Other radiation hypersensitivity/chromosome breakage syndromes[c]											
Generic	-	-	+	+	+	-	-	(+)	(+)	(+)	+
Conley (V$_2$) [1986]	-	-	+	-	+	-	?	-	+	+	+
Wegner (V$_2$) [1988]	-	-	+	+	+	-	-	+	+	+	+
Seemanova #5 [1985]	-	-	?	+	?	?	-	+	-	-	+

[a] Letter in parentheses denotes AT Complementation Group assignment

[b] Personal communication

[c] Despite the absence of ataxia or telangiectasia, these could also become "AT variants" if an AT complementation group assignment were made.

(+) Usually positive

(-) Usually negative

Discussion

The existence of five different complementation groups and numerous clinical variants suggest caution in approaching the question of genetic heterogeneity in A-T. On the other hand, the troublesome scenario of multiple independent A-T loci scattered throughout the genome is inconsistent with the linkage data. The evidence for a locus in the STMY – D11S424 interval is compelling. Almost all A-T pedigrees (148 out of 150) show linkage to this interval. The available linkage data do not lend much support to the contention that there is another A-T locus in the interval D11S147 – D11S133, to which the ATDC gene maps [Kapp et al. 1992]. In fact, the likelihood ratio statistics and posterior probabilities suggest the opposite. It is possible that our data contain very few group D pedigrees; certainly none of the assigned pedigrees belong to group D. The preponderance of linkage evidence points to genetic homogeneity, not heterogeneity. This conclusion is supported as well by the independent linkage study of Cornelis et al. [this volume].

Despite this general conclusion, we are unwilling to rule out genetic heterogeneity altogether. We have not applied a significance test to the data in the strict sense because the two models considered do not fit the usual large sample paradigm of one hypothesis smoothly nested inside another. There are also one or two classical A-T pedigrees that appear not link to 11q at all. These may represent new mutations in one parent or mistaken identifications of specimens. The latter is being checked.

Finally, there is the question of A-T variants. The boundaries separating typical A-T patients from variant A-T patients are sometimes vague. Ultimately, understanding the molecular genetics of A-T will clarify these boundaries and lead to reliable tests for detecting carriers and compound heterozygotes. Meanwhile, we must continue to perform linkage analyses with sensitivity to the clinical variability of A-T. Positional cloning requires a clear location assignment for at least the first A-T gene.

Acknowledgements

This research was supported by USPHS Grants CA 16042, CA 57569, DOE Grant FGD3 87ER60548, and grants from the A-T Medical Research Foundation and the Thomas Appeal A-T Medical Research Trust.

52

References

Aicardi J, Barbosas C, Andermann E, Andermann F, Morcos R, Ghanem Q, Fukuyama Y, Awaya Y, Moe P (1988) Ataxia-ocular motor apraxia: a syndrome mimicking ataxia-telangiectasia. *Ann Neurol* 24:497-502

Byrne E, Hallpike JF, Manson JI, Sutherland GR, Thong YH (1984) Progressive multisystem degeneration with IgE deficiency and chromosomal instability. *J Neurol Sci* 66:307-317

Charmley P, Foroud T, Wei S, Concannon P, Weeks DE, Lange K, Gatti RA (1990) A primary linkage map of the human chromosome 11q22-23 region. *Genomics* 6:316-323

Conley ME, Spinner MB, Emanuel BS, Nowell PC, Nichols WW (1986) A chromosome breakage syndrome with profound immunodeficiency. *Blood* 67:1251-1256

Curry CJR, O'Lague P, Tsai J, Hutchinson HT, Jaspers NGJ, Wara D, Gatti RA (1989) AT_{Fresno}: A phenotype linking ataxia-telangiectasia with the Nijmegen breakage syndrome. *Amer J. Hum Genet* 45:270-275

Dausset J, Cann H, Cohen D, Lathrop M, Lalouel J-M, White R (1990) Centre d'Etude du Polymorphisme Humain (CEPH): Collaborative genetic mapping of the human genome. *Genomics* 6:575-577

Fiorilli M, Businco L, Pandolfi F, Paganelli R, Russo G, Aiuti F (1983) Heterogeneity of immunological abnormalities in ataxia-telangiectasia. *J Clin Immunol* 3:135-141

Foroud T, Wei S, Ziv Y, Sobel E, Lange E, Chao A, Goradia T, Huo Y, Tolun A, Chessa L, Charmley P, Sanal O, Salman N, Julier C, Concannon P, McConville C, Taylor AMR, Shiloh Y, Lange K, Gatti RA (1991) Localization of an ataxia-telangiectasia locus to a 3 cM interval on chromosome 11q23: Linkage analysis of 111 families by an international consortium. *Am J Hum Genet* 49:1263-1279

Gatti RA, Berkel I, Boder E, Braedt G, Charmley P, Concannon P, Ersoy F, Foroud T, Jaspers NGJ, Lange K, Lathrop GM, Leppert M, Nakamura Y, O'Connell P, Paterson M, Salser W, Sanal O, Silver J, Sparkes RS, Susi E, Weeks DE, Wei S, White R, Yoder F (1988a) Localization of an ataxia-telangiectasia gene to chromosome 11q22-23. *Nature* 336:577-580

Gatti RA, Shaked R, Wei S, Koyama M, Salser W, Silver J (1988b) DNA polymorphism in the human Thy-1 gene. *Hum Immunol* 22:145-150

Goradia TM, Lange K, Miller PL, Nadkarni PM (1992) Fast computation of genetic likelihoods on human pedigree data. *Hum Hered* 42:42-62

Hecht F, McCaw BK (1977) Chromosome instability syndromes, in Genetics of Human Cancer. (eds. Mulvihill JJ, Miller RW, Fraumeni JF). *Raven Press* ,New York pp 105-123

Jaspers NGJ, Gatti RA, Baan C, Linssen PCML, Bootsma D (1988) Genetic complementation analysis of ataxia-telangiectasia and Nijmegen breakage syndrome: a survey of 50 patients. *Cytogenet Cell Genet* 49:259-263

Jaspers NGJ, Taalman RDFM, Baan C (1988) Patients with an inherited syndrome characterized by immunodeficiency, microcephaly, and chromosomal instability: genetic relation to ataxia-telangiectasia. *Amer J. Hum Genet* 42:66-73

Julier C, Nakamura Y, Lathrop M, O'Connell P, Leppert M, Litt M, Mohandas T, Lalouel JM, White R (1990) A detailed map of the long arm of chromosome 11. *Genomics* 7:335-345

Kapp LN, Painter RB (1989) Stable radioresistance in ataxia-telangiectasia cells containing DNA form normal human cells. *Int J Radiat Biol* 56:667-675

Kapp LN, Painter RB, Yu L-C, van Loon N, Richard CW, James MR, Cox DR, Murnane JP (1992) Cloning of a candidate gene for ataxia-telangiectasia group D. *Am J Hum Genet* 51:45-54

Komatsu K, Kodama S, Okumura Y, Koi M, Oshimura M (1990) Restoration of radiation resistance in ataxia-telangiectasia cells by the introduction of normal human chromosome 11. *Mutat Res* 235:59-63

Lander ES, Green P (1987) Construction of multilocus genetic linkage maps in humans. *Proc Natl Acad Sci USA* 84:2363-2367

Lange K, Matthysse S (1989) Simulations of pedigree genotypes by random walks. *Amer J Hum Genet* 45:959-970

Lange K, Sobel E (1991) A random walk method for computing genetic location scores. *Am J Hum Genet* 49:1320-1334

Lange K, Weeks DE (1989) Efficient computation of lod scores: Genotype elimination, genotype redefinition, and hybrid maximum likelihood algorithms. *Ann Hum Genet* 53:67-83

Lathrop GM, Lalouel J-M, Julier C, Ott J (1984) Strategies for multilocus linkage analysis in humans. *Proc Natl Acad Sci USA* 81:3443-3446

Lathrop GM, Lalouel J-M, White RL (1986) Construction of human linkage maps: likelihood calculations for multilocus linkage analysis. *Genet Epidem* 3:39-52

McConville CM, Formstone CJ, Hernandez D, Thick J, Taylor AMR (1990a) Fine mapping of the chromosome 11q22-23 region using PFGE, linkage and haplotype analysis; localization of the gene for ataxia telangiectasia to a 5cM region flanked by NCAM/DRD2 and STMY/CJ52.75, phi 2.22. *Nucleic Acids Res* 18: 4335-4343

McConville CM, Woods CG, Farrall M, Metcalfe JA, Taylor AMR (1990b) Analysis of 7 polymorphic markers at chromosome 11q22-23 in 35 ataxia- telangiectasia families: further evidence of linkage. *Human Genet* 85:215-220

Maserati E, Ottoline A, Veggiatti P, Lanzi G, Pasquali F (1988) Ataxia without telangiectasia in two sisters with rearrangements of chromosomes 7 and 14. *Clin Genet* 34:283-287

Maslen CL, Jones C, Glaser T, Magenis RE, Sheehy R, Kelogg J, Litt M (1988) Seven polymorphic loci mapping to human chromosome region 11q22-qter. *Genomics* 2:66-75

Ott J (1991) *Analysis of Human Genetic Linkage, Rev. Ed.* Johns Hopkins, Baltimore.

Sanal O, Wei S, Foroud T, Malhotra U, Concannon P, Charmley P, Salser W, Lange K, Gatti RA (1990) Further mapping of an ataxia-telangiectasia locus to the chromosome 11q23 region. *Am J Hum Genet* 47: 860-866

Seemanova E, Passarge E, Beneskova D, Houstek J, Kasal P, Sevcikova M. (1985) Familial microcephaly with normal intelligence, immunodeficiency, and risk for lymphoreticular malignancies: a new autosomal recessive disorder. *Am J Med Genet* 20:639-648

Sobel E, Lange E, Jaspers NGJ, Chessa L, Sanal O, Shiloh J, Taylor AMR, Weemaes CMA, Lange K, Gatti RA (1992) Ataxia-telangiectasia: linkage evidence for genetic heterogeneity. *Am J Hum Genet* 50:1343-1348

Taylor AMR, Flude E, Laher B, Stacer M, McKay E, Watt J, Green SH, Harding AE (1987) Variant forms of ataxia-telangiectasia. *J Med Genet* 24: 669-677

Weemaes CMR, Hustinx TWJ, Scheres JMJC, Van Munster PJJ, Bakkeren JAJM, Taalman RDFM (1981) A new chromosomal instability disorder: the Nijmegen breakage syndrome. *Acta Paediatr. Scand.* 70:557-562

Wegner RD, Metzger M, Hanefeld NG, Jaspers J, Baan C, Magdorf K, Kunze J, Sperling K (1988) A new chromosomal instability disorder confirmed by complementation studies. *Clin Genet* 33:20-32

Wei S, Rocchi M, Archidiacono N, Sacchi N, Romeo G, Gatti RA (1990) Physical mapping of the human chromosome 11q23 region containing the ataxia-telangiectasia locus. *Cancer Genet Cytogenet* 46:1-8

Ying KL, Decoteau WE (1981) Cytogenetic anomalies in a patient with ataxia, immune deficiency and high alpha-fetoprotein in the absence of telangiectasia. *Cancer Genet Cytogenet* 4: 311-317

Ziv Y, Amiel A, Jaspers NGJ, Berkel AI, Shiloh Y (1989) Ataxia-telangiectasia: a variant with altered in vitro phenotype of fibroblast cells. *Mut Res* 210:211-219

Ziv Y, Frydman M, Lange E, Zelnik N, Rotman G, Julier C, NGJ Japsers, Dagan Y, Abeliovicz D, Dar H, Borochowitz Z, Lanthrop M, Gatti RA, Shiloh Y (1992) Ataxia-telangiectasia: linkage analysis in highly inbred Arab and Druze families and differentiation from an ataxia-microcephaly-cataract syndrome. *Hum Genet* 88:619-626

Ziv Y, Rotman G, Frydman M, Dagan J, Cohen T, Foroud T, Gatti RA, Shiloh Y (1991) The ATC (ataxia-telangiectasia group C) locus localizes to chromosome 11q22-q23. *Genomics* 9:373-375

ISOLATION OF HUMAN cDNAS THAT COMPLEMENT THE ATAXIA-TELANGIECTASIA PHENOTYPE IN CULTURED FIBROBLASTS

M. Stephen Meyn, Jennifer M. Lu-Kuo and Laura B. K. Herzing
Department of Genetics
Yale University School of Medicine
333 Cedar Street, New Haven, CT 06510
USA

INTRODUCTION

The autosomal recessive disease ataxia-telangiectasia (A-T) represents an important model system for the study of immunodeficiency, cancer and neurologic degeneration as well as for cellular responses to induced and spontaneous DNA damage. However, despite extensive investigation, no A-T gene has been identified to date and the site of action of the A-T gene product(s) is unknown.

One aspect of the A-T phenotype, sensitivity to the killing effects of ionizing radiation and radiomimetic chemicals, offers the possibility of cloning A-T genes as well as other genes involved in the same pathway by complementation of the A-T phenotype in culture. As detailed by Shiloh *et al.* (this volume), previous efforts to isolate these genes by complementation after transfection of genomic human DNA have been impeded by low transfection frequencies, a tendency to integrate relatively small segments of DNA, instability of integrated DNA and difficulties in recovering transfected genes from complemented cells.

To circumvent these difficulties we are using a human cDNA expression library constructed in an Epstein-Barr virus (EBV)-based cDNA expression vector (pRep5) for expression cloning of candidate A-T genes. The pRep5 vector confers hygromycin resistance to human cells and is maintained episomally both in human cells and in bacteria (Groger *et al.*, 1989). As a result, plasmids containing cDNAs can be rescued from complemented cells by direct transfection of nuclear DNA into *E. coli,* thus enhancing transfection efficiency and ease of recovery as well as eliminating the need to reclone complementing cDNAs (Strathdee *et al.*, 1992).

In our cloning scheme a human cDNA library is electroporated into a population of A-T cells. Cells which have been stably transformed are selected for by growth in hygromycin and then subjected to treatment with streptonigrin, a DNA-damaging agent that preferentially kills A-T cells. Cells that survive streptonigrin selection are then cloned and screened to identify complemented cells and transfected vectors rescued from those cells which have acquired a normal phenotype. Further analysis then can identify complementing cDNAs and candidate disease genes contained within the rescued vectors. Using this approach we have isolated 9 unrelated cDNAs from SV40-transformed group D A-T fibroblasts that had acquired mutagen-resistance after transfection with a human fibroblast cDNA library. Five of these cDNAs partially complemented the mutagen-sensitivity of A-T D fibroblasts, but none of the cDNAs we have mapped to date localize to the known A-T locus at 11q23.

CHOICE OF A RECIPIENT CELL LINE

Although lymphoblasts may be more efficiently transformed by EBV-based vectors than fibroblasts, we chose to use the SV40-transformed fibroblast line GM5849 (AT5BIVI), because fibroblasts form colonies. This allows selection for colony survival rather than survival of individual cells. Selection for survival of a colony of streptonigrin-resistant cells can be more powerful than selection of individual resistant cells, because the probability of a colony's survival is a multiplicative product of the likelihood of survival of its member cells. Thus, a colony that is composed entirely of streptonigrin-resistant complemented cells is far more likely to survive and grow in a given time than a colony composed of sensitive non-complemented cells.

In an attempt to improve the efficiency of stable transfection of GM5849 fibroblasts, we electroporated them with the plasmid pNeoA/EBNA-1, constructed by insertion of the EBV nuclear antigen-1 gene (EBNA-1) from pCEGE into the BamH1 and Pst1 cloning sites of pCMIneoA (Meyn, unpublished data). pNeoA/EBNA-1 contains the EBNA-1 gene and the dominant selectable marker *neo* transcribed from independent promoters, and can be used to create fibroblast lines that constitutively express the EBV nuclear antigen-1, a protein required to maintain EBV-based plasmids as episomes. Six GM5849 clones that had acquired G418-resistance after being transfected with pNeoA/EBNA-1 did not show increased frequencies of stable transformation to hygromycin-resistance when subsequently electroporated with pRep5. We concluded that providing EBNA-1 *in trans* did not improve the efficiency of transfection of GM5849 with pRep5 and did not use EBNA-1-expressing GM5849 derivatives as recipients for cDNA library transfections.

GM5849-5L20, the A-T cell line ultimately used for the cDNA library transfections, is a derivative of GM5849 that contains a single copy of the recombination vector pLrec integrated in its genomic DNA. This vector contains two mutant copies of an SV40 promoter-driven *E. coli lacZ* gene that serve as recombination substrates. Recombination events involving the *lacZ* genes are detected by histochemical staining for β-Galactosidase activity, and spontaneous intrachromosomal recombination rates determined by fluctuation analysis (Herzing and Meyn, submitted).

cDNA LIBRARY TRANSFECTION OF A-T FIBROBLASTS AND PHENOTYPIC CHARACTERIZATION OF PRIMARY TRANSFORMANTS

We have carried out a series of electroporations of the group D A-T fibroblast line GM5849-5L20 with LN, a human cDNA library constructed using mRNA from SV40-transformed fibroblasts (GM847) and the pRep5 expression vector. The transfections yielded ~610,000 primary transformants, 68 of which survived streptonigrin selection (10-21 days exposure to 0.1-0.3 ng/ml streptonigrin). 43/68 surviving clones were at least partially streptonigrin-resistant, showing >20% survival after 24 hr exposure to 0.5ng/ml streptonigrin as compared to 1-3% survival for the 5L20 parent (data not shown). Figure 1a shows theresults of a quantitative evaluation of streptonigrin resistance for three of these primary

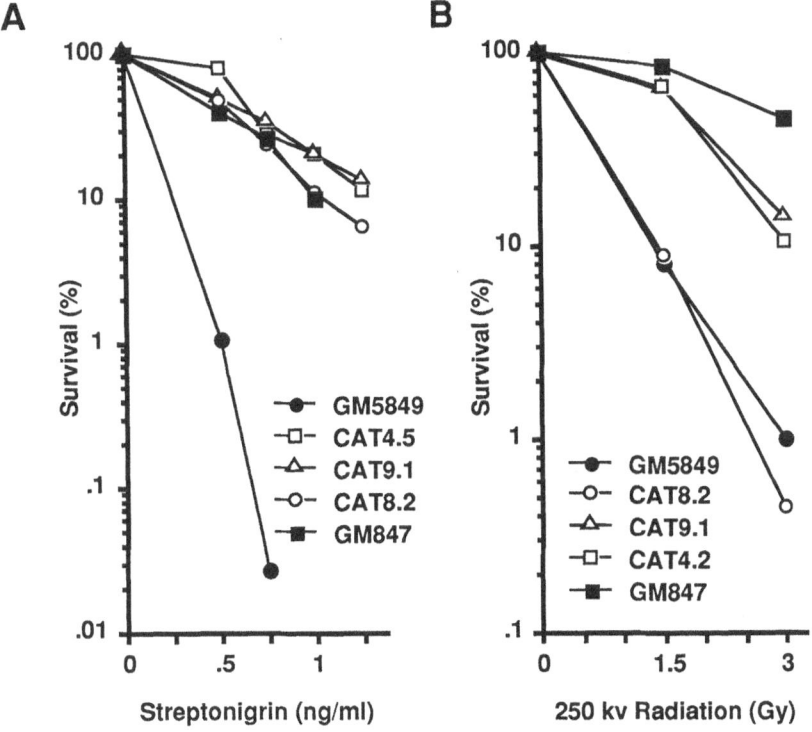

Figure 1. Survival after (A) 24 hrs exposure to streptonigrin or (B) exposure to 250 kv ionizing radiation. CAT4.5, CAT8.2, CAT4.2 and CAT9.1 are A-T D fibroblasts transfected with the LN cDNA library; GM5849 is the parent A-T D cell line and GM847 is a control cell line. Survival was measured by colony-forming ability, and points represent averages of duplicate plates. cDNA library construction, transfection and selection of recipient A-T fibroblasts and phenotypic characterization of primary transformants were carried out as described in Meyn, *et al.*, submitted.

transformants along with appropriate controls. Fifteen of the streptonigrin[R] transformants demonstrated >30% survival after 1.5 Gy irradiation and were classified radiation-resistant. Figure 1b shows survival after irradiation for control cell lines along with three streptonigrin[R] transformants that arose independently on separate dishes. The parent vector, pRep5, also was tested and found not to affect the streptonigrin- and radiation-sensitivity of the A-T D fibroblasts (data not shown).

GM5849 has a high spontaneous rate of intrachromosomal recombination (Meyn, submitted) and the primary transformants were tested for suppression of this aspect of the A-T phenotype. Figure 2 summarizes measurements of spontaneous recombination rates for a control cell line (GM847), the A-T cell line used for library transfections (GM5849-5L20) and a

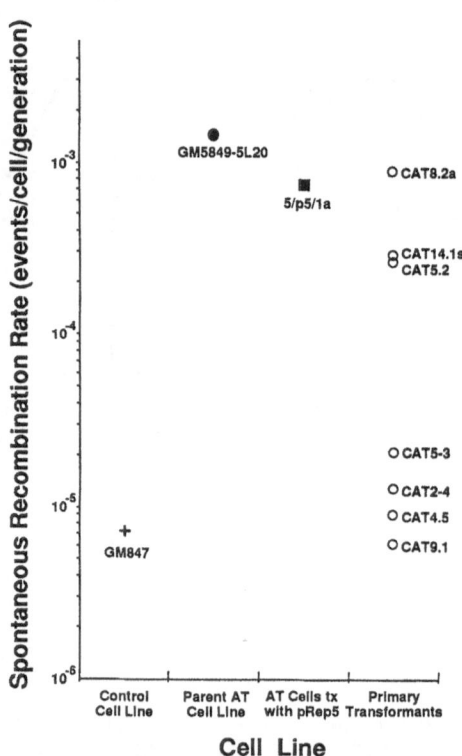

Figure 2. Spontaneous rates of intrachromosomal recombination between tandem *lacZ* genes contained in the pLrec vector integrated in the chromosomal DNA of GM847, GM5849-5L20 and transfected derivatives of GM5948-5L20. Rates were measured by fluctuation analysis as described in Herzing and Meyn, submitted.

derivative of 5L20 transfected with the pRep5 vector (5/p5/1a) as well as for seven of the streptonigrin[R] primary transformants. The spontaneous recombination rates of 3 of the primary transformants, CAT8.2a, CAT14.1s and CAT5.2 were only slightly less than that of 5L20, while four of the primary transformants tested, CAT5-5, CAT9.1, CAT4.5 and CAT4.4, had lost the hyper-recombination phenotype of their parent.

Table 1. Episomal plasmids recovered from streptonigrin[R] primary transformants

Size of rescued cDNA (name of cDNA)	Primary Transformant	colonies + for cDNA inserts total screened*	*size of other rescued plasmids*				
			3.8kb	7.2kb	10kb	parent†	other
8.6kb (pCAT6-4)	CAT6-4	1/7	0	5	0	0	1
4.5kb (pCAT4.4)	CAT4.4	1/6	1	0	3	1	0
	CAT2.1	14/93	20	2	13	0	0
	CAT9.1	13/82	52	1	16	0	0
	CAT6-1s	5/13	0	0	8	0	0
	CAT3-3	1/18	13	4	0	0	0
	CAT6-3	5/23	14	0	4	0	0
	CAT2-1	1/15	14	0	0	0	0
	CAT2-4	1/8	7	0	0	0	0
4.2kb (pCAT4.5)	CAT4.5	17/22	1	1	3	0	0
	CAT4-7	1/13	12	0	0	0	0
2.7kb (pCAT5.2)	CAT5.2	19/19	0	0	0	0	
2.1kb (pCAT8.2)	CAT8.2	13/13	0	0	0	0	0
	CAT14.1s	2/80	0	0	43	0	35
1.9kb (pCAT4.2)	CAT4.2	5/6	1	0	0	0	0
	CAT19.1	1/26	2	0	21	0	2
1.7kb (pCAT5-3)	CAT5-3	12/12	0	0	0	0	0
1.4kb (pCAT5-5)	CAT5-5	1/1	0	0	0	0	0
0.9kb (pCAT4-2)	CAT4-2	19/19	0	0	0	0	0

Low molecular weight nuclear DNA from streptonigrin[R] A-T fibroblasts transfected with the LN cDNA library was electroporated into E. coli and plasmids from the resultant Amp[R] colonies recovered and analysed as described in Meyn, et al., submitted. *The number of bacterial colonies that harbored a vector with a cDNA insert/the total number of bacterial colonies analysed. †10.5 kb in size and identified as the parent vector by restriction enzyme analysis.

cDNA RESCUE AND ANALYSIS

cDNAs were rescued by electroporating *E. coli* with low-molecular-weight nuclear DNA isolated from 28 of the streptonigrin^R primary transformants. Plasmids were recovered from all 28, but only 20 yielded vectors containing cDNA inserts (Table 1). 5 of 20 primary transformants contained only a single vector with a cDNA insert while 14 of the remaining 15 carried additional plasmids along with a cDNA-containing vector. These passengers were always smaller than the parent vector and generally fell into three distinctive size classes: 3.8 kb, 7 kb and 10 kb. In one case, we recovered a cDNA-containing vector along with the parent plasmid used to construct the library. Screening an average of 40 rescued plasmids from each of the 8 remaining streptonigrin^R primary transformants yielded only plasmids that were smaller than the parent vector and contained no discernible cDNA inserts (data not shown).

Analysis of the 20 vectors that contained cDNAs by restriction enzyme digestion and Southern hybridization revealed that they represented 9 unrelated cDNAs ranging in size from 0.8 kb to 8.6 kb. Four of the cDNAs were rescued from more than one independent transformant. For example, pCAT 4.2 was isolated from two drug-resistant clones of AT fibroblasts that arose independently on separate dishes. Primary transformants harboring the same cDNA were concordant for phenotype and fell into two broad groups: streptonigrin^R, radiosensitive cells with high spontaneous rates of recombination (CAT6-4, CAT5.2, CAT8.2, CAT5-3 and CAT4-2) and streptonigrin^R, radioresistant cells with near normal rates of recombination (CAT4.5, CAT4.2, CAT5-5 and CAT4.4).

MAPPING OF cDNAS

The pCAT4.2 insert was hybridized to a human-rodent somatic cell hybrid mapping panel and unambiguously mapped to chromosome 6 (data not shown). Four of the remaining cDNAs were mapped by FISH: pCAT5-5 mapped to 15q22, pCAT6-4 mapped to 18q21, pCAT5-3 mapped to 7p13 and pCAT4.5 mapped to 17p11.1 (data not shown).

PHENOTYPIC CHARACTERIZATION OF SECONDARY TRANSFORMANTS

cDNAs were individually transfected into GM5849 fibroblasts and stable transformants tested for streptonigrin and/or radiation resistance. Five of 8 pCAT4.4 transformants, three of 7 pCAT5-5 transformants, six of 10 pCAT4.5 transformants and two of 3 pCAT5.2 transformants were partially resistant to streptonigrin and/or radiation exposure (data not shown). A cDNA rescued from the streptonigrin^R, radiation^R primary transformant pCAT4.2 has been tested more extensively for its ability to complement the phenotypic defects of A-T D fibroblasts. Three of 4 pCAT4.2 transformants demonstrated partial resistance to streptonigrin

61

and radiation, with all transformants concordant for either resistance or sensitivity. Survival after exposure to streptonigrin is shown in Figure 3a for CAT4.2/4d, a representative streptonigrin[R] secondary transformant of pCAT4.2, while Figure 3b documents the partial radiation resistance of this transformant. Spontaneous recombination of the *lacZ* genes contained in the pLrec plasmid carried by pCAT4.2/4d was found to be 5.2 x 10^{-5} events/cell/generation, more than 20-fold lower than that of the parent line (data not shown).

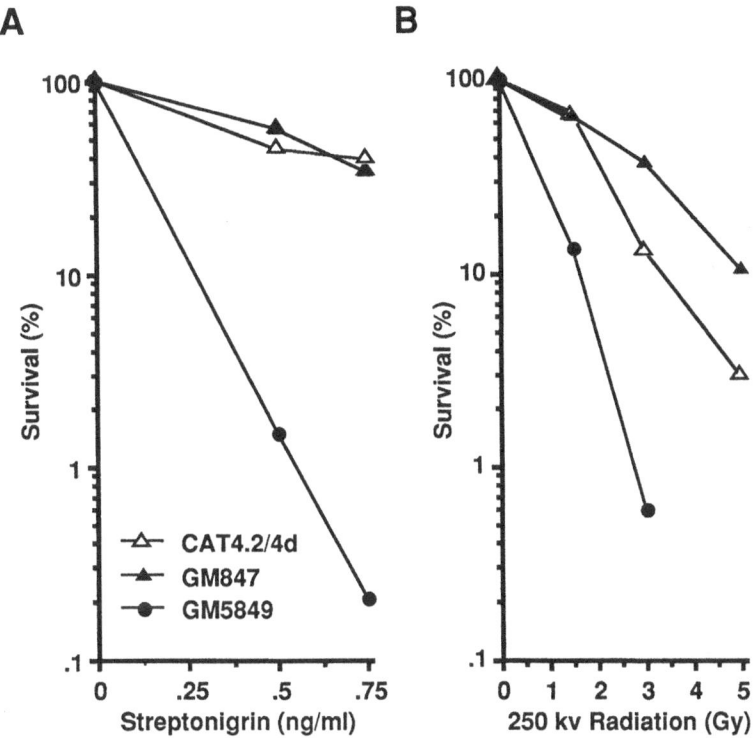

Figure 3. Survival after (A) 24 hrs exposure to streptonigrin or (B) exposure to 250 kv ionizing radiation. CAT4.2/4d is a A-T D fibroblast clone transfected with the pCAT4.2 cDNA, GM5849 is the parent A-T D cell line and GM847 is a control cell line. Survival was measured by colony-forming ability, and points represent averages of duplicate plates.

DISCUSSION

As detailed above, our initial experience with expression cloning illustrates several of the advantages and problems associated with the use of EBV-based episomal vectors. By transfecting the immortalized A-T D fibroblast line GM5849-5L20 with LN, a human cDNA library constructed using the EBV-based episomal expression vector pRep5, we achieved stable transfection frequencies of 0.5-2%. This is 50-100 fold better than transfection frequencies obtained when transforming GM5849 with genomic DNA (Lohrer *et al.;* 1988) and demonstrates the high transfection efficiency possible using EBV-based episomal vectors even when the recipient cell is not expressing the EBNA-1 gene *in trans*. Selection against streptonigrin sensitivity resulted in survival of only 68 out of ~610,000 stable LN transformants but allowed recovery of clones that had been complemented for several aspects of the A-T phenotype. Only 43 of the 68 colonies demonstrated streptonigrin-resistance upon further testing, suggesting that some colonies survived not because of acquired drug resistance, but because they failed to sustain lethal damage from the streptonigrin treatment. Fifteen of the streptonigrin^R transformants exhibited partial correction of radiation sensitivity and those radiation-resistant clones that were tested had correction of high spontaneous recombination rates. The radiation-sensitive streptonigrin^R clones may have acquired cDNAs that interfered with the uptake, metabolism or action of streptonigrin, rather than cDNAs that complemented the underlying defect in A-T cells. Correction of the A-T phenotype was not due to the presence of pRep5 vector sequences.

A major advantage of EBV-based episomal vectors over transfection of genomic DNA for complementation cloning is the relative ease of rescuing complementing sequences. We successfully rescued plasmids containing cDNAs from 20 of 28 streptonigrin^R primary transformants. However, we frequently recovered deleted plasmids without cDNA inserts from the same cells and in many cases these deleted passengers represented the majority of the plasmids recovered. The rescue of multiple deleted episomes from the same primary transformant may reflect the inherent genetic instability of the recipient A-T cells. In eight cases we only recovered deleted plasmids despite extensive screening. Those clones may have integrated the transfected cDNA that was responsible for mutagen-resistance or they may be revertants. The 20 cDNA-containing vectors recovered represented nine unrelated cDNAs, including several that were rescued multiple times from independently-arising clones. Only 5 of the 9 cDNAs came from streptonigrin^R clones that also had acquired partial radiation resistance, including two that expressed normal rates of intrachromosomal recombination.

Because electroporation can result in individual fibroblasts being transfected with more than one episomal vector it is possible that rescued cDNAs may be "passengers" rather than complementing cDNAs. Alternatively, reversion could confer mutagen-resistance to primary transformants. Consequently, it is important to verify that rescued cDNAs are able to complement the mutant phenotype upon secondary transfection. Five of the rescued cDNAs, pCAT4.4, pCAT5-5, pCAT5.2, pCAT4.2 and pCAT4.5, did confer partial mutagen-resistance to A-T D cells on secondary transformation. These complementing cDNAs were derived from mRNAs isolated from cells that had not been treated with ionizing radiation or chemical mutagens, indicating that, at least in transformed fibroblast lines, there is a constitutive level of expression of these cDNAs.

The chromosomal location of the A-T D gene is not known, but indirect evidence is consistent with a location on 11q23 telomeric to the A-T A and C loci (Gatti *et al.;* 1988; Ziv *et al.;* 1991; Sobel, *et al.,* 1992) and a candidate gene has been isolated from that region (Kapp *et al.,* 1992; Kapp *et al.,* this volume). This would suggest that the complementing cDNAs that we isolated may represent genes whose overexpression suppresses the A-T phenotype. Although the underlying abnormality in A-T is unknown, A-T cells lack several normal cellular responses to DNA damage (Hilgers *et al.;* 1988; Bates and Lavin 1989; Kasten *et al.;* 1992), findings that are consistent with the hypothesis that the primary defect in A-T results in an inability to properly activate these damage-sensitive functions (Meyn, manuscript in preparation). The complementing cDNAs that we have recovered may be involved in control of DNA repair and/or cell cycle damage-sensitive checkpoints, perhaps at a step in the A-T pathway downstream of the site of A-T gene action. Alternatively, overexpression of these cDNAs may facilitate functioning of the defective A-T D gene product. No cDNA completely complemented the sensitivity of A-T cells to ionizing radiation. This may be the result of having obtained only partial clones, rearrangement of the vector or unregulated expression from the RSV promoter of the pRep5 vector.

Combining episomal expression vector complementation with FISH mapping of rescued cDNAs offers a rapid and efficient method for obtaining candidate A-T disease genes as well as secondary suppressors that could shed light on the nature of the A-T defect and the cellular processes it affects. Our approach can readily be adapted for use with other A-T complementation groups. Multiple attempts to clone human DNA repair genes by complementing the mutagen sensitivity of A-T and other human diseases using genomic DNA transfection have only rarely succeeded (Green *et al.,* 1987; Lohrer *et al.,* 1988; Kapp and Painter, 1989). EBV-based episomal expression vectors were designed to circumvent problems associated with genomic DNA transfection. The present study, along with recent reports of cloning candidate XP and FA genes using EBV-based episomal expression vectors (Strathdee, *et al.,* 1992; Legerski and Perterson, 1992), documents the utility of this approach in isolating putative DNA repair genes and suggests that these vectors may facilitate the cloning of cDNAs that complement defects in mutant human cells for which there is strong selection or sorting.

ACKNOWLEDGMENTS

We wish to thank Dr. Michael Tykocinski for the gift of the pRep5 vector, Dr. Teresa Yang-Feng for providing the somatic cell mapping panel data for the pCAT4.2 cDNA, and Dr. David Ward for cDNA mapping by FISH, as well as Drs. R. Michael Liskay and Richard Gatti for many helpful discussions. This work was supported in part by grants from the American Cancer Society and the A-T Medical Research Foundation.

REFERENCES

Bates PR and Lavin MF (1989) Comparison of gamma-radiation-induced accumulation of ataxia telangiectasia and control cells in G2 phase. Mut Res 218: 165-170

Gatti RA, Berkel I, Boder E, Braedt G, Charley P, Concannon P, Ersoy F, Foroud T, Jaspers NGJ, Lange K, Lathrop,GM, Leppert M, Nakamura Y, O'Connell P, Paterson M, Salser W, Sanal O, Silver J, Sparkers RS, Susi E, Weeks DE, Wei S, White, R and Yoder F (1988) Localization of an ataxia-telangiectasia gene to chromosome 11q22-23. Nature 336: 577-580

Green MH, Lowe JE, Arlett CF, Harcourt SA, Burke JF, James MR, Lehmann AR and Povey SM (1987) A gamma-ray-resistant derivative of an ataxia telangiectasia cell line obtained following DNA-mediated gene transfer. J Cell Sci Suppl 6: 127-137

Groger RK, Morrow DM and Tykocinski ML (1989) Directional antisense and sense cDNA cloning using Epstein-Barr virus episomal expression vectors. Gene 81: 285-294

Herzing LHK and Meyn MS (1993) Novel lacZ-based recombination vectors for mammalian cells. (submitted)

Hilgers G, Abrahams PJ, Chen YQ, Schouten R, Cornelis JJ, Lowe JE, van der Eb AJ and Rommelaere J (1989) Impaired recovery and mutagenic SOS-like responses in ataxia telangiectasia cells. Mutagenesis 4: 271-276

Kapp LN and Painter RB (1989) Stable radioresistance in ataxia-telangiectasia cells containing DNA from normal human cells. Int J Radiat Biol 56: 667-675

Kapp LN, Painter RB, Yu L-C, van Loon N, Richard III CW, James MR, Cox DR and Murnane JP (1992) Cloning of a candidate gene for ataxia-telangiectasia group D. Am J Hum Genet 51: 45-54

Kastan MB, Zhan Q, el Deiry WS, Carrier F, Jacks T, Walsch WV, Plunkett BS and Vogenstein B (1992) A mammalian cell cycle checkpoint pathway utilizing p53 and GADD45 is defective in ataxia-telangiectasia. Cell 71: 587-597

Legerski R and Peterson C (1992) Expression cloning of a human DNA repair gene involved in xeroderma pigmentosum group C. Nature 359: 70-73

Lohrer H, Blum M, and Herrlich P (1988) Ataxia telangiectasia resists gene cloning: an account of parameters determining gene transfer into human recipient cells. Mol Gen Genet 212: 474-480

Meyn MS (1993) High spontaneous intrachromosomal recombination rates: A new facet of genetic instability in ataxia-telangiectasia. (submitted)

Meyn MS, Lu-Kuo JM and Herzing LBK (1993) Expression cloning of human cDNAs that complement the mutant phenotypes of ataxia-telangiectasia group D fibroblasts. (submitted)

Strathdee CA, Gavish H, Shannon WR, and Buchwald M (1992) Cloning of cDNAs for Fanconi's anaemia by functional complementation. Nature 356: 763-767

Sobel E, Lange E, Jaspers NGJ, Chessa L, Sanal O, Shilow Y, Taylor AMR, Weemaes CMA, Lange K and Gatti R (1992) Ataxia-telangiectasia: linkage evidence for genetic heterogeneity. Am J Hum Genet 50: 1343-1347

Ziv Y, Rotman G, Frydman M, Dagan J, Cohen T, Foroud T, Gatti RA and Shiloh Y (1991) The ATC (ataxia-telangiectasia complementation group C) locus localizes to 11q22-q23. Genomics 9: 373-375

Complementation of the Cellular A-T Phenotype by Gene Transfer

Yael Ziv[1], Tsafi Danieli[1], Galit Rotman[1], Adam Sartiel[1], Anat Bar-Shira[1], N.G.J. Jaspers[2], Richard Swirski[3], Robert T. Schimke[3], Roger L. Eddy[4], Thomas B. Shows[4] and Yosef Shiloh[1]

[1] Department of Human Genetics
Sackler School of Medicine
Tel Aviv University
Ramat Aviv 69978, Israel

The identification of the genes responsible for the chromosomal breakage syndromes by their function has been discussed since the discovery of the common feature of these diseases, cellular sensitivity to specific DNA damaging agents. The advent of gene transfer methods supplied the experimental system for this approach, which is apparently simple and straightforward: Exogenous DNA is introduced in vitro into the patient's cells, and selection is applied to identify cell clones showing increased resistance to the lethal action of the DNA damaging agent. An attempt is then made to rescue the piece of DNA responsible for this phenotypic change, which is expected to represent a candidate gene.

This strategy, often referred to as "expression cloning" or "complementation cloning", has been particularly rewarding when human DNA was used to complement the sensitivity to DNA damaging agents of mutant rodent cells. The high DNA uptake by rodent cell lines, and the relative ease with which human DNA can be identified on the background of the rodent's genome, led to the identification of a series of human genes involved in DNA repair processes (Hoeijmakers and Bootsma, 1992). Two of these genes turned out to be involved in the disease xeroderma pigmentosum,

[2] Department of Cell Biology and Genetics, Erasmus University, 3000 DR Rotterdam, Netherlands; [3] Department of Biological Sciences, Stanford University, Stanford, CA 94305-5020; [4] Department of Human Genetics, Roswell Park Cancer Institute, Buffalo, NY 14263.

NATO ASI Series, Vol. H 77
Ataxia-Telangiectasia
Edited by R. A. Gatti and R. B. Painter
© Springer-Verlag Berlin Heidelberg 1993

characterized by cellular sensitivity to UV light (Weeda et al., 1990; Fletjer et al., 1992). Another gene associated with this disease was isolated by complementing the UV sensitivity of human xeroderma pigmentosum (group A) cells using mouse genomic DNA (Tanaka et al., 1990).

Despite these successes, obtaining stable phenotypic complementation in mutant human cells transfected with human DNA has proven to be exceedingly difficult in most cases, due mainly to the low DNA uptake of human cells and their poor ability to integrate and maintain exogenous DNA in their genome (Debenham et al., 1984). The unstable genome of A-T cells adds an additional obstacle to this difficulty (Lohrer et al., 1988).

The limited life span of diploid fibroblast lines precludes their use in long-term complementation experiments. A number of "immortalized" A-T fibroblast lines have been obtained in several laboratories by transformation of diploid strains using replication-defective SV40 (Murnane et al., 1985; Hashimoto et al., 1986; Ziv et al., 1989). In general, these permanent cell lines have retained the characteristics of the parent cells and have not shown any detectable reversion to the normal phenotype. While this renders them apparently suitable for complementation attempts, the actual history of these attempts demonstrates the experimental complexity associated with a full cycle of transfection, integration expression and rescue of a piece of DNA when A-T cells are involved.

Extensive complementation experiments using human genomic DNA and the A-T(D) cell line AT5BIVA were performed by Lehmann et al (1986) and Green et al. (1987). These experiments resulted in a cell clone with a considerable and stable reduction in radiosensitivity, but radioresistant DNA synthesis typical of A-T cells was retained. Attempts to isolate the DNA fragment responsible for this phenomenon were not successful. Similar experiments by Lohrer et al. (1988) did not yield radioresistant clones. More encouraging results were recently obtained by Kapp et al. (1989, 1992), who transfected AT5BIVA cells with a genomic library in a cosmid vector, and were able to rescue from a radioresistant cell clone a gene (ATDC) that might be involved in A-T

(Group D). Further analysis of this gene is reported in this volume.

An important caveat associated with the use of genomic DNA in such experiments is the limitation on the size of fragments that can integrate into the cellular genome, since the desired gene may span tens or even hundreds kb of DNA. A possible solution to this problem is to use cDNA libraries rather than genomic DNA. We began our complementation experiments using a cDNA library cloned in the expression vector pCD (Okayama and Berg, 1985). The recipient was a permanent cell line, AT22IJE-T, obtained in our laboratory by transforming diploid A-T(A) fibroblasts using ori⁻ SV40 DNA (Ziv et al., 1989). The library was co-transfected into the cells with a plasmid containing a neomycin-resistance marker, and the cells were subjected to two selections: with the neomycin analog G418 and with several doses of the radiomimetic drug neocarzinostatin (NCS) (Shiloh et al., 1982). Out of 200,000 G418-resistant cell clones, two survived the radiomimetic selection and showed partial complementation of two central features of the A-T phenotype: radiomimetic sensitivity and radioresistant DNA synthesis (Fig. 1). This phenotypic change was found to be stable over a wide range of time and passage levels. However, attempts to rescue the cDNA clone(s) integrated in the chromosomal DNA of these cells either by screening genomic libraries with pCD sequences or by PCR with vector-based primers were not successful. Southern blotting experiments indicated possible dissociation between the insert and vector sequences, partly explaining the difficulties in releasing these sequences from the cellular genome.

A possible way to circumvent genomic instability is to use cDNA libraries cloned in episomal vectors that remain in the cells as extrachromosomal elements. Plasmids carrying the oriP sequence of Epstein-Barr virus (EBV) replicate autonomously in mammalian cells in the presence of EBV nuclear antigen-1 (EBNA-1) (Sugden et al., 1985; Yates et al., 1985). The advantages of such vectors are high transfection rates, independence of genomic stability of the host cells and a relatively simple mode of rescue (Belt et

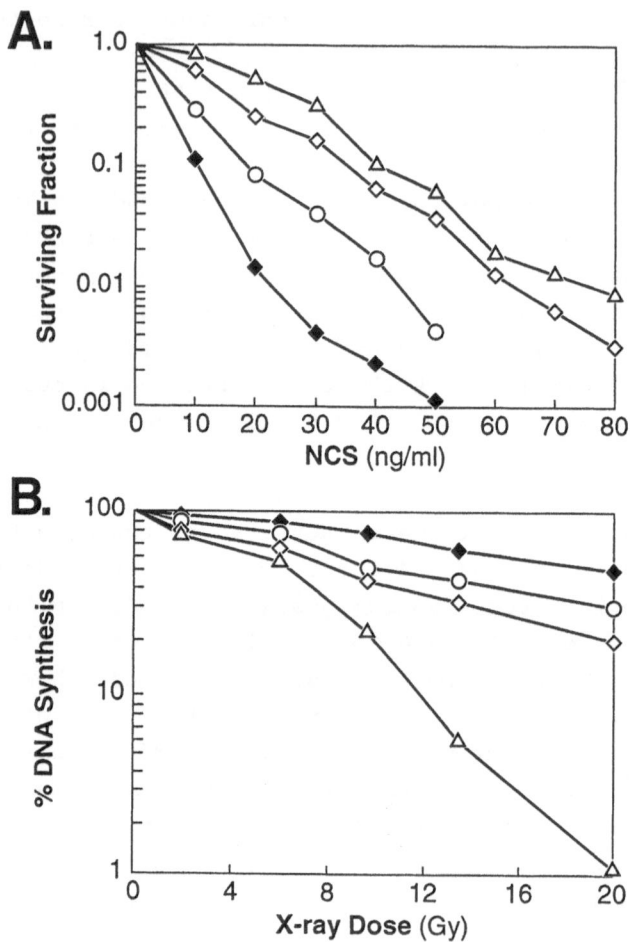

Partial complementation of the A-T cellular phenotype in two
clones of the cell line AT22IJE-T (Group A) following
transfection with a cDNA library in the vector pCD. A:
Survival curves after treatment with various doses of the
radiomimetic drug neocarzinostatin (NCS). B: Inhibition of
DNA synthesis by ionizing radiation. △ : a normal cell
line, GM537B. ◆ : the parent cell line, AT22IJE-F.
◇,○ : transfectant cell clones, AT22-pCD1 and
AT22-pCD2, respectively.

al., 1989; Groger et al., 1989; Hammarskjold et al., 1989; Margolskee et al., 1988). Phenotypic complementation experiments using cDNA libraries in such vectors have recently led to the isolation of the genes for tumor necrosis factor (Heller et al., 1990), O^6-methylguanine transferase (Hayakawa et al., 1990), Fanconi's anemia (Group C) (Strathdee et al., 1992) and xeroderma pigmentosum (Group C) (Legerski et al., 1992).

We are using several cDNA libraries cloned in the episomal vectors pDR2 (Swirski et al., 1993), pEBS7 (Peterson and Legersky, 1991) and pREP4 (Strathdee wt al., 1992) to complement the radiomimetic sensitivity of A-T(A) and A-T(C) cell lines. The cells were made permissive to these vectors by prior transfection with the plasmid CMV-EBNA in which the EBNA-1 gene is promoted by the CMV promoter (Swirski et al., 1993). These vectors endow the cells with resistance to the antibiotic hygromycin, which is used for primary selection of transformants. Secondary selection is done using the radiomimetic drugs streptonigrin (SN) and neocarzinostatin (NCS). The plasmids are isolated from resistant cell clones and propagated in bacteria for further analysis.

It should be noted that even genes that truly complement the cellular phenotype may not be the disease genes. A typical example was reported by Teitz et al. (1990) who found that the gene for the beta subunit of casein kinase II complements UV sensitivity of xeroderma pigmentosum cells. The preliminary test of authenticity of candidate cDNAs should be based, therefore, on their chromosomal location. This simple test became possible following the recent localization of the A-T(A) and A-T(C) genes to chromosome 11, region q22-23 (Gatti et al., 1988; McConville et al., 1990; Foroud et al., 1991; Ziv et al., 1991, 1992), and is used to exclude cDNA clones irrelevant to the disease.

In a typical experiment, 5×10^6 AT22IJE-T cells were transfected with a HeLa cDNA library in the vector pDR2 (Swirski et al., 1993), and 3×10^4 hygromycin-resistant clones were obtained. Ten of these clones survived the radiomimetic selection with SN and 4 cDNAs were rescued from these cell clones. While 3 cDNAs mapped to chromosomes other than 11, one clone appeared to represent an extensive gene family scattered over 7 different chromosomes, including chromosome 11. In further large-scale experiments, a normal fibroblast cDNA library in the episomal vector pEBS17 (Peterson and Legersky, 1991) was introduced into this cell line, and 10⁶ hygromycin-resistant colonies were obtained and are currently under radiomimetic selection.

The localization of a major A-T locus at chromosome 11q22-23 set the scene for positional cloning of the A-T genes. This strategy calls for the isolation of all the genes contained in the disease locus and the identification of the one involved in the disease by searching for mutations in patients (Collins, 1992). In spite of being so different, positional and functional cloning can and should interact and reinforce each other. For example, candidate genes isolated via phenotypic complementation may be mapped using genomic contigs constructed at the disease locus. More important, candidate genes identified by positional cloning should be examined using the functional test, complementation of the cellular phenotype. In view of this experimental paradigm, we initiated in parallel with the experiments described above the construction of a genomic contig in yeast artificial chromosomes (YACs) spanning the A-T locus at chromosome 11. Identification of cDNA clones in the episomal libraries using these YAC clones should expedite the search for the elusive A-T genes.

ACKNOWLEDGMENTS

This work was supported by research grants from the Ataxia-Telangiectasia Medical Research Foundation, The Thomas Appeal (A-T Medical Research Trust) and the Fund for Basic Research of the Israel Academy of Sciences and Humanities.

REFERENCES

Belt, P.B.G.M., Groeneveld, H., Teubel, W.J., van der Putte, P. and Backendorf, C. (1989) Construction and properties of an Epstein-Barr-virus-derived cDNA expression vector for human cells. Gene, 84:407-417.

Collins, F.S. (1992) Positional cloning: Let's not call it reverse anymore. Nature Genet., 1:3-6.

Debenham, P.G., Webb, M.B.T., Masson, W.K., and Cox, R. (1984) DNA-mediated gene transfer into human diploid fibroblasts derived from normal and ataxia-telangiectasia donors: parameters for DNA transfer and properties of DNA transformants. Int. J. Radiat. Biol., 45:525-536.

Fletjer, W.L., McDaniel, L.D., Johns, D., Friedberg, E.C. and Schultz, R. (1992) Correction of xeroderma pigmentosum complementation group D mutant cell phenotypes by chromosome and gene transfer: Involvement of the human ERCC2 DNA repair gene. Proc. Natl. Acad. Sci. USA, 89:261-265.

Foroud, T., Sobel, E., Ziv, Y., (1991) Localization of an ataxia-telangiectasia locus to an 4 cM interval on chromosome 11q23 by linkage analysis of an international consortium of 111 families. Am. J. Hum. Genet. 49:1263-1279.

Gatti, R.A., Berkel, I., Boder, E. et al. (1988) Localization of an ataxia-telangiectasia gene to chromosome 11q22-23. Nature, 336:577-580.

Green, M.H.L., Lowe, J.E., Arlett, C.F., Harcourt, S.A., Burke, J.F., James, M.R. and Lehmann, A.R. (1987) A gamma-ray resistant derivative of an ataxia-telangiectasia cell line obtained following DNA mediated gene transfer. J. J. Cell Sci. Suppl. 6:127-137.

Groger, R.K., Morrow, D.M. and Tykocinski, M.L. (1989) Directional antisense and sense cDNA cloning using Epstein-Barr virus episomal expression vectors. Gene, 81:285-294.

Hammarskjold, M.-L., Wang, S.-C. and Klein G. (1986) High-level expression of the Epstein-Barr virus EBNA-1 protein in CV1 cells and human lymphoid cells using a SV40 late replacement vector. Gene, 43:41-50.

Hashimoto, T., Nakano, Y., Owada, M.K., Kakunaga, T., and Furuyama, J.-I. (1986) Establishment of cell lines derived from ataxia telangiectasia and xeroderma pigmentosum patients with high radiation sensitivity. Mutat. Res., 166:215-220, 1986.

Hayakawa, H., Kioke, G. and Sekiguchi, M. (1990) Expression and cloning of complementary DNA for a human enzyme that repairs O^6-methylguanine in DNA. J. Mol. Biol., 213:739-747.

Heller, R.A., Song, K., Villaret, D., Margolskee, R., Dunne, J., Hayakawa, H. and Ringold, G.M. (1990) Amplified expression of tumor necrosis factor receptor in cells transfected with Epstein-Barr virus shuttle vector cDNA libraries. J. Biol. Chem., 265:5708-5717.

Hoeijmakers, J.H.J. and Bootsma, D. (1992) DNA repair: two pieces of the puzzle. Nature Genetics, 1:313-314.

James, M.R., Stary, A., Daya-Grosjean, A., Drougard, C., and Sarasin, A. (1989) Comparative study of Epstein-Barr virus and SV40-based shuttle expression vectors in human repair deficient cells. Mutat. Res., 220:169-185.

Kapp, L.N. and Painter, R. (1989) Stable radioresistance in ataxia-telangiectasia cells containing DNA from normal human cells. Int. J. Radiat. Biol., 56:667-675.

Kapp, L.N., Painter, R.B., Yu, L-C., van Loon, N., Richard, C.W., James, M.R., Cox, D.R. and Murnane, J.P. (1992) Cloning of a candidate gene for ataxia-telangiectasia group D. Am. J. Hum. Genet., 51:45-54.

Legersky, R. and Peterson, C. (1992) Expression cloning of a human DNA repair gene involved in xeroderma pigmentosum group C. Nature, 359:70-73.

Lehmann, A.R., Arlett, C.F., Burke, J.F., Green, M.H. L., James, M.R. and Lowe, J.E. (1986) A derivative of an ataxia-telangiectasia (A-T) cell line with normal radiosensitivity but A-T-like inhibition of DNA synthesis. Int. J. Radiat. Biol., 49:639-643.

Lohrer, H., Blum, M. and Herrlich, P. (1988) Ataxia telangiectasia resists gene cloning: an account of parameters determining gene transfer into human recipient cells. Mol. Gen. Genet., 212:474-480.

Margolskee, R.F., Kavathas, P. and Berg, P. (1988) Epstein-Barr virus shuttle vector for stable episomal replication of cDNA expression libraries in human cells. Mol. Cell. Biol., 8:2837-2847.

McConville, C.M., Formstone, C.J., Hernandez, D. et al. (1990) Fine mapping of the chromosome 11q22-23 region using PFGE, linkage and haplotype analysis; localization of the gene for ataxia telangiectasia to a 5cM region flanked by NCAM/DRD2 and STMY/CJ52.75, $m2.22$. Nucleic Acids Res., 18:4335-4343.

Murnane, J.P., Fuller, L.F. and Painter, .B. (1985) Establishment and characterization of a permanent pSVori-transformed ataxia-telangiectasia cell line. Exp. Cell. Res., 158:119-126, 1985.

Okayama, H. and Berg, P. (1985) A cDNA vector that permits

expression of cDNA inserts in mammalian cells. Mol. Cell. Biol., 3:280-289.

Peterson, C. and Legersky, R. (1991) High-frequency transformation of human repair-deficient cell lines by an Epstein-Barr virus-based expression vector. Gene, 107:279-284.

Shiloh, Y., Tabor, E. and Becker, Y. (1982) The response of ataxia-telangiectasia homozygous and heterozygous skin fibroblasts to neocarzinostatin. Carcinogenesis, 3:815-820.

Strathdee, C.A., Gavish, H., Shannon, W.R. and Buchwald, M. (1992) Cloning of cDNAs for Fanconi's anaemia by functional complementation. Nature, 356:763-767.

Sugden, B., Marsh, K. and Yates, J. (1985) A vector that replicates as a plasmid and can be efficiently selected in B-lymphoblasts transformed by Epstein-Barr virus. Mol. Cell. Biol., 5:410-413.

Swirski, R.A., Van den Berg, D., Murphy, A.J., Lambert, C.M., Friedberg, E.C., and Schimke, R.T. (1993) Improvements in the Epstein-Barr-based shuttle vector system for direct cloning in human tissue culture cells. Methods: A Companion to Methods in Enzymology, Vol. 4 (in press).

Tanaka, K., Miura, N., Satokata, I., Miyamoto, I., Yoshida, M.C., Satoh, Y., Kondo, S., Yasui, A., Okayama, H. and Okada, Y. (1991) Analysis of a human DNA excision repair gene involved in group A xeroderma pigmentosum and containing a zinc-finger domain. Nature, 348:73-76.

Teitz, T., Eli, D., Penner, M., Bakhanashvili, M., Naiman, T., Timme, T.L., Wood, C.M., Moses, R.E. and Canaani, D. (1990) Expression of the cDNA for the beta subunit of human casein kinase II confers partial UV resistance on xeroderma pigmentosum cells. Mutat. Res., 236:85-97.

Weeda, G., Van Hamm, R.C.A., Vermeulen, W., Bootsma, D., van der Eb, A.J. and Hoeijmakers, J.H.J. (1990) A presumed DNA helicase encoded by ERCC-3 is involved in the human repair disorders xeroderma pigmentosum and Cockayne's syndrome. Cell, 62:777-791.

Yates, J.L., Warren, N. and Sugden, B. (1985) (1985) Stable replication of plasmids derived from Epstein-Barr virus in various mammalian cells. Nature, 313:812-815.

Ziv, Y., Etkin, S., Danieli, T., Amiel, A., Ravia, Y., Jaspers, N.G.J. and Shiloh, Y., (1989) Cellular and biochemical characteristics of an immortalized ataxia-telangiectasia (group AB) cell line. Cancer Res., 49:2495-2501.

Ziv. Y., Rotman, G., Frydman, M., Foroud, T., Gatti, R.A. and Shiloh, Y. (1991) The ATC (ataxia-telangiectasia

complementation group   C) locus   localizes   to   11q22-q23.
Genomics, 9:373-375.

Ziv, Y., Frydman, M., Lange, E.,   et al. (1992) (1991)
Ataxia-telangiectasia: linkage   analysis   in highly   inbred
Arab and Druze   families   and   differentiation   from   an
ataxia-microcephaly-cataract   syndrome.   Hum.   Genet.,
88:619-626.

Use of Microcell Hybrids for Analysis of the 11q23 Region and Improved Localization of the A-T Group A/C Genes

Y. Ejima, M. Oshimura*, and M. S. Sasaki
Radiation Biology Center
Kyoto University
Yoshida-konoecho
Sakyo-Ku
Kyoto 606
Japan

INTRODUCTION

Ataxia-telangiectasia (A-T) is a human autosomal recessive disease; hypersensitivity to ionizing radiation has been a consistent cellular hallmark of this disease (Taylor et al. 1975). Localization of the A-T gene to chromosome 11q22-23 was first suggested from a genetic linkage study (Gatti et al. 1988) and this has been followed by recent additional reports confirming that the genes responsible for A-T complementation groups A and C are located at the 11q23 region (McConville et al. 1990; Ziv et al. 1991; Foroud et al. 1991). A candidate gene for A-T complementation group D has recently been cloned and was also shown to localize at 11q23 (Kapp et al. 1992). Studies using microcell hybrids (Komatsu et al. 1990; Ejima et al. 1990; Lambert et al. 1991) have substantiated this A-T gene localization for group D as well since the introduction of chromosome 11 or 11q segments produced radioresistant group D A-T cells. Our recent studies with microcell hybrids led to the finding that the loss of radioresistance in an A-T-derived microcell hybrid was associated with a minute deletion in the 11q23 region (Ejima et al. 1991).   This 11q23-deleted chromosome could thus be useful for the molecular dissection of

---

*Department of Molecular and Cell Genetics, School of Life Sciences, Tottori University, Nishimachi 86, Yonago 683, Japan

NATO ASI Series, Vol. H 77
Ataxia-Telangiectasia
Edited by R. A. Gatti and R. B. Painter
© Springer-Verlag Berlin Heidelberg 1993

the 11q23 region and provide additional information on the exact A-T locus. Here we describe the construction of a micro-cell hybrid carrying the 11q23-deleted chromosome and on its possible use in the analysis of the 11q23 region.

MATERIALS AND METHODS

An immortalized A-T cell line established by transfection of pSVori$^-$ DNA, AT2KYSV (Ejima et al. 1990), and its 6thioguanine-resistant derivative, AT2KYSVTG, were used. The five mouse A9 strains, A9(neo11)-1, A9(7149)-5, A9(2859)-3, A9(3322)-3, A9(3552)-2, carry a single human 11, X or X/11 recombinant chromosome derived from human diploid fibroblasts. The chromosome regions carried by the latter three A9 strains were Xqter→Xq11::11p11→11qter, Xqter→Xq22::11q13→11pter, Xqter → Xq26::11q23→11pter, respectively (Koi et al., 1989). The cells were cultured in alpha-modified MEM supplemented with 100 u/ml Penicillin, 100 μg/ml Streptomycin and 10% heat-inactivated fetal bovine serum at 37°C in a humidified incubation with 5% CO_2.

Microcell-mediated chromosome transfer was performed as described previously (Oshimura et al. 1989). Either G418(400 μg/ml) or HAT(100 μM hypoxanthine, 0.4 μM aminopterin, 16μM thymidine) was added to the medium for selection of microcell hybrids. Chromosomes were analyzed by the conventional trypsin-Giemsa banding method of Seabright (1971). Cellular radiosensitivity was estimated from colony forming ability after X-irradiation as described previously (Ejima et al. 1990).

PCR was performed using an *Alu* primer, TC-65, described by Nelson et al.(1989). A 100 μl reaction mixture contained 1 μg DNA and 1 μM of primer in 50mM KCl/10mM Tris HCl,pH8.0/1.5mM MgCl$_2$/0.01% gelatin/250 μM dNTPs and 2.5 units of *Taq* polymerase(Perkin-Elmer/Cetus). PCR was carried out for 35 cycles with 94°C denaturation (1min), 55°C annealing (45sec), and 68°C extension (5min) in an automated thermal cycler

(Perkin-Elmer/Cetus) with initial denaturation for 4 min at 94°C.

DNA was visualized with ethidium bromide after electrophoresis in 1.3% agarose gels. Size markers were a mixture of λ DNA digested with HindIII and ϕ X174 DNA digested with HaeIII. Southern transfers to nylon membranes (Nytran, Schleicher & Shuell) were done using standard protocols (Sambrook et al. 1989). DNA probes were labeled with ^{32}P using the nick-translation method and were incubated with human placental DNA (0.5 mg/ml) at 65°C for 2 hours prior to use in hybridization (Patel et al. 1990). Hybridization was carried out in 1M NaCl/1% SDS/10% dextran sulfate/0.5 mg/ml human placental DNA at 65°C overnight. Post hybridization washes were with 2XSSC/0.1% SDS, 1XSSC/0.1% SDS and 0.1XSSC/0.1% SDS at 65°C. To clone the PCR products, they were digested with NotI, ligated into NotI-digested pUCBM20 vector (Boeringer-Mannheim) and used to transform Escherichia coli DH5α competent cells.

RESULTS

The microcell hybrids obtained from the fusion of AT2KYSVTG with A9(2859)-3, carrying an X/11 chromosome containing the 11p11→qter region, showed an increased radioresistance when compared with parental AT2KYSVTG cells. One variant clone, 2859/4, displayed partial radioresistance, and one of the clones derived from 2859/4, designated 2859/4-1, had completely lost its radioresistance and contained an interstitial deletion at 11q23 in the transferred X/11 chromosome (Fig. 1(A)). In order to construct a microcell hybrid carrying the 11q23-deleted X/11 chromosome, microcells were prepared from 2859/4-1 and transferred back into mouse A9 cells. Of the three HAT-resistant hybrids obtained, the deleted X/11 chromosome was recognized in one clone, A9(2859/4)-2, but three other human chromosomes were also present (Fig. 1(B)). Microcells were prepared again from A9(2859/4)-2 and fused with A9 cells. One of the six HAT-resistant hybrids obtained after this second round of microcell fusions, designated A9(2859/4/2)-1, had a single X/11 chromosome with an 11q23 deletion (Fig. 1(C)).

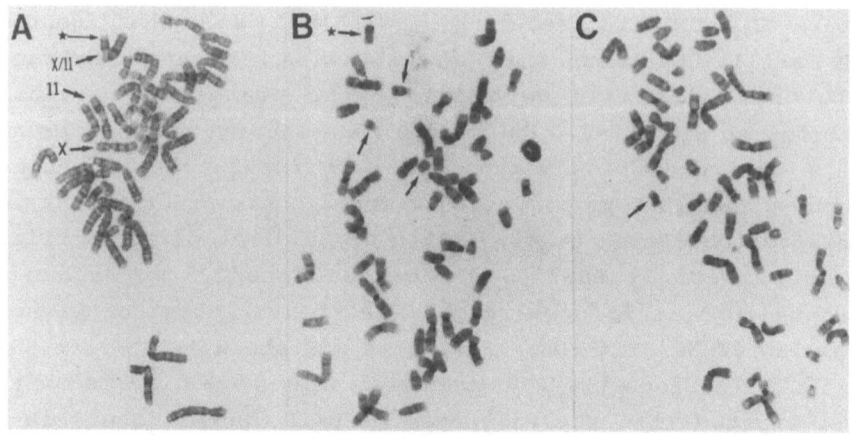

Fig. 1. GTG-banded chromosomes in microcell hybrids. (A) 2859/4-1. Star indicates deleted 11q23 region. (B) A9(2859/4)-2. Arrows indicate human chromosomes. Star indicates deleted X/11 chromosome. (C) A9(2859/4/2)-1. Arrow indicates deleted X/11 chromosome.

In order to visualize human DNA present in these human/mouse microcell hybrids, human DNA was selectively amplified by PCR using human specific *Alu* sequences as a primer. Fig. 2 shows the amplified DNA seen in various cell strains using the TC65 primer. Amplification was not seen in mouse cells, and results in a smear when used with human DNA. Amplifications of different microcell hybrids containing overlapping regions show similar patterns of bands (Fig. 2(A)). Amplification products from 2859/4-1-derived microcell hybrids are shown in Fig. 2(B). PCR fragments found in A9(2859/4/2)-1, which has the 11q23-deleted X/11 chromosome, are nearly identical to those in its parental hybrid A9(2859)-3 which contains no deletion.

To identify PCR products originating from the deleted 11q23 region, PCR products from each of the deletion-containing microcell hybrids were subjected to Southern analysis. Probes

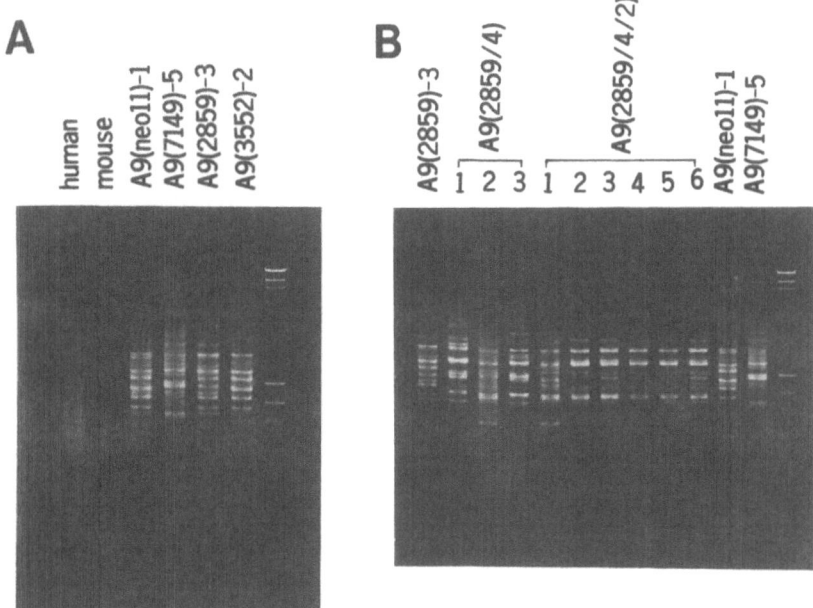

Fig. 2. Amplification of human DNA from microcell hybrids using the TC-65 *Alu* primer. (A) PCR with DNA from human, mouse and microcell hybrids containing chromosome 11, X or X/11 translocated chromosomes. (B) PCR with DNA from microcell hybrids constructed from 2859/4-1.

were made from slices from each of the amplification products found in A9(neo11)-1, a hybrid containing a single human chromosome 11 (Fig. 3(A)). Some fragments seen in slice 3 were found to be missing in A9(2859/4/2)-1 (Fig. 3(B)). Individual fragments included in this slice were further analyzed (Fig. 4). Two fragments (1.8kb and 1.7kb) were found to be missing in A9(2859/4/2)-1, the deletion-containing hybrid. The 1.8kb fragment was present in A9(3552)-2 while the 1.7kb fragment was also missing in A9(3552)-2. A9(3552)-2 carries the pter→q23 region of chromosome 11 and this segment has been shown to

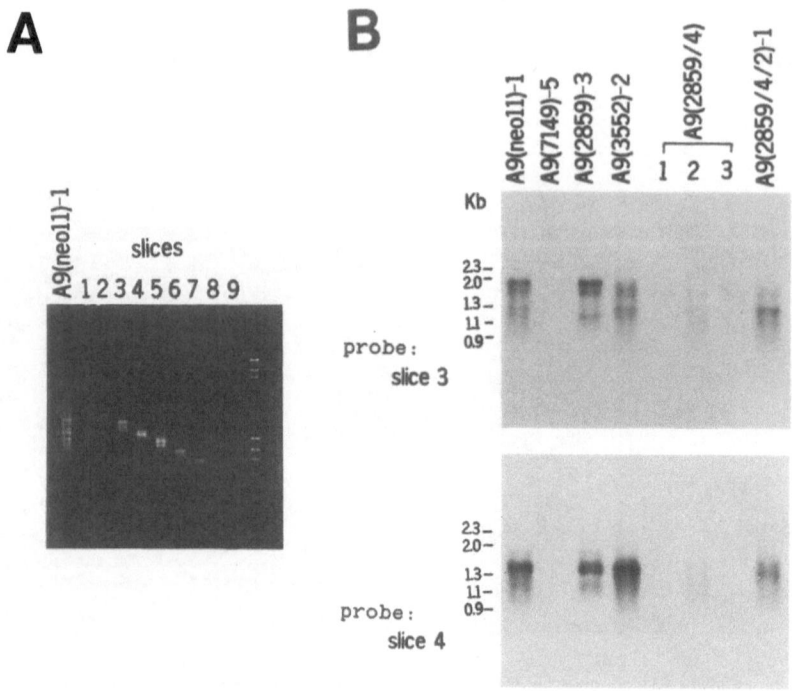

Fig. 3. Southern analysis of PCR products from microcell hybrids. (A) Ethidium bromide-stained gel of size-fractionated PCR products obtained from A9(neo11)-1 DNA. (B) Autoradiograph of Southern blot using size-fractionated PCR products as probes.

correct A-T radiosensitivity (Ejima et al. 1991). This indicates that the X/11 breakpoint in A9(3552)-2 lies within the minute 11q23 deletion. This also implies that the PCR products missing in A9(2859/4/2)-1 but not in A9(3552)-2 (e.g. the 1.8kb fragment) could serve as markers located very close to the A-T locus. Two such PCR products were cloned and Southern analysis using them as probes indicated that they were missing in A9(2859/4/2)-1 but not in A9(3552)-3 (Fig. 5). Several more such PCR fragments which originate from the

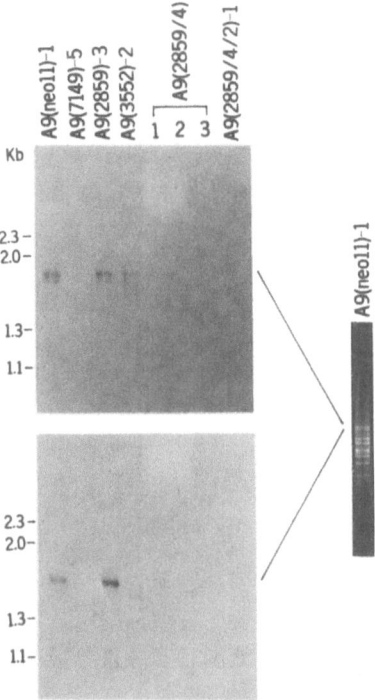

Fig. 4. Southern analysis of PCR products from microcell hybrids using two individual *Alu* PCR fragments as probes.

deleted 11q23 region have been identified and cloned, and are now being characterized.

DISCUSSION

Construction of a microcell hybrid which carries a human chromosome with a minute deletion in 11q23 was described here. The amplification of human sequences by an *Alu* primer and differential analysis of PCR products was shown to be a feasible tool to identify markers that are located within the deleted 11q23 region. Characterization of the DNA markers obtained here should reveal their precise chromosomal location relative to the A-T locus and some of these markers should be potential probes to screen genomic libraries. Efforts are also being made to construct somatic cell hybrids which carry 11q23-

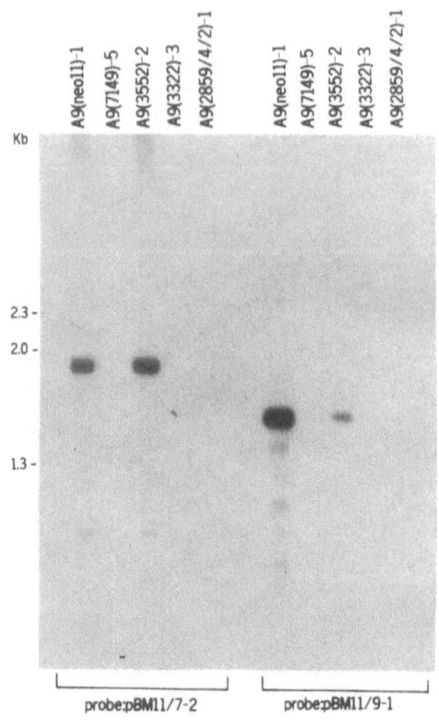

Fig. 5. Southern analysis of PCR products from microcell hybrids using two cloned *Alu* PCR fragments, pBM11/7-2 and pBM11/9-1, as probes.

containing minute chromosome fragments created by radiation-induced fragmentation of human chromosome 11. The mouse A9(3552)-2 strain is particularly useful for the generation of such hybrids because it carries an X/11 chromosome that has the pter→q23 segment of chromosome 11 and the X/11 breakpoint lies between D11S144 and THY1, and a linkage to A-T has been shown for both of these markers (Gatti et al. 1988; Foroud et al. 1991). Also the presence of the *hprt* locus on the X chromosome close to the X/11 junction would favor the selection of stable hybrids. Such radiation hybrids could be useful for dissection of the 11q23 region and as a source to generate genomic libraries specific for the 11q23 region including the A-T locus.

Recently a candidate gene for A-T complementation group D

has been cloned (Kapp et al. 1992) and shown to be located at 11q23, telomeric to THY1. This location is discrete from the loci for group A or C which are located 25 cM centromeric to THY1 (Foroud et al. 1991). The complementation group of AT2KY used here is not known; however, because the A9(3552)-2-derived X/11 chromosome contains the 11pter→q23 region and does not contain the region telomeric to THY1, but does complement the phenotype of AT2KY (Ejima et al. 1991), it seems likely that this cell line should belong to group A or C.

Radioresistant DNA synthesis is another cellular hallmark of A-T which is consistently associated with radiation hypersensitivity (Painter and Young, 1980). However, an enhanced cellular radioresistance without the correction of A-T-like DNA synthesis has occasionally been observed in A-T-derived DNA transfectants (Lehmann et al. 1986; Kapp and Painter, 1989) or in somatic cell hybrids (Komatsu et al. 1989), raising a question about the possible link between radioresistant DNA synthesis and enhanced cellular radiosensitivity. The A-T-derived microcell hybrids which we have constructed by introducing chromosome 11 or its derivatives into A-T cells (Ejima et al. 1991) should help to examine the relationship between these two A-T hallmarks as well as to study the regulation of gene expression by externally introduced DNA or chromosomes.

REFERENCES

Ejima Y, Oshimura M, Sasaki MS (1990) Establishment of a novel immortalized cell line from ataxia telangiectasia fibroblasts and its use for the chromosomal assignment of radiosensitivity gene. Int J Radiat Biol 58:989-997

Ejima Y, Oshimura M, Sasaki MS (1991) Determination of the chromosomal site for the human radiosensitive ataxia telangiectasia gene by chromosome transfer. Mutation Res 250:337-343

Foroud T, Wei S, Ziv Y, Sobel E, Lange E, Chao A, Goradia T, Huo Y, Tolun A, Chessa L, Charmley P, Sanal O, Salman N, Julier C, Concannon P, McConville C, Taylor AMR, Shiloh Y, Lange K, Gatti RA (1991) Localization of an ataxia-telangiectasia locus to a 3-cM interval on chromosome 11q23:

Linkage analysis of 111 families by an international consortium. Am J Hum Genet 49:1263-1279

Gatti RA, Berkel I, Boder E, Braedt G, Charmley P, Concannon P, Ersoy F, Foroud T, Jaspers NGJ, Lange K, Lathrop GM, Leppert M, Nakamura Y, O'Connell P, Paterson M, Salser W, Sanal O, Silver J, Sparkes RS, Susi E, Weeks DE, Wei S, White R, Yoder F (1988) Localization of an ataxia-telangiectasia gene to chromosome 11q22-23. Nature 36:577-580

Kapp LN, Painter RB (1989) Stable radioresistance in ataxia-telangiectasia cells containing DNA from normal human cells. Int J Radiat Biol 56:667-675

Kapp LN, Painter RB, Yu LC, van Loon N, Richard CW 3d, James MR, Cox DR, Murnane JP (1992) Cloning of a candidate gene for ataxia-telangiectasia group D. Am J Hum Genet 51:45-54

Koi M, Morita H, Shimizu M, Oshimura M (1989) Construction of mouse A9 clones containing a single human chromosome (X/autosome translocation) via micro-cell fusion. Jpn J Cancer Res 80:122-125

Komatsu K, Okumura, Y, Kodama S, Yoshida M, Miller RC (1989) Lack of correlation between radiosensitivity and inhibition of DNA synthesis in hybrids (A-T x HeLa). Int J Radiat Biol 56:863-867

Komatsu K, Kodama S, Okumura Y, Koi M, Oshimura M (1990) Restoration of radiation resistance in ataxia telangiectasia cells by the introduction of normal human chromosome 11. Mutation Res 235:59-63

Lambert C, Schultz RA, Smith M, Wagner-McPherson C, McDaniel LD, Donlon T, Stanbridge EJ, Friedberg EC (1991) Functional complementation of ataxia-telangiectasia group D (ATD) cells by microcell-mediated chromosome transfer and mapping of the AT-D locus to the region 11q22-23. Proc Natl Acad Sci, USA 88:5907-5911

Lehmann AR, Arlett CF, Burke JF, Green MHL, James MR, Lowe JE (1986) A derivative of an ataxia-telangiectasia (A-T) cell line with normal radiosensitivity but A-T like inhibition of DNA synthesis. Int J Radiat Biol 49:639-643

McConville CM, Woods CG, Farrall M, Metcalfe JA, Taylor AMR (1990) Analysis of 7 polymorphic markers at chromosome 11q22-23 in 35 ataxia-telangiectasia families; further evidence of linkage. Hum Genet 85:215-220

Nelson DL, Ledbetter SA, Corbo L, Victoria MF, Ramiréz-Solis R, Webster TD, Ledbetter DH, Caskey CT (1989) Alu polymerase chain reaction: A method for rapid isolation of human-specific sequences from complex DNA sources. Proc Natl Acad Sci, USA 86:6686-6690

Oshimura M, Kugoh H, Koi M, Shimizu M, Yamada H, Satoh H, Barrett JC (1989) Transfer of a normal human chromosome 11 suppresses tumorigenicity of some but not all tumor cell lines. J Cell Biochem 42:135-142

Painter RB, Young BR (1980) Radiosensitivity in ataxia-telangiectasia: A new explanation. Proc Natl Acad Sci, USA 77:7315-7317

Patel PI, Garcia C, de Oca-Luna RM, Malamut RI, Franco B, Slaugenhaupt S, Chakravarti A, Lupski JR (1990) Isolation of a marker linked to the Charcot-Marie-Tooth disease type1A by differential *Alu*-PCR of human chromosome 17-retaining hybrids. Am J Hum Genet 47:926-934

Sambrook J, Fritsch EF, Maniatis T (1989) Molecular cloning: a laboratory manual, 2nd ed. Cold Spring Harbor Laboratory, Cold Spring Harbor, New York

Seabright M (1971) A rapid banding technique for human chromosomes. Lancet 2:971-972

Taylor AMR, Harnden DG, Arlett CF, Harcourt SA, Lehmann AR, Stevens S, Bridges BA (1975) Ataxia-telangiectasia:a human mutation with abnormal radiation sensitivity. Nature 258:427-429

Ziv Y, Rotman G, Frydman M, Dagan J, Cohen T, Foroud T, Gatti RA (1991) The ATC (ataxia-telangiectasia group C) locus localizes to chromosome 11q22-q23. Genomics 9:373-375

AT-like Radiosensitive Rodent Cell Mutants: An Alternative Approach to the Isolation of the A-T Gene(s)

M.Z. Zdzienicka[1], G.W.C.T. Verhaegh, W. Jongmans, N.G.J. Jaspers[2], M.Oshimura[3], M.R. James[4] and P.H.M. Lohman

MGC-Department of Radiation Genetics and Chemical Mutagenesis, State University of Leiden and J.A. Cohen Institute, Interuniversity Research Institute for Radiopathology and Radiation Protection, Wassenaarseweg 72 2333 AL Leiden, The Netherlands

INTRODUCTION

Ataxia-telangiectasia (A-T) is a human autosomal recessive multisystem disorder characterized by progressive cerebellar ataxia, oculocutaneous telangiectasia, immunodeficiency, hypersensitivity to ionizing radiation and predisposition to cancer (for review see Sedgwick and Boder, 1991). Despite extensive investigation, the molecular defect responsible for these pleiotropic abnormalities in A-T remains unknown.

Clinical radiosensitivity was confirmed *in vitro*, as cultured cells from A-T patients are hypersensitive to lethal and clastogenic effects of ionizing radiation (Taylor et al., 1975) and some radiomimetic drugs such as bleomycin. A-T cells appear to rejoin DNA double- and single-strand breaks at normal rates (Fornace and Little, 1980; van der Schans et al., 1980; Hariharan et al., 1981; Jaspers et al., 1982; Coquerelle and

---

[1]To whom correspondence should be addressed (Tel. 31-71-276175 and Fax 31-71-221615)

[2]MGC-Department of Cell Biology and Genetics, Erasmus University, Rotterdam, The Netherlands

[3]Department of Molecular and Cell Genetics, Tottori University, Japan

[4]CEPH, Paris, France

NATO ASI Series, Vol. H 77
Ataxia-Telangiectasia
Edited by R. A. Gatti and R. B. Painter
© Springer-Verlag Berlin Heidelberg 1993

Weibezahn 1982). Another characteristic feature of A-T cells is a less pronounced inhibition of DNA synthesis after exposure to ionizing radiation or radiomimetic agents (for review see Lavin and Schroeder, 1988). This phenomenon, called radioresistant DNA synthesis (RDS) has been used as a marker in complementation analysis of A-T. So far, four complementation groups (A, C, D and E) have been identified in this disorder (Jaspers et al., 1989). Genetic linkage analysis (Gatti et al., 1988; McConville et al., 1990, Sanal et al., 1990; Ziv et al., 1991) and chromosome transfer studies (Lambert et al., 1991) have shown that the genes associated with three complementation groups (A, C and D) are located at the chromosomal region 11q22-q23. Recently, a gene partially correcting the defect in A-T group D cells has been isolated (Kapp et al., 1992) which appears to be located in this region.

Nijmegen Breakage Syndrome (NBS), a human recessive disorder with microcephaly, immunodeficiency, cancer susceptibility and chromosomal instability but not ataxia or telangiectasia, shares with A-T the cellular characteristics of radiosensitivity, radioresistant DNA synthesis and chromosomal abnormalities (Weemaes et al., 1981; Seemanova et al., 1985; Conley et al., 1986; Wegner et al., 1988). In this disorder two complementation groups have been identified (Jaspers et al., 1989).

Mutants of rodent cell lines with an abnormal cellular response to DNA damaging agents have contributed to our knowledge of mammalian DNA repair processes, because they provide a tool for the isolation of human genes complementing the defect in rodent cell mutants and for comparative biochemical studies of DNA repair. Recently, using Chinese hamster cell UV-sensitive mutants, three human genes complementing the defects in xeroderma pigmentosum (group B and group D) and Cockayne's syndrome (group B) have been cloned (Weeda et al., 1990; Flejter et al., 1992; Troelstra et al., 1992). These studies demonstrate the similarity at the genetic level between the artificially produced rodent cell mutants and the inherited human disorders associated with the increased sensitivity to UV. It has also been shown that one of the Chinese hamster V79 cell mutants sensitive to cross-linking agents is impaired in the gene homologous to Fanconi anemia - group A (Zdzienicka et al., 1990; Arwert et al., 1991).

During the past few years a wide variety of ionizing radiation-sensitive rodent cell mutants has been isolated and classified into at least nine complementation groups (Jeggo et al., 1991; Thacker and Wilkinson, 1991; Zdzienicka et al., 1992), indicating great complexity for the cellular defence mechanisms against ionizing radiation. In a search for rodent mutants homologous to A-T we have isolated several X-ray-sensitive Chinese hamster cell mutants, some properties of which are presented here.

RESULTS

Rodent ionizing radiation-sensitive Chinese hamster V79 cell mutants

To expand the existing collection of mutants with defective responses to ionizing radiation, several clones of V79 cells showing hypersensitivity to X-rays have been isolated (Zdzienicka and Simons, 1987; Zdzienicka et al., 1988; Zdzienicka et al., 1989; Zdzienicka et al., 1992).

Table 1.   X-ray-sensitive mutants of Chinese hamster V79 cell

Mutant cells	Sensitivity[a] to X-rays	Bleomycin	DNA repair defect	Complementation group	Reference
V-C4	~3	5	?	one group	Zdzienicka and Simons, 1987
V-E5	~3	2	?		Zdzienicka et al., 1989
V-G8	~2	2	?		
irs 2	2.5	n.d.	?		Jones et al., 1987, 1990
					Thacker and Ganesh, 1990
XR-V15B	8	3	DSB	the same as xrs[*]	Zdzienicka et al., 1988
XR-V9B	4	17	DSB	different than XR-V15B, V-3 and XR-1	Zdzienicka et al.,1992

[a] - the increased sensitivity based on D_{10} values

[*] Jeggo and Kemp, 1983

The mutants display a 2-8 fold increase in cell killing by ionizing radiation and they are cross-sensitive to an array of free radical-producing agents (Table 1). Without any further selection pressure, this phenotype was stably maintained in all mutants during culture for a period of at least 3 months. Complementation analysis by cell fusion followed by radiation exposure revealed that these X-ray-sensitive mutants belong to three distinct complementation groups. In representatives of two groups (XR-V9B and XR-V15B) a defect in the rejoining of double-strand DNA break (DSB) repair was observed, as measured by the sensitive DNA filter elution technique (see Table 1). The third group, however, represented by mutant cell lines V-C4, V-E5 and V-G8, was completely normal in both DSB and single-strand DNA break (SSB) repair, and therefore, in this respect resembled A-T cells.

Radioresistant DNA synthesis

To further investigate the apparent resemblance of V-C4, V-E5 and V-G8 to A-T cells, we have measured the initial rates of DNA synthesis after various exposures to gamma-rays. As shown at Fig. 1a, all three cell lines displayed less inhibition of DNA replication, whereas this RDS phenotype was not apparent in XR-V9B and XR-V15B cells. Instead, the mutants that were defective in DSB rejoining showed a more pronounced gamma-ray-induced DNA synthesis inhibition compared to the parental V79B cells (Fig. 1b).

RDS behaves as a recessive phenotype in cultured A-T human fibroblasts as has been shown by complementation studies of A-T. The results of our previous studies, where the X-ray sensitivity of AT-like mutants was used as marker in complementation analysis, indicated that V-C4, V-E5 and V-G8 belong to one complementation group (Zdzienicka et al., 1989). Therefore, it was of interest to determine whether hybrids between these mutants also show the same degree of RDS or whether the phenotype of RDS can be complemented in these mutants in the absence of complementation for X-ray sensitivity. The various hybrid cell lines obtained after fusion between the V-C4, V-E5 and V-G8 mutants not only remained sensitive, in terms of survival, but also showed RDS; this is in agreement with our previous assignment of these mutants to one complementation group (Verhaegh et al., 1993). The results suggest that, as in A-T cells, the two phenomena of X-ray sensitivity and RDS are the pleiotropic effects of the same genetic defect.

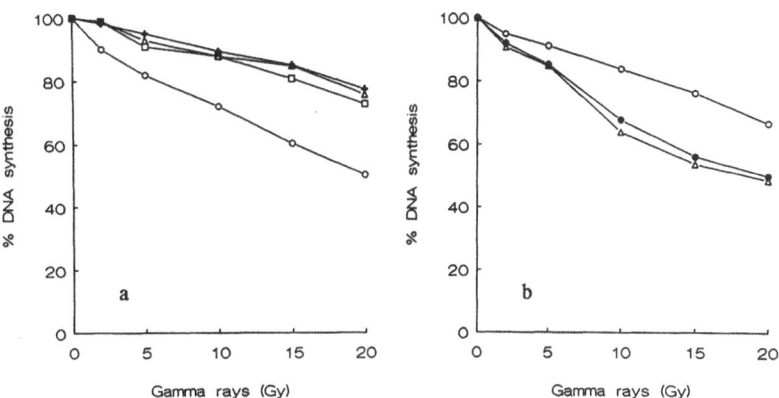

Figure 1. Inhibition of DNA synthesis after γ-rays: a/ in V79 (o), V-C4 (+), V-E5 (□) and V-G8 (Δ); b/ in V79B (o), XR-V9B (●) and XR-V15B (Δ) cells.

Studies on chromosome assignment of the AT-like mutants

If the AT-like mutants (V-C4, VE5 and V-G8) are defective in one of the genes homologous to ATA, ATC or ATD, it is expected that introduction of a normal human chromosome 11 will result in complementation of the radiosensitive phenotype, as has been shown for AT-D cells (Komatsu et al., 1990; Lambert et al., 1991). To investigate this possibility, human chromosome 11 was introduced into the V-E5 and V-G8 mutants by the micro-cell-mediated chromosome transfer technique as described by Komatsu et al., (1990). After fusion of microcells with V-E5 or V-G8 cells, forty hybrid clones growing in medium with G418 were obtained. The presence of human chromosome 11 was verified in these hybrids by *in situ* hybridization. The presence of the relevant chromosomal region 11q22-23, which carries the gene(s) involved in ATA, ATC or ATD, was determined by PCR using polymor-phic DNA markers specific for the ATA and ATC loci (CJ52.75, CJ52.3, CJ52.114) and the putative ATDC locus (Thy 1) (Kapp et al., 1992). In twelve hybrids this whole region was found (Fig. 2).

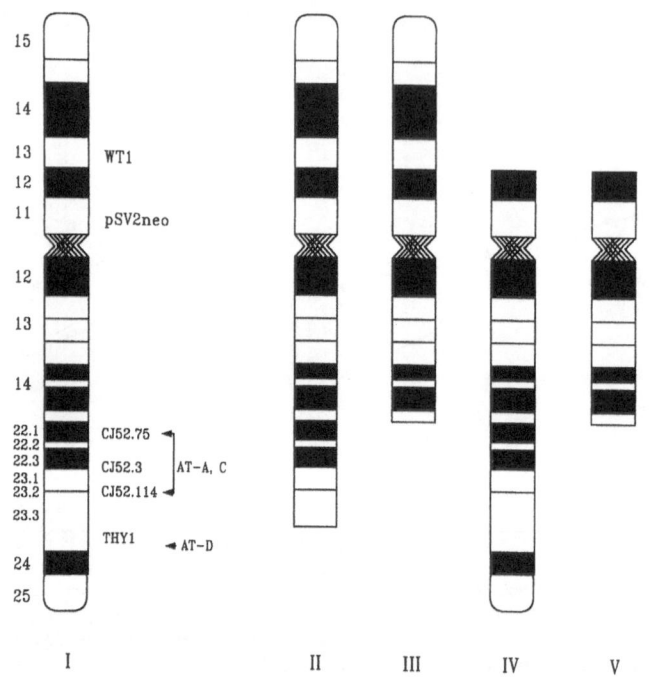

Figure 2. A single human chromosome 11 tagged with one copy of pSV2neo
(11p11 region) present in monochromosomal human - AT-like
hamster cell (V-E5 and V-G8) mutants hybrids: I/ V-E5(neo)-1,
10, 17, 18, 20, 23, 25 and V-G8(neo)-2, 5, 11, 15; II/ V-E5
(neo)-6; III/ V-E5(neo)-2, 13, 6, 7; IV/ V-G8(neo)-10; V/ V-
E5(neo)-5. The rest of hybrids contained only a very small part
of chromosome 11.

Finally, X-ray survival of these hybrids was determined. The results
show that despite the unequivocal presence of the human 11q22-23 region,
none of these hybrid clones showed complementation of the X-ray-
sensitivity, whereas fusion to human HeLa cells frequently resulted in
correction of the defective phenotype (Jongmans et al., submitted). These
results indicate that the AT-like hamster cell mutants probably are not
defective in one of the ATA, ATC or ATD genes, and that the underlying
genetic defect is not located on human chromosome 11 but on another
chromosome. Work to identify this human chromosome is in progress.

DISCUSSION

The XR-V9B and XR-V15B mutants which belong to two different complementation groups, do not show a radioresistant DNA synthesis but do show a
defect in DSB repair (Zdzienicka et al., 1988; Zdzienicka et al., 1992),
indicating that the defect in these mutants differs substantially from that
of A-T cells. On the other hand, the V-C4, V-E5 and V-G8 mutants show all
typical features of A-T cells, inasmuch as they are hypersensitive to both
X-rays and radiomimetic chemical agents such as bleomycin, streptonigrin
and VP16 (Jongmans et al., submitted), have normal rates of DSB and SSB
rejoining, show chromosomal instability and the characteristic feature of
RDS (Zdzienicka et al., 1989). Another X-ray-sensitive mutant (*irs 2*) of
Chinese hamster V79 cells, which belongs to the same complementation group
as the V-C4, V-E5 and VG8 mutants, has similar characteristics (Thacker and
Ganesh, 1990; Jones et al., 1990). Amongst nine complementation groups,
that have been identified in ionizing-radiation-sensitive rodent cell
mutants (Jeggo et al., 1991; Thacker and Wilkinson, 1991; Zdzienicka at
al., 1992), this is the only group bearing such a close resemblance to
cells from A-T and NBS patients. Therefore, it is likely that mutants of
this group are defective in the same pathway as A-T/NBS cells. As such,
these AT-like mutants can serve as a rodent cell model for studies of this
pathway.

Further genetic characterization of this complementation group has
revealed that the underlying defect is distinct from that in A-T group A ,
group C and group D, because human chromosome 11 does not complement the
defect in the AT-like mutants. However, the involvement of the less
frequent A-T group E or the two NBS genes (V1 and V2) has not been investigated, because the genes for these complementation groups have not been
localized. An A-T family showing apparent non-linkage to chromosome 11q22-
23 has also been reported (Hernandez et al., 1991), but the family was not
assigned to a complementation group. Besides the chromosome assignment of
the defect in the AT-like mutants, we are currently expanding the collection of radiosensitive mutants, in hope of obtaining a hamster homologue to
other A-T groups.

It has become evident that repair deficient mutants of rodent cells
provide an important tool for the isolation of human genes involved in DNA
repair. Chinese hamster cell lines, in contrast to transformed human

fibroblasts, are good recipients of human DNA in transfection experiments, and have been used successfully for the isolation of human genes complementing their defects (Westerveld et al., 1984; Weber et al., 1988; Thompson et al., 1990; Weeda et al., 1990; Troelstra et al., 1992). Cloning and characterization of the correcting gene in the AT-like mutants described here will also enhance our understanding of the molecular defect in the A-T and NBS disorders.

ACKNOWLEDGMENTS

This work was supported by Grants IKW 90-03 and 91-01 from the Dutch Cancer Society and the Ataxia-telangiectasia Medical Research Foundation, Los Angeles, U.S.A.

REFERENCES:

Arwert F, Rooimans MA, Westerveld A, Simons JWIM, Zdzienicka MZ (1991) The Chinese hamster V79 cell mutant V-H4 is homologous to Fanconi anemia (complementation group A). Cytogenetics and Cell Genet 56:23-26

Conley ME, Spinner MB, Emmanuel BS, Nowell PC, Nichols WW (1986) A chromosome breakage syndrome with profound immunodeficiency. Blood 67:1251-1256

Coquerelle TM, Weibezahn KW (1981) Rejoining of DNA double-strand breaks in human fibroblasts and its impairment in one AT and two Fanconi strains. J Supramol Struct Cell Biochem 17:369-376

Flejter WL, McDaniel LD, Johns D, Friedberg EC, Schultz RA (1992) Correction of xeroderma pigmentosum complementation group D mutant cell phenotypes by chromosome and gene transfer: involvement of the human ERCC2 DNA repair gene. Proc Nat Acad Sci USA 89:261-265

Fornace AJ, Little JB (1980) Normal repair of DNA single strand breaks in patients with AT. Biochim Biophys Acta 607:432-437

Gatti RA et al (1988) Localization of an ataxia-telangiectasia gene to chromosome 11q22-23. Nature 336:577-580

Hariharan PV, Eleczko S, Smith BP, Paterson MC (1981) Normal rejoining of DNA strand breaks in AT fibroblast lines after low X-ray exposure.

Radiat Res 86:589-597

Hernandez D, McConville CM, Taylor AMR (1991) Failure to map the AT gene to 11q22-23 in a large inbred family. Cytogenet Cell Genet 58:1962-1963

Jaspers NGJ, de Wit J, Regulski MR, Bootsma D (1982) Abnormal regulation of DNA replication and increased lethality in AT cells exposed to car- cinogenic agents. Cancer Res 42:335-341

Jaspers NGJ, Gatti RA, Baan C, Linssen CML, Bootsma D (1989) Genetic com- plementation analysis of ataxia telangiectasia and Nijmegen breakage syndrome: a survey of 50 patients. Cytogenet. Cell Genet 49:259-263

Jeggo PA, Kemp LM (1983) X-ray-sensitive mutants of Chinese hamster ovary cell line. Isolation and cross-sensitivity to other DNA damaging agents. Mutation Res 112:313-327

Jeggo PA, Tesmer J, Chen DJ (1991) Genetic analysis of ionising radiation- sensitive mutants of cultured mammalian cell lines. Mutation Res 254: 125-133

Jones NJ, Cox R, Thacker J (1987) Isolation and cross-sensitivity of X-ray- sensitive mutants of V79-4 hamster cells. Mutation Res 183:279-286

Jones NJ, Stewart SA, Thompson LH (1990) Biochemical and genetic analysis of the Chinese hamster mutants *irs1* and *irs2* and their comparison to cultured ataxia telangiectasia cells. Mutagenesis 5:15-23

Jongmans W, Wiegant J, Oshimura M, James MR, Lohman PHM, Zdzienicka MZ. Human Chromosome 11 complements ataxia-telangiectasia cells but does not complement the defect in the AT-like Chinese hamster cell mutants. Human Genet subm

Jongmans W, Verhaegh GWCT, Sankarayanan K, Lohman PHM, Zdzienicka MZ. Cellular Characteristics of AT-like Chinese hamster cells. Mutation Res subm

Kapp LN, Painter RB, Yu L-C, van Loon N, Richard III CW, James MR, Cox DR, Murnane JP (1992) Cloning of a candidate gene for Ataxia-telangiectasia group D. Am J Hum Genet 51:45-54

Komatsu K, Kodama S, Okumura Y, Koi M, Oshimura M (1990) Restoration of radiation resistance in ataxia telangiectasia cells by the introduction of normal human chromosome 11. Mutation Res 235:59-63

Lambert C, Schultz RA, Smith M, Wagner-McPherson C, McDaniel LD, Donlon T, Stanbridge EJ, Friedberg EC (1991) Functional complementation of ataxia- telangiectasia group D (AT-D) cells by microcell-mediated chromosome transfer and mapping of the AT-D locus to the region 11q22-23. Proc Nat Acad Sci USA 88:5907-5911

Lavin MF, Schroeder AL (1988) Damage-resistant DNA synthesis in eukaryotes.

Mutation Res 193:193-206

McConville C, Woods CG, Farrell M, Metcalfe JA, Taylor AMR (1990) Analysis of 7 polymorphic markers at chromosome 11q 22-23 in 35 ataxia telangiectasia families: further evidence of linkage. Hum Genet 85:215-220

Sanal et al (1990) Further mapping of an ataxia-telangiectasia locus to the chromosome 11q23 region. Am J Hum Genet 47:860-866

Schans GP van der, Centen HB, Lohman PHM (1980) Studies on the repair defect(s) of ataxia-telangiectasia fibroblasts. Radiat Environ Biophys 17:351

Sedgwick RP, Boder E (1991) Ataxia-telangiectasia, in : Handbook of Clinical Neurology 16 pp 347-423, Elsevier Science Publishers, Amsterdam, New York (eds Vinken PJ, Bruyn GW, Klawans HL)

Seemanova EE, Passarge E, Beneskova D, Houstek J, Kasal P, Sevcikova M (1985) Familial microcephaly with normal intelligence, immunodeficiency and risk for lymphoreticular malignancies. Am J med Genet 20:639-648

Taylor AMR, Harnden DG, Arlett CF, Harcourt SA, Lehmann A, Stevens R, Bridges BA (1975) Ataxia telangiectasia: a human mutation with abnormal radiation sensitivity. Nature 285:427-429

Thacker J, Wilkinson RE (1991) The genetic basis of resistance to ionising radiation damage in cultured mammalian cells. Mutation Res 254: 135-142

Thacker J, Ganesh AN (1990) DNA-break repair, Radioresistance of DNA synthesis, and camptothecin sensitivity in the radiation-sensitive *irs* mutants: Comparison to ataxia-telangiectasia cells. Mutation Res 235: 49-58

Thompson LH, Brookman KW, Jones NJ, Allen SA, Carrano AV (1990) Molecular cloning of the human *XRCC1* gene, which corrects defective DNA strand break repair and sister chromatide exchange. Mol Cell Biol 10:6160-6171

Troelstra C, van Gool A, de Wit J, Vermeulen W, Bootsma D, Hoeijmakers JHJ (1992) *ERCC6*, a member of a subfamily of putative helicases, is involved in Cockayne's syndrome and preferential repair of active genes. Cell in press

Verhaegh GWCT, Jaspers NGJ, Lohman PHM, Zdzienicka MZ. Co-dominance of radioresistant DNA synthesis in a group of AT-like Chinese hamster cell mutants. Cytogenet Cell Genet accepted

Weber CA, Salazar EP, Stewart SA, Thompson LH (1988) Molecular cloning and biological characterization of a human gene, *ERCC2*, that corrects the nucleotide excision repair defect in CHO UV5 cells. Mol Cell Biol 8:1137-1146

Weeda G, van Ham RCA, Vermeulen W, Bootsma D, van der EB AJ, Hoeijmakers
    JHJ (1990) A presumed DNA helicase, encoded by the excision repair gene
ERCC3 is involved in the human repair disorders xeroderma pigmentosum   and
Cockayne's syndrome. Cell 62:777-791

Weemaes CMR, Hustinx TWJ, Scheres JMJC, van Munster PJJ, Bakkeren JAJM,
    Taalman RDFM (1981) New chromosome instability disorder: the Nijmegen
    breakage syndrome. Acts pediat scand 70:557-562

Wegner RD, Metzger M, Hanefelt F, Jaspers NGJ, Baan C, Magdorf K, Kunze J,
    Sperling K (1988) A new chromosome instability disorder confirmed by
    complementation studies. Clin Genet 33:20-32

Westerveld A, Hoeijmakers JHJ, van Duin M, de Wit J, Odijk H, Pastink A,
    Wood RD, Bootsma D (1984) Molecular cloning of a human DNA repair gene.
    Nature 310:425-428

Zdzienicka MZ, Simons JWIM (1987) Mutagen-sensitive cell lines are obtained
    with a high frequency in V79 Chinese hamster cells. Mutation Res 178:
    235-244

Zdzienicka MZ, Tran Q, van der Schans GP, Simons JWIM (1988) Characteriza-
    tion of an X-ray-sensitive mutant of V79 Chinese hamster cells. Mutation
    Res 194:239-249

Zdzienicka MZ, Jaspers NGJ, van der Schans GP, Natarajan AT, Simons JWIM
    (1989) Ataxia telangiectasis-like Chinese hamster V79 cell mutants with
    radioresistant DNA synthesis, chromosomal instability and normal DNA
    strand break repair. Cancer Res 49:1481-1485

Zdzienicka MZ, Arwert F, Neuteboom I, Rooimans M, Simons JWIM (1990) The
    Chinese hamster V79 cell mutant V-H4 is phenotypically like Fanconi
    anemia cells. Somatic Cell Mol Genet 16:575-581

Zdzienicka MZ, van Wessel N, van der Schans GP (1992) A fourth complementa-
    tion group among ionizing radiation-sensitive Chinese hamster cell
    mutants defective in DNA double-strand break repair. Radiation Res 131:
    309-314

Ziv Y et al., (1991) The AT-C (ataxia-telangiectasia complementation group
    C) locus localize to 11q22-23. Genomics 9:373-375

III. A–T Heterozygotes and Complementation

Identification of A-T heterozygotes

D. Scott[1], L.A. Jones[1], S.A.G. Elyan[2], A. Spreadborough[1], R. Cowan[3]
and G. Ribiero[3]
CRC Departments of Cancer Genetics[1] and Experimental Radiation
Oncology[2]
Paterson Institute for Cancer Research and Department of Clinical
Oncology[3]
Christie Hospital NHS Trust
Manchester
M20 9BX
UK

Introduction

Since the discovery of the abnormal response of cells from
ataxia-telangiectasia (A-T) homozygotes to ionising radiation and
free radical-generating chemicals (reviewed in Bridges and
Harnden, 1982) the response of cells from heterozygotes has been
investigated with many procedures (summarised by Weeks *et al.*,
1991). Most techniques are able to detect a shift in the *average*
response of heterozygote cells compared with normals but with
considerable overlap between the two groups. The assay that has
been reported to provide the best discrimination has been devised
by K.K. Sanford and colleagues at the National Cancer Institute
(NCI) and involves X-irradiating cells in the G_2 phase of the
cell cycle and quantifying radiation-induced chromosome damage
in these cells when they undergo mitosis. In comparisons between
52 controls and 29 obligate heterozygotes, 50 of the controls had
lower chromosome aberration frequencies than any of the
heterozygotes. These studies were on cultured skin fibroblasts
(20 heterozygotes and 17 controls for which there was complete
discrimination; Parshad *et al.*, 1985; Shiloh *et al.*, 1986; Shiloh
et al., 1989) and peripheral blood lymphocytes (9 heterozygotes
and 35 controls with overlap of 2 controls; Sanford and Parshad,
1990). Since it has been estimated that A-T heterozygotes
constitute approximately 1% of the US white population (Swift *et
al.*, 1986), it is possible that the 2 controls that had a
chromosomal sensitivity similar to obligate heterozygotes were
carriers of the A-T gene. The NCI group has also reported that
this assay will detect many other cancer-prone syndromes
including basal cell naevus syndrome, familial polyposis and

NATO ASI Series, Vol. H 77
Ataxia-Telangiectasia
Edited by R. A. Gatti and R. B. Painter
© Springer-Verlag Berlin Heidelberg 1993

xeroderma pigmentosum (XP), as well as XP heterozygotes and putative carriers of cancer-predisposing genes in "cancer families" (see Sanford and Parshad, 1990). In view of these reports we have utilised the NCI protocol on blood lymphocytes from a number of cancer-prone individuals, including members of A-T families; the latter are reported here.

Of the many other assays that have been used to try to identify A-T heterozygotes, another which has been reported to give good, but not complete discrimination, involves the use of low dose rate gamma rays on skin fibroblasts with colony-forming ability as the endpoint (Paterson et al., 1985; Weeks et al., 1991).

Even with a relatively simple radiosensitivity assay that would completely discriminate A-T gene carriers from non-carriers it would still be a formidable task to screen the general population with the frequency of carriers being only about 1%. The screening could be more focused if restricted to cancer families or cancer patients, since the A-T gene confers an increased risk of cancer, particularly breast cancer, for which the relative risk is 5.1 compared with spouse controls (i.e. non A-T gene carriers), leading to the provocative estimate that between 9-18% of breast cancer cases are A-T heterozygotes (Swift et al., 1986, 1991). An even higher proportion of carriers might be found amongst breast cancer patients who have shown excessive normal tissue damage ("overreaction") after radiotherapy if the moderately elevated radiosensitivity of heterozygote cells is reflected in their normal tissue response. For homozygotes, who show extreme cellular radiosensitivity (Taylor et al., 1975; Bridges and Harnden, 1982) conventional radiotherapy produces devastating, life-threatening tissue necrosis (Gotoff et al., 1967; Cunliffe et al., 1975).

As a first step towards possible heterozygote identification amongst cancer patients we have addressed the question of whether or not overreaction to radiotherapy in breast cancer patients is associated with abnormal response of their lymphocytes to irradiation in vitro. Regardless of considerations of A-T heterozygote detection, the demonstration of a relationship between clinical overreaction and lymphocyte radiosensitivity could provide a simple predictive test for normal tissue

tolerance and lead to appropriate adjustment of radiotherapy
doses (Norman *et al.*, 1988; Burnet *et al.*, 1992).

In addition to our studies with the NCI G_2 chromosomal
radiosensitivity assay, we have investigated the radiation
response of lymphocytes of obligate A-T heterozygotes (and
homozygotes from the same families) and overreacting breast
cancer patients using three other techniques: 1) a modification
of the NCI assay 2) lymphocyte survival after low dose rate
irradiation of G_0 cells and 3) chromosome aberration induction by
low dose irradiation of G_0 cells. The studies are not complete
and the available results are somewhat unbalanced in the sense
that, in a particular assay, the majority of results may be
biased towards A-T families or overreactors and that relatively
few cases have been studied in more than one assay. When
complete, this study will allow us to evaluate the relative
merits of each assay for detecting abnormal radiation response
in A-T heterozygotes and overreacting breast cancer patients.

Materials and Methods

Chromosomal radiosensitivity in G_2

The NCI assay. Unless otherwise stated, we adhered strictly to
the NCI protocol (Parshad *et al.*, 1990). Briefly, at 72h after
phytohaemagglutin (PHA) stimulation, whole blood cultures in RPMI
1640 medium with 15% foetal bovine serum (FBS) were aliquotted
into pyrex centrifuge tubes, spun at 150 g, most of the medium
removed, cell pellets irradiated and then fresh prewarmed medium
added. Thirty minutes later, colcemid (0.1 μg ml^{-1}) was added
for 60 minutes and the harvesting procedure (including hypotonic
treatment) begun. Fixative was added to the cells at 140 mins
post-irradiation. All procedures, including irradiation,
centrifugation and hypotonic treatments were performed at 37°C.

We did not have access to the same Torrex 150 kV X-ray
source as used at the NCI (Sanford *et al.*, 1987). Ours is a
Pantak unit operating at 300 kV, 10 mA, dose rate 1.2 Gy min^{-1}
with HVT = 2.3 mm Cu. We did not anticipate that the difference
between the sources would lead to different results because, for
their fibroblast studies, the NCI group have used a number of
radiation sources giving X-rays of differing qualities with no

difference in results (Sanford et al., 1989). We did, however, find that the NCI's recommended exposure of 100R resulted in almost complete elimination of mitotic activity. For reasons that will be explained in detail elsewhere (Scott et al., 1993) we decided to use biological dosimetry i.e. a radiation dose which gave us a yield of aberrations similar to that obtained at the NCI. This dose was 0.25 Gy.

One hundred cells were scored for each datum point in Figures 1 and 2. Aberrations were mainly chromatid gaps and breaks. A low frequency of chromatid exchanges was induced but this is not included in the Figures.

Cell Survival

Survival was assessed by a limiting dilution assay in which lymphocytes are irradiated in G_0 and then stimulated with PHA and interleukin-2 (James et al., 1983). In most cases lymphocytes had been cryopreserved before use in the survival assay. Lymphocytes were exposed to 4 Gy ^{60}Co gamma rays at low dose rate (0.0098 Gy min^{-1}) to obtain SF4 values (surviving fraction at 4 Gy). Further technical details are given in Elyan et al (1993).

Chromosomal radiosensitivity in G_0

The low dose-rate irradiation procedure was based upon the method of Paterson et al (1985) for fibroblasts and modified by C.J. Roberts (Harwell, England; personal communication) for blood samples. One ml aliquots of whole blood were added to 3 ml medium (RPMI 1640 with 15% FBS, without PHA) in plastic screw-topped centrifuge tubes, which were rotated at 25 rpm in a 37°C incubator in the radiation field (^{60}Co gamma rays at 0.0031 Gy min^{-1}) for 16h 8m to give a total dose of 3.0 Gy. One hour after irradiation the contents of the tubes were transferred to tissue culture flasks and additional medium was added to give a final blood:medium ratio of 1:10. PHA (Wellcome, reagent grade; final concn. 1%) was then added to stimulate proliferation and cells were harvested at 50h post stimulation after a 2h treatment with colcemid (0.1 μg ml^{-1}). Unirradiated controls were similarly rotated prior to culturing and bromodeoxyuridine (final concentration 5 μg ml^{-1}) was added to the cultures to determine the proportion of second division cells at 50h; this never exceeded 6% so the majority of irradiated cells analysed would have been at their first mitosis (Scott and Lyons, 1979). One hundred cells were scored for each of the datum points shown in Fig. 4.

Results

Chromosomal radiosensitivity in G_2

The NCI assay

A-T families: Chromosomal radiosensitivity of members of A-T families (homozygotes and obligate heterozygotes) was compared with a normal control (in one case two controls) within each experiment. The results of six experiments are presented in Fig. 1. For all but two experiments (symbols O and Δ) a different control was used. All homozygotes gave aberration yields significantly higher than the highest control value (Fig 1a). For heterozygotes, whereas the average value was somewhat higher than the average control value there was considerable overlap; only 6/10 were higher than all controls. The horizontal lines in Fig 1a represent the range of values obtained with the NCI protocol from 42 experiments on 19 controls (range 29-82 aberrations per 100 cells). Using the upper limit, only 2/10 heterozygotes are above the highest control value. Repeat studies on the same normal individuals have shown that the observed variability in aberration yields for controls is *inter-experimental variability* rather than individual-to-individual variation. This variability can be removed by expressing the aberration yields in homozygotes and heterozygotes relative to the control value within each experiment. When this is done (Fig 1b) 9/10 heterozygotes are more sensitive than their parallel controls; the relative sensitivities range from 0.93 to 1.65 (mean 1.27).

The Paterson G_2 assay. The main problems we have experienced with the NCI assay are: considerable experimental variability (see above), and failure to obtain complete discrimination between A-T heterozygotes and controls. We have found that experimental variability can be reduced by omitting the

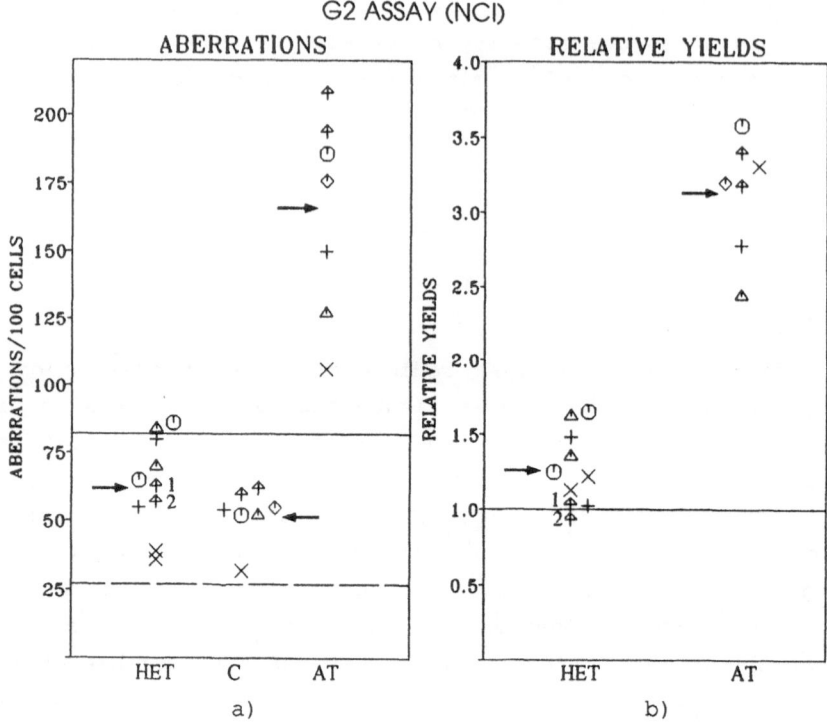

Fig 1. G_2 chromosomal radiosensitivity (0.25 Gy) of controls (C), A-T patients and obligate A-T heterozygotes (HET). Samples handled within the same experiment are shown with the same symbol. Experiments O, +, ♠ and X were performed strictly according to the NCI protocol. In experiments ∆ and ◊ medium was changed without centrifugation, one hour before irradiation. Numbered symbols represent individuals studied also in other assays (see Fig. 4). Horizontal arrows indicate mean values.

1a: Primary data.
1b: Each value expressed relative to the control sample within the same experiment i.e. each control is given a value of 1.0 (horizontal line).

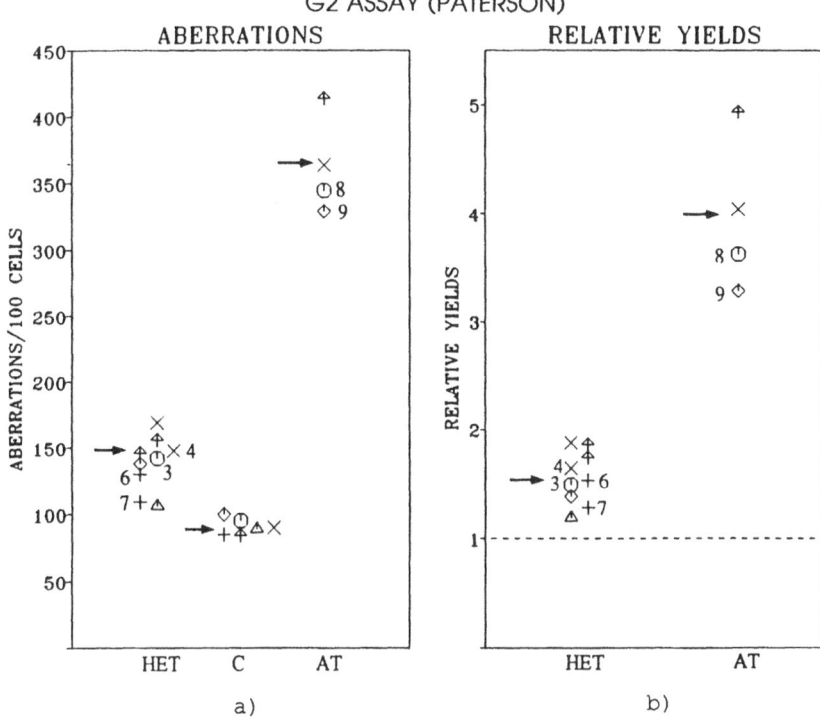

Fig 2. As for Figure 1 but using the Paterson G_2 assay (0.5
        Gy). Two overreacting breast cancer patients (cases
        6 and 7) are also shown. Horizontal arrows indicate
        mean values. The left-hand horizontal arrows in Figs
        2a and 2b represent the mean value for heterozygotes
        (overreactors excluded).

centrifugation of cells prior to irradiation (medium can be
changed by removal of old medium with a Pasteur pipette since the
cells are at the bottom of the flask) and by harvesting the cells
at low temperature (this stops repair as soon as harvesting
begins).   Weincke *et* *al* (1992) have obtained better
discrimination between heterozygotes and controls with increasing
radiation dose in a G_2 radiosensitivity assay.   We therefore
increased our radiation dose from 0.25 to 0.50 Gy.   This
"Paterson G_2 assay" has been applied to A-T families and
overreactors and results are available for 4 A-T homozygotes, 7
heterozygotes and 2 overreactors (Fig 2).

These modifications to the G_2 assay have, so far, markedly reduced the experimental variability and given better heterozygote detection. The range of values for controls is only from 85–100 aberrations per 100 cells (5 individuals, repeat on one). All 7 heterozygotes had yields higher than 100 aberrations per 100 cells although for one case the yield was only 106 per 100 cells. Expressed as relative yields (Fig 2b), the values range from 1.12 to 1.88 (mean 1.60); this is an improvement on our results with the NCI assay (mean 1.27). This improvement is also reflected in the increased relative sensitivities of the homozygotes, 2.44–3.40 (mean 3.13) with the NCI assay, 3.29–4.93 (mean 3.97) with the Paterson G_2 assay.

Both overreactors (cases 6 and 7 in Fig. 2) were more sensitive than their parallel normal controls; relative yields were 1.28 and 1.53. These overreactors could, of course, be A-T heterozygotes.

Cell survival (SF4) in A-T families

In each experiment an aliquot from a large store of cryopreserved lymphocytes from a single normal control individual was used in parallel with lymphocytes from A-T homozygotes and/or heterozygotes. Results from 7 experiments are shown in Fig. 3. SF4 values for the control ranged from 5.6 –14.3 (mean 10.3%) which represents inter-experiment variability. Mean survival for homozygotes was only 0.4% (ratio control: homozygotes = 1.00:0.04) and for heterozygotes was 8.5% (ratio control:heterozygotes = 1.00:0.83). Three of 7 heterozygotes had survival levels lower than the lowest value obtained for the common control. When inter-experiment variability is eliminated by expressing survival of homozygotes and heterozygotes relative to their parallel control sample (Fig 3b) 5/7 heterozygotes were significantly more sensitive than the control. Two of the 5 (designated 3 and 4 in Fig 3) were also assessed in the Paterson G_2 assay and were radiation sensitive (Fig 2, cases 3 and 4). One heterozygote ($\times$ in Fig 3) gave an unexpected SF4 value, showing a survival value (13%) more than twice as high as the parallel control sample (5.6%).

LOW DOSE RATE ASSAY (SURVIVAL)

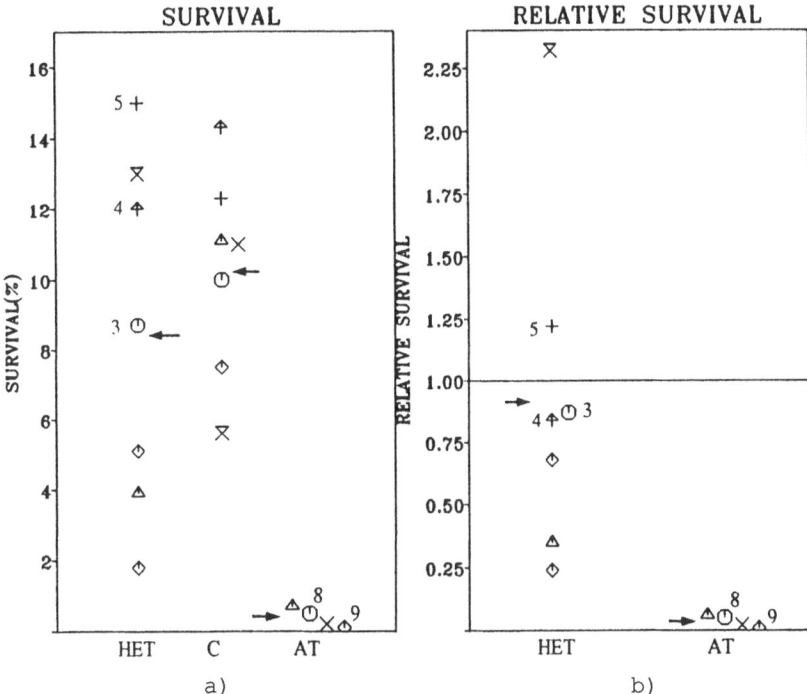

a)

b)

Fig 3. Surviving fraction after 4 Gy (SF4) gamma rays were
delivered at a low dose rate to lymphocytes of one
normal control (C), A-T patients and obligate
heterozygotes (HET). Samples handled within the same
experiment are shown with the same symbol. Numbered
symbols represent individuals studied also with other
assays (see Figs 2 and 4). Horizontal arrows indicate
mean values.

3a: Primary data.
3b: Survival expressed in relation to the parallel control
      sample.
      Note that, unlike the chromosome aberration data in
      Figs 1, 2 and 4, *sensitive* individuals have low values
      (i.e. low cell survival).

In separate studies (Elyan *et al.*, 1993), the mean SF4 value in 16 experiments that used stored lymphocytes from the one control donor used in these studies was found to be very similar to the mean SF4 values for 23 separate individuals. This control individual is therefore a good representative of normal radiosensitivity.

Chromosomal radiosensitivity in G_0

A-T families

In the first experiment, a homozygote, the father and a normal control were compared (Fig. 4, symbol O). In additional experiments 3 obligate heterozygotes were compared with 3 controls. Yields of dicentric aberrations are given in Fig. 4 because these are the most easily identified aberrations. The homozygote was 2.5 times more sensitive to aberration induction than the parallel control but the average yield of heterozygotes was the same as that of the controls; only 2/4 heterozygotes were more sensitive than their controls, and none was outside the normal range (26-51 dicentrics/100 cells). The two heterozygotes that were not more sensitive than their parallel controls were similarly insensitive in the G_2 NCI assay (cases 1 and 2 in Figs 1 and 4), but one of the sensitive heterozygotes (case 5) was not detected as sensitive in the cell survival assay (Fig. 3).

Breast cancer overreactors

Nine overreactors were compared with 12 controls (Fig. 4) and in each experiment an overreactor was tested together with 1 or 2 controls. The mean aberration frequency of the overreactors (45.7) was higher than the mean control value (38.8) and 3/9 overreactors were above the normal range. When compared with parallel controls, 7/9 overreactors were more sensitive (Fig. 4b). Two of the sensitive overreactors (cases 6 and 7) had also been tested in the Paterson G_2 assay (Fig. 2) and found to be more sensitive than their controls.

It is conceivable that the chromosomal radiosensitivity observed in the majority of our breast cancer overreactors may simply have been a consequence of their disease or their prior radiotherapy. It is essential therefore to examine chromosomal

LOW DOSE RATE ASSAY (ABERRATIONS)

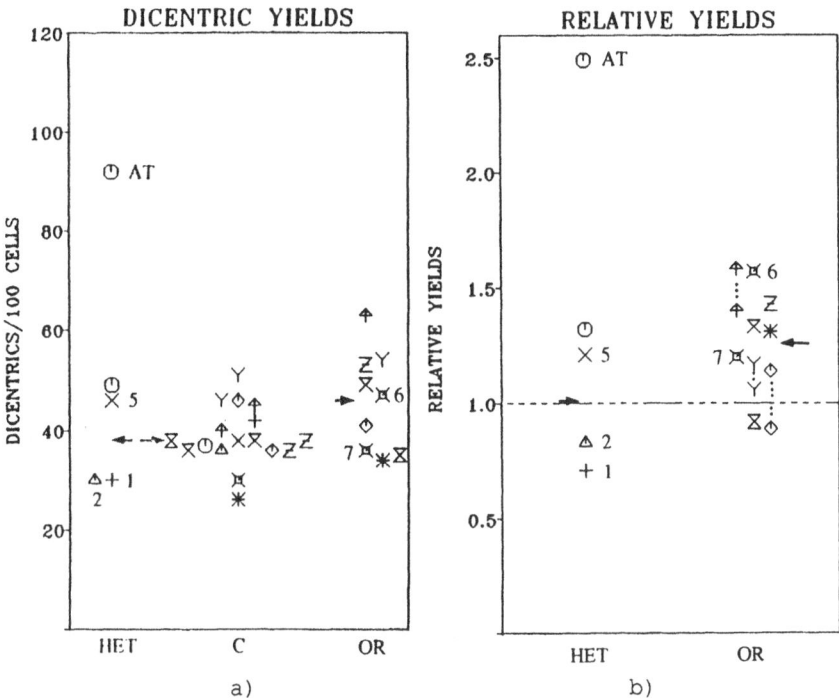

Fig 4. G_0 chromosomal radiosensitivity. Frequencies of dicentrics scored after 3 Gy gamma rays were delivered at a low dose rate to lymphocytes of an A-T patient, obligate heterozygotes (HET) and overreacting breast cancer patients (OR). Samples handled within the same experiment are shown with the same symbol. Numbered symbols represent individuals studied also with other assays (see Figs 1, 2 and 3). Horizontal arrows indicate mean values; those in the column designated HET do not include the homozygote.

4a: Primary data

4b: Yields expressed relative to control samples within the same experiment. For 5 of the overreactors there were 2 parallel controls; for 3 cases the calculated relative yields of patients to controls differed by more than 10% so both relative yield values are plotted using the same symbol (⚡◊Y) joined by a dotted line.

radiosensitivity of breast cancer patients who have not shown any untoward response to radiotherapy. We have results available on two such cases, both of whom showed no evidence of radiosensitivity in the G_0 chromosomal assay. Dicentric yields in the two patients and a control within the same experiment were, respectively, 50, 45 and 47 per 100 cells.

Discussion

Our first study in which we investigated the efficacy of the NCI G_2 assay in detecting cancer-prone individuals, including A-T heterozygotes, is now complete and will be reported in detail elsewhere. The second study of A-T heterozygotes and overreacting breast cancer patients using 3 different assays is not yet complete and only tentative conclusions are therefore possible.

A-T heterozygotes

Even though we have attempted to follow the NCI G_2 protocol as closely as possible, we have by no means obtained complete discrimination between heterozygotes and controls (Fig 1a). Even when results are expressed relative to the parallel control sample (Fig. 1b), not all heterozygotes are identified. Another major difference between our results and those at the NCI is that our range of values for controls is considerably greater and this is attributable to experimental variability. We have identified the reasons for this variability, modified the assay accordingly and, so far, with the Paterson G_2 technique, we have obtained complete discrimination between 5 controls and 7 heterozygotes (Fig. 2a). However, the difference in the mean aberration frequencies is not as great as that found by the NCI group using their own procedure and we anticipate some overlap between controls and heterozygotes when we have studied additional cases, although we would expect better discrimination than we have obtained with the NCI technique.

As with the NCI G_2 assay, we observed considerable overlap between control and heterozygote values with the cell survival (SF4, low dose rate) technique (Fig. 3a). We obtained better, though not complete discrimination, when results were expressed relative to the parallel control (Fig. 3b). The discrimination was probably better than it would have been if a number of different controls had been used because the inter-experimental variability for the single control donor who was used (cryopreserved lymphocytes used on different occasions) was less than that for different donors, indicating real and reproducible differences between normal individuals (Elyan et al 1993).

The limited results available from the low dose rate G_0 chromosomal radiosensitivity assay are not encouraging because none of the 4 cases was outside the normal range (Fig. 4).

Breast cancer overreactors

Even from the relatively little data available, it appears that, on average, the cellular radiosensitivity of overreactors is greater than controls (Figs. 2 and 4). We have most data from the G_0 chromosomal radiosensitivity technique and, in this, 7/9 overreactors were more sensitive than parallel controls (Fig. 4b). More breast cancer cases who have not shown an overreaction will need to be tested before we can be confident that there is a correlation between clinical and in vitro cellular hypersensitivity.

Future studies

Our immediate aim is to complete the study of the relative effectiveness of the 3 assays in detecting A-T heterozygotes and overreacting breast cancer patients. Even at this stage, however, it is apparent that complete discrimination from controls will not be achieved with any of these procedures. Nevertheless, better discrimination than we have achieved so far should be possible with modifications of these techniques. For example, preliminary results with the G_0 chromosome aberration assay suggest that the use of an even lower dose rate (0.001 Gy min^{-1}) is an improvement. A limitation of our cytogenetic assays is the time taken to analyse metaphase cells for aberrations, such that analysis is usually restricted to 100 cells. We find that, in the same time, it is possible to analyse 1000 cells for the presence or absence of micronuclei that are derived from metaphase aberrations. We are therefore converting our metaphase assays to the cytochalasin-B micronucleus technique (Fenech and

Morley, 1985) to improve quantification of radiation-induced chromosome damage.

An important question that arises in relation to these assays is whether or not reproducible results can be obtained for a given individual. We have found that this is the case for control individuals with the low dose rate survival technique (Elyan *et al.*, 1993) but it is important to establish whether this is the case for the other assays and for A-T heterozygotes and overreactors. It is important to know whether there are consistent and reproducible differences in radiosensitivity between different heterozygotes and different overreactors because if complete discrimination from controls is not possible, as seems likely, it would still be of value to identify the most radiosensitive heterozygotes and the most radiosensitive cancer patients who are to receive radiotherapy. The most radiosensitive heterozygotes would be advised to minimise their exposure to diagnostic X-rays because of the suggestion that such exposure leads to cancers in A-T gene carriers (Swift *et al.*, 1991). Reduction of radiotherapy doses could be envisaged for those cancer patients at the upper end of the cellular radiosensitivity spectrum; confirmation of whether or not these are A-T heterozygotes must await cloning of the A-T genes.

Acknowledgements

We wish to thank the following individuals for their co-operation in this study: Dr K.K. Sanford and colleagues at the National Cancer Institute, Bethesda, USA; Dr A.M.R. Taylor of the CRC Department of Cancer Studies, Birmingham, England; Mike Kirby of our Radiation Physics Department; the A-T families, breast cancer patients and controls who have given blood samples and the phlebotomists who have been involved, including Miss Lisa Burnell (Paterson Institute), Mrs Diane Averill (Institute of Cancer Research, Surrey, England) and Mrs M. Alcock (ICRF Genetic Epidemiology Laboratory, Leeds, England). This work was supported by grants from the Cancer Research Campaign and the UK Co-ordinating Committee on Cancer Research.

References

Bridges BA, Harnden DG (eds) (1982) Ataxia-telangiectasia: A cellular and molecular link between cancer, neuropathology and immune deficiency. John Wiley, Chichester.

Burnet NG, Nyman J, Turesson I, Wurm MD, Yarnold JR, Peacock JH (1992) Potential for improving tumour cure rates by predicting normal tissue tolerance to radiotherapy from *in vitro* cellular radiation sensitivity. Lancet i: 1570-1571.

Cunliffe PN, Mann JR, Cameron AH, Roberts KD, Ward HWC (1975) Radiosensitivity in ataxia telangiectasia. Br J Radiol 48: 374-376.

Elyan SAG, West CML, Roberts SA, Hunter RD (1993) Reproducible ranking of human T-lymphocyte intrinsic radiosensitivity. Submitted to Int J Radiat Biol.

Fenech M, Morley AA (1985) Solutions to the kinetic problem in the micronucleus assay. Cytobio 43: 233-246.

Gotoff SP, Amirnokri E, Liebnor EJ (1967) Ataxia-telangiectasia, neoplasia, untoward response to X-irradiation and tuberous schlerosis. Am J Dis Child 114: 617-627.

James SE, Arlett CF, Green MHL, Bridges BA (1983) Radiosensitivity of human T-lymphocytes proliferating in long term culture. Int J Radiat Biol 44: 417-422.

Norman A, Kagan AR, Chan SL (1988) The importance of genetics for the optimisation of radiation therapy. Am J Clin Oncol 11: 84-88.

Parshad R, Sanford KK, Jones GM (1985) Chromosomal radiosensitivity during the G_2 cell-cycle period of skin fibroblasts from individuals with familial cancer. Proc Natl Acad Sci USA 82: 5400-5403.

Paterson MC, MacFarlane SJ, Gentner NE, Smith BP (1985) Cellular hypersensitivity to chronic γ-radiation in cultured fibroblasts from ataxia-telangiectasia heterozygotes. In: Ataxia-telangiectasia: Genetics, neuropathology and immunology of a degenerative disease of childhood. Gatti RA, Swift M (eds) Liss New York 73-87.

Sanford KK, Parshad R (1990) Detection of cancer-prone individuals using cytogenetic response to X-rays. In: Chromosome aberrations, basic and applied aspects. Obe G, Natarajan AT (eds) Springer-Verlag 113-120.

Sanford KK, Parshad R, Green MH, Tarone RE, Tucker MA, Jones GM (1987) Hypersensitivity to G_2 chromatid damage in familial dysplastic naevus syndrome. Lancet ii: 1111-1115.

Sanford KK, Parshad R, Gantt R, Tarone RE, Jones GM, Price FM (1989) Factors affecting and signficance of G_2 chromatin radiosensitivity in predisposition to cancer. Int J Radiat Biol 55: 963-981.

Scott D, Lyons CY (1979) Homogeneous sensitivity of human peripheral blood lymphocytes to radiation-induced chromosome damage. Nature 278: 756-758.

Scott D, Spreadborough AR, Jones LA (1993) Chromosomal radiosensitivity in G_2 lymphocytes as an indicator of cancer predisposition: Experience with the National Cancer Institute technique. In preparation.

Shiloh Y, Parshad R, Frydman M, Sanford KK, Portnoi S, Ziv Y, Jones GM (1989) G_2 chromosomal radiosensitivity in families with ataxia-telangiectasia. Hum Genet 84: 15-18.

Shiloh Y, Parshad R, Sanford KK, Jones GM (1986) Carrier
    detection in ataxia-telangiectasia. Lancet i: 689-690.
Swift M, Morrell D, Cromartic E, Chamberlin AR, Skolnick MH,
    Bishop DT (1986) The incidence and gene frequency of ataxia-
    telangiectasia in the United States. Am J Hum Genet 39:
    573-583.
Swift M, Morrell D, Massey RB, Chase CL (1991) Incidence of
    cancer in 161 families affected by ataxia-telangiectasia. New
    Eng J Med 325: 1831-1836.
Taylor AMR, Harnden DG, Arlett CF, Harcourt SA, Lehman AR,
    Stevens S, Bridges BA (1975) Ataxia-telangiectasia: a human
    mutation with abnormal radiation sensitivity. Nature 258:
    427-429.
Weeks DE, Paterson MC, Lange K, Andrais B, Davis RC, Yoder F,
    Gatti RA (1991) Assessment of chronic γ-radiosensitivity as
    an *in vitro* assay for heterozygote identification in ataxia-
    telangiectasia. Radiat Res 128: 90-99.
Weincke JR, Wara DW, Little JB, Kelsey KT (1992) Heterogeneity
    in the clastogenic response to X-rays in lymphocytes from
    ataxia-telangiectasia heterozygotes and controls. Cancer
    Causes and Control 3: 237-245

Correction of Post-γ Ray DNA Repair Deficiency in Ataxia-Telangiectasia Complementation Group A Fibroblasts by Cocultivation with Normal Fibroblasts

M.C. Paterson and R. Mirzayans
Molecular Oncology Program
Department of Medicine
Cross Cancer Institute
11560 University Avenue
Edmonton, Alberta T6G 1Z2
Canada

INTRODUCTION

Ataxia-telangiectasia (A-T) is a rare human recessively-inherited disorder characterized by, among other symptoms, a devastating and sometimes fatal reaction to conventional radiotherapy (Boder, 1985; Sedgwick and Boder, 1991). Radiation intolerance *in vitro*, as manifested by impaired colony-forming ability and exessive chromosomal instability, is universally displayed by cultured dermal fibroblasts and peripheral blood lymphocytes derived from A-T donors (Lehmann, 1982; Taylor, 1982; Paterson et al., 1984). As an extension of these radiobiological studies on A-T, we have recently conducted a detailed study on the deleterious effects of 4-nitro-quinoline 1-oxide (4NQO), a partially radiomimetic carcinogen, on A-T fibroblast strains and have demonstrated that representative strains belonging to complementation groups A (AT2BE and AT3BI) and C (AT4BI) are defective in removal of a class of alkali-stable 4NQO-DNA adducts, whereas a group D strain (AT5BI) exhibits normal repair capacity (Mirzayans et al., 1989; Mirzayans and Paterson, 1991a). In this investigation, repair was monitored with the aid of 1-β-D-arabinofuranosylcytosine (araC), a potent inhibitor of DNA polymerases α and δ (Wist, 1979; Cleaver, 1984; Keeney and Linn, 1990). In this widely used approach, the extent of DNA strand breaks accumulating in cultures incubated with araC, following carcinogen treatment, becomes a measure of the efficiency to perform long-patch excision repair (Snyder et al., 1984; Cleaver, 1989; Mirzayans and Paterson, 1991b). In the present study we compared the ability of AT3BI (group A) and normal

NATO ASI Series, Vol. H 77
Ataxia-Telangiectasia
Edited by R. A. Gatti and R. B. Painter
© Springer-Verlag Berlin Heidelberg 1993

fibroblast strains to repair DNA lesions induced by ^{60}Co γ radiation. We observed that the incidence of araC-detectable DNA lesions undergoing repair during 2 h after exposure to 150 Gy was markedly reduced in the A-T cells, and that this repair deficiency could be corrected completely by cocultivation with normal fibroblasts.

MATERIALS AND METHODS

Cells and their cultivation

The fibroblast strain AT3BI, derived from the skin of a 4-year-old male patient with A-T (group A), was kindly provided by Dr. A.R. Lehmann (University of Sussex, Brighton, UK). The normal fibroblast strains GM38 (9-year-old female) and GM323 (11-year-old male) were purchased from NIGMS Human Genetic Cell Repository (Camden, NJ). The absence of *Mycoplasma* contamination was confirmed for all strains, as assayed by relative incorporation of exogenous [³H]uridine/[³H]uracil in cellular RNA (Schneider et al., 1974). Cells were cultivated at 37°C in Ham's F12 medium supplemented with 10% (v/v) fetal bovine serum, 1 mM glutamine, 100 units penicillin G/ml, and 100 µg streptomycin sulphate/ml in a humidified atmosphere of 5% CO_2 in air. All cell culture supplies were purchased from GIBCO Laboratories (Grand Island, NY).

Gamma irradiation

^{60}Co γ-irradiation was delivered under oxia (i.e., in equilibrium with air) in a Gammacell 220 unit (Atomic Energy of Canada Limited, Ottawa, Ontario) at a dose rate ranging from 60 to 65 Gy/min, as calibrated by Fricke colorimetry (Fricke and Hart, 1966).

Radioactive labelling of cellular DNA

Cellular DNA was prelabeled by incubating exponentially growing cultures for 24 h in medium containing 6.7 Ci/mmol [*methyl*-^{3}H]thymidine (New England Nuclear Canada, Lachine, PQ) at 0.5 µCi/ml.

Analysis of DNA damage and its repair by alkaline-sucrose velocity sedimentation

Prelabeled cultures were seeded in 60-mm Petri dishes at ~100,000 cells/dish and incubated at 37°C overnight. The cells were then incubated for ~15 min in the absence or in the presence of repair inhibitors (0.1 mM araC plus 2 mM hydroxyurea), irradiated (without removal of the medium) with ^{60}Co γ rays at room temperature, and re-incubated at 37°C for appropriate times. Cell monolayers were scraped into ice-cold phosphate-buffered saline (~0.2 ml/dish), and single-cell suspensions were prepared, after which a 50-µl sample of each suspension was lysed and subjected to velocity sedimentation in alkaline sucrose gradients as detailed elsewhere (Mirzayans et al., 1988; 1992). Analysis of the radioactivity distributions in the gradient profiles yielded the weight-average-molecular-weight values of DNA from which the number of DNA single-strand breaks was computed (for details, see Hiss and Preston, 1977). The amount of repair of araC-detectable sites was calculated from the difference in molecular weights of DNA from identically irradiated cultures that were incubated in the presence and in the absence of araC (Hiss and Preston, 1977; Mirzayans et al., 1988).

RESULTS

Repair of araC-detectable sites

Incubation of γ irradiated normal (GM38) and A-T (AT3BI) fibroblasts in the presence of araC resulted in the accumulation of single-strand scissions, which were measured retrospectively by alkaline-sucrose velocity sedimentation analysis (Figure 1). These araC-accumulated breaks are known to represent DNA lesions abortively operated on by the long-patch excision repair process, due to the inhibitory action of araC on

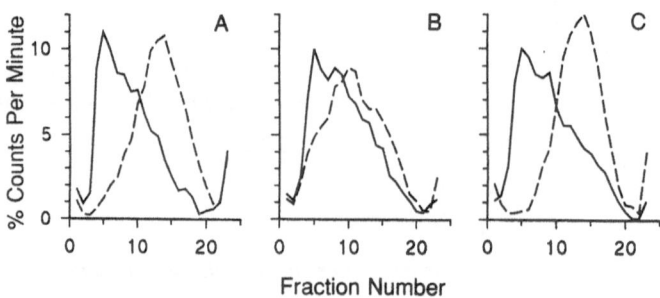

Figure 1. Alkaline sucrose sedimentation profiles of DNA from GM38 (panel *A*) and AT3BI (*B* and *C*) fibroblasts that were prelabeled with ^{3}H-thymidine, exposed to 150 Gy of ^{60}Co γ radiation, and subsequently incubated for 2 h in the absence (solid lines) or presence (dashed lines) of araC plus hydroxyurea. Experimental (prelabeled) cells were cocultivated with unlabeled GM38 (panels *A* and *C*) or AT3BI (*B*) cells.

DNA polymerases α and δ (Wist, 1979; Cleaver, 1989; Mirzayans et al., 1992); the rate of appearance of these additional breaks thus serves as an index of the DNA repair capability of each strain in response to radiation treatment.

The ability of AT3BI and the two normal strains (GM38 and GM323) to repair araC-detectable DNA lesions induced by γ rays (150 Gy) is compared in Figure 2. The results obtained from six independent experiments (over 20 determinations for AT3BI and GM38 cells) are averaged. The amount of repair in the A-T strain was ~30% of that found in the control strains. As shown in Table I, the rates of both the initial induction and the disappearance of γ ray-induced strand breaks were identical in the A-T and control strains, indicating that those araC-detectable γ radioproducts not repaired by A-T cells are alkali-stable lesions.

In all aforementioned experiments, the various strains were prelabeled with ^{3}H-dThd and plated in separate dishes. However, in some studies, ^{3}H-dThd prelabeled AT3BI cells were mixed and coplated with ^{14}C-dThd labeled GM38 cells prior to monitoring DNA repair following γ irradiation. In these latter experiments, the amount of repair of araC-detectable sites arising in the A-T cells proved to be close to that seen in the normal strain (data not shown). This unexpected observation prompted us to carry out the cocultivation experiments described below in order to test the possibility that the

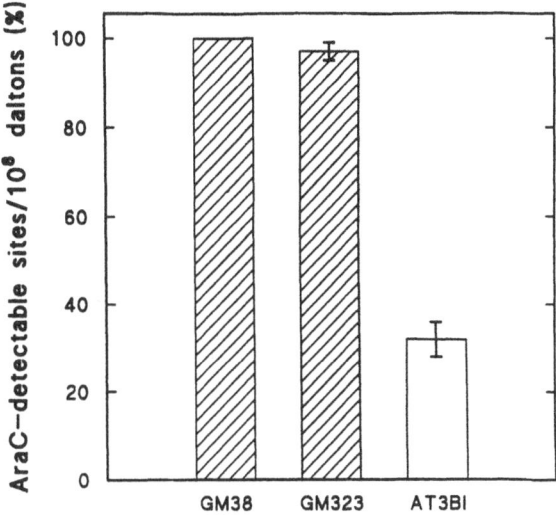

Figure 2.   Repair of araC-detectable DNA lesions in the indicated normal and A-T fibroblast strains during 2 h after exposure to 150 Gy of γ radiation. The extent of repair in each strain is expressed as a percentage of that observed in GM38 cells, which were included in all experiments as an internal control. The data represent the mean (± SE) of 4-6 independent experiments.

Table I. Induction and repair of DNA radioproducts in human fibroblasts[a]

γ ray dose (Gy)	Post-treatment incubation conditions	Strain	Strand breaks per 10^8 daltons
0	2 h with araC	GM38	0
		AT3BI	0
150	No incubation	GM38	7.1
		AT3BI	7.9
150	1 h w/o araC	GM38	0.6
		AT3BI	0.7
150	2 h w/o araC	GM38	0.1
		AT3BI	0.1
150	2 h with araC	GM38	1.8
		AT3BI	0.4

[a] Results of a typical experiment

repair deficiency in A-T may be corrected by a putative diffusible factor secreted by normal cells.

Effect of cocultivation on repair of araC-detectable sites

AT3BI cells were prelabeled with ^{3}H-dThd, mixed with unlabeled GM38 cells at a ratio of 1 A-T to 10 normals, and coplated in 60 mm dishes (2×10^{5} cells/dish). When the mixed cultures were incubated for 24 h before they were γ irradiated and araC site repair measured, the amount of repair in the A-T cells ranged from 70 to 80% of normal (as opposed to 10 to 40% repair when incubated alone or coincubated with unlabelled

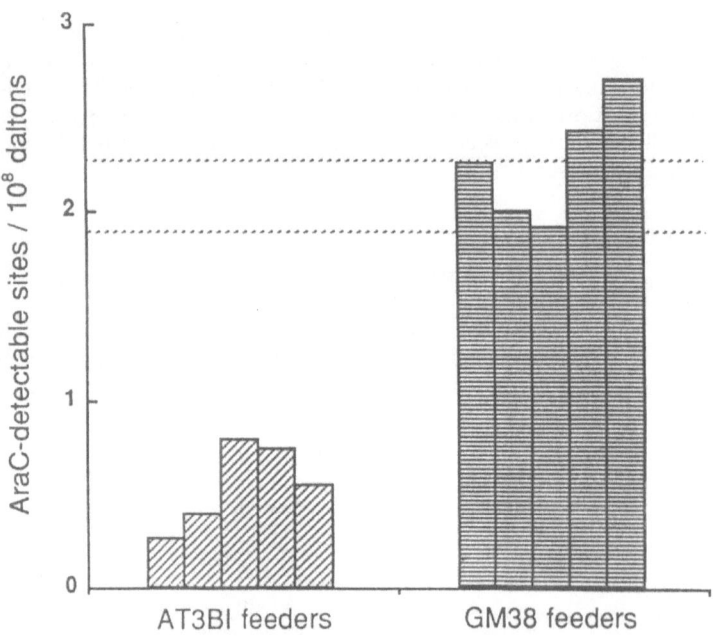

Figure 3. Repair of araC-detectable sites during 2 h of post-γ ray (150 Gy) incubation of ^{3}H-labeled AT3BI cells preincubated for 48 h in the presence of unlabeled AT3BI (left) or GM38 (right) feeder cultures. Each histogram represents an independent result. Dotted lines bracket the range of araC-detectable site repair observed in normal (GM38) cells processed in parallel.

cells of the same A-T strain) (data not shown). However, when these same cultures were incubated for a further 24 h prior to irradiation (i.e., 48 h in total), the amount of repair in the A-T cells cocultivated with GM38 cells increased to the level displayed by GM38 cells themselves (Figures 1C and 3).

DISCUSSION

We have demonstrated that AT3BI (group A) fibroblasts are defective in the repair of araC-detectable DNA lesions induced by ^{60}Co γ radiation and that this anomaly can be completely restored to normalcy by cocultivation (i.e. cell mixture) with normal fibroblasts. In addition, in a follow-up investigation to be published elsewhere, coincubation with normal cells, acting as feeders, was found to significantly decrease the susceptibility of the A-T cells to γ ray-induced inactivation and to rectify completely their failure to undergo inhibiton of DNA synthesis following γ irradiation. On the other hand, pretreatment of normal human fibroblasts with inhibitors of signal transduction pathways (H-7, W-7 and W-13) conferred radioresistant, "A-T-like" DNA synthesis (unpublished observations). We are therefore led to speculate that post γ-ray DNA metabolism (repair and replication) in normal human cells is mediated by a signal transduction pathway, a component of which is malfunctional in A-T group A cells.

Several other recent studies also implicate signal transduction pathways in the regulation of DNA metabolism in response to ionizing radiation: (i) Haimovitz-Friedman et al. (1991) have demonstrated that basic fibroblast growth factor (bFGF) serves as a potent inducer of repair of potentially lethal damage in bovine endothelial cells exposed to ^{137}Cs radiation. (ii) Primary rat embryo fibroblasts cotransfected with H-*ras* and v-*myc* oncogenes exhibit abnormally enhanced inhibition of DNA synthesis following X-irradiation (Wang and Iliakis, 1992), i.e., the antithesis of that displayed by A-T cells. The products of these genes are proposed to be key components of a transduction pathway(s) that controls DNA replication in irradiated cells (Wang and Iliakis, 1992). (iii) Nontransformed skin fibroblast strains, derived from affected members of a family with diverse malignancies and documented anomalies in recessive (p53) and dominant (c-*myc*) proto-oncogenes (Chang et al., 1987; Srivastava et al., 1990), display enhanced resistance to radiation toxicity which is associated with a novel pattern of DNA synthesis following

124

exposure to γ rays (Paterson et al., 1989). (iv) Recent observations of Kastan et al. (1992) indicate that the product of one of the genes conferring the A-T phenotype plays a role upstream in the p53-mediated signal transduction circuitry known to control the progression from G_1-to-S phase in response to radiation exposure.

The effects of various modulators of transduction pathways, including phorbol esters (protein kinase C activator; Catagna et al., 1982) and bFGF (inducer of potentially lethal damage repair; Haimovitz-Friedman et al., 1991), on cell survival and DNA synthesis in γ irradiated normal and A-T fibroblasts are currently under investigation. In addition, we are in the process of monitoring the expression of various relevant genes in these two cell types, including: (i) the PKC gene family and the cascade of genes activated by their products, e.g., c-*myc*, c-*sis*, c-*rel* and members of the *fos* and *jun* family (Varmus, 1984; Weinberg, 1985); (ii) genes encoding bFGF and its receptor; and (iii) genes whose products also play an essential role in cell division, e.g., p53, RB, TGF-b, cyclin genes (A, D, G1) and cdc2 (Cantley et al., 1991; Marshall, 1991; Xing et al., 1991). These cellular and molecular studies should enable us to identify the signal transduction pathway(s) mediating the suppression of DNA synthesis in irradiated cells and the component(s) of the pathway presumed to be defective in ataxia-telangiectasia.

REFERENCES

Boder E (1985) Ataxia-telangiectasia: An overview. *In*: RA Gatti and M Swift (eds) Ataxia-Telangiectasia: Genetics, Neuropathology and Immunology of a Degenerative Disease of Childhood. pp. 1-63, Liss, New York
Cantley LC, Auger KR, Carpenter C, Duckworth B, Graziani A, Kapeller R and Soltoff S (1991) Oncogenes and signal transduction. Cell 64:281-302
Catagna M, Takai Y, Kaibuchi K, Sano K, Kikkawa U and Nishizuka Y (1982) Direct activation of calcium-activated phospholipid dependent protein kinase by tumour promoting phorbol esters. J Biol Chem 257:7847-7851
Chang EH, Pirollo KF, Zou ZQ, Cheung H-Y, Lawler EL, Garner R, White E, Bernstein WB, Fraumeni JF Jr and Blattner WA (1987) Oncogenes in radioresistant, noncancerous skin fibroblasts from a cancer-prone family. Science 237:1036-1039
Cleaver JE (1984) Completion of excision repair patches in human cell preparations: identification of a probable mode of excision and resynthesis. Carcinogenesis 5:325-330
Cleaver JE (1989) DNA damage and repair in normal, xeroderma pigmentosum and XP revertant cells analysed by gel electrophoresis: excision of cyclobutane dimers from the whole genome is not necessary for cell survival. Carcinogenesis 10:1691-1696
Fricke H and Hart EJ (1966) Chemical dosimetry. *In*: Attix EH and Roesch EJ (eds) Radiation Dosimetry, Vol. 2, 2nd ed., pp. 167-239, Academic Press, New York

Haimovitz-Friedman A, Vlodavsky I, Chaudhuri A, White L and Fuks Z (1991) Autocrine effects of fibroblast growth factor in repair of radiation damage in endothelial cells. Cancer Res 51:2552-2558

Hiss, EA and Preston RJ (1977) The effect of cytosine arabinoside on the frequency of single-strand breaks in DNA of mammalian cells following irradiation or chemical treatment. Biochim Biophys Acta 478:1-8

Kastan MB, Zhan Q, El-Deiry WS, Carrier F, Jacks T, Walsh V, Plunkett B, Vogelstein B and Fornace AJ Jr (1992) A mammalian cell cycle checkpoint pathway utilizing p53 and ADD45 is defective in ataxia-telangiectasia. Cell 71:587-597

Keeney S and Linn S (1990) A critical review of permeabilized cell systems for studying mammalian DNA repair. Mutat Res 236:239-252

Lehmann AR (1982) The cellular and molecular responses of ataxia-telangiectasia cells to DNA damage. In: Bridges BA and Harnden DG (eds) Ataxia-Telangiectasia - A Cellular and Molecular Link Between Cancer, Neuropathology, and Immune Deficiency, pp. 83-101, Wiley, Chichester

Marshall CJ (1991) Tumor suppressor genes. Cell 64:313-326

Mirzayans R and Paterson MC (1991a) Lack of correlation between hypersensitivity to cell killing and impaired inhibition of DNA synthesis in ataxia telangiectasia fibroblasts treated with 4-nitroquinoline 1-oxide. Carcinogenesis 12:19-24

Mirzayans R and Paterson MC (1991b) Differential repair of 1-β-D-arabinofuranosyl-cytosine-detectable sites in DNA of human fibroblasts exposed to ultraviolet light and 4-nitroquinoline 1-oxide. Mutat Res 255:57-65

Mirzayans R, Waters R and Paterson MC (1988) Induction and repair of DNA strand breaks and 1-β-D-arabinofuranosylcytosine-detectable sites in 40-75 kVp X-irradiated compared to ^{60}Co γ-irradiated human cell lines. Radiat Res 114:168-185

Mirzayans R, Smith BP and Paterson MC (1989) Hypersensitivity to cell killing and faulty repair of 1-β-D-arabinofuranosylcytosine-detectable sites in ataxia-telangiectasia fibroblasts treated with 4-nitroquinoline 1-oxide. Cancer Res :5523-5529

Mirzayans R, Andrais B and Paterson MC (1992) Synergistic effect of aphidicolin and 1-β-D-arabinofuranosylcytosine on the repair of γ-ray-induced DNA damage in normal human fibroblasts. Int J Radiat Biol 62: 417-425

Paterson MC, Bech-Hansen NT, Smith PJ and Mulvihill JJ (1984) Radiogenic neoplasia, cellular radiosensitivity, and faulty DNA repair. In: Boice JD Jr and Fraumeni JF Jr. (eds) Radiation Carcinogenesis: Epidemiology and Biological Significance, pp. 319-336, New York: Raven Press

Paterson MC, Aubin RA, Fourney RM and Mirzayans R (1989) Survey of post-γ ray colony-forming ability, DNA metabolism and oncogene status in nonmalignant fibroblast strains from cancer-prone families and individual cancer patients. In: Baverstock KF and Stather JW (eds) 14th L.H. Grey Conference on Low ose Radiation Risk Assessment, pp. 227-239, Taylor & Francis, London

Schneider EL, Stanbridge EJ and Epstein CJ (1974) Incorporation of [³H]uridine and [³H]uracil into RNA: a simple technique for the detection of mycoplasma contamination of cultured cells. Exp Cell Res 84:311-318

Sedgwick RP and Boder E Ataxia-Telagiectasia (1991) In: de Jong JMBV (ed) Handbook of Clinical Neurology: Hereditary Neuropathies and Spinocellular Atrophies. Vol. 16(60), pp. 347-423, Elsevier Science Publ., Amesterdam

Snyder RD, Van Houten B and Regan JD (1984) The accumulation of DNA breaks due to incision; comparative studies with various inhibitors. In: Collins A, Downes CS and Johnson RT (eds) DNA Repair and Its Inhibition, pp. 13-43, IRL Press, Oxford, England

Srivastava S, Zou Z, Pirollo K, Blattner W and Chang EH (1990) Germ-line transmission of a mutated p53 gene in a cancer-prone family with Li-Fraumeni syndrome. Nature 348:747-749

Taylor AMR (1982) Cytogenetics of ataxia-telangiectasia. *In*: Bridges BA and Harnden DG (eds) Ataxia-Telangiectasia - A Cellular and Molecular Link Between Cancer, Neuropathology, and Immune Deficiency, pp. 53-81, Wiley, Chichester

Varmus HE (1984) The molecular genetics of cellular oncogenes. Ann Rev Genet 18: 553-612

Wang Y and Iliakis G (1992) Prolonged inhibition of DNA synthesis in cells obtained by transformation of primary rat embryo fibroblasts with oncogenes H-*ras* and v-*myc*. Cancer Res 52:508-514

Weinberg RA (1985) The action of oncogenes in the cytoplasm and nucleus. Science 230:770-776

Wist E (1979) The role of DNA polymerases α, β and γ in nuclear DNA synthesis. Biochim Biophys Acta 562:62-69

Xing Y, Connolly T, Futcher B and Beach D (1991) Human D-type cyclin. Cell 65:691-699

The A-T gene does not make a major contribution to familial breast cancer

Richard Wooster[1], Douglas F. Easton[2], Deborah Ford[2], Jonathan Mangion, Bruce A.J. Ponder[3], Julian Peto[2], and Michael R. Stratton.
Section of Molecular Carcinogenesis
Institute of Cancer Research
15 Cotswold Road
Sutton
Surrey SM2 5NG
United Kingdom

Introduction

Breast cancer is known to have a strong familial component, consistent in some families with autosomal dominant inheritance. It has been estimated that approximately 5% of breast cancers may be the result of a highly penetrant autosomal dominant gene (Claus *et al.*, 1991). Such individuals tend to develop breast cancer at an early age, have a high prevalence of bilaterality and are at an elevated risk of other neoplasms (Lynch and Hirayam, 1989). Recently the location of a gene predisposing to both breast and ovarian cancer on chromosome 17q (BRCA1) has been established by genetic linkage analysis (Hall *et al.*, 1990). In an analysis of 214 breast cancer families worldwide, the proportion of families linked to this locus was estimated to be 100% for breast-ovarian cancer families and 45% for families with multiple cases of breast cancer only (Easton *et al.*, 1993). Among breast cancer families without cases of ovarian cancer, a small minority have features of the Li-Fraumeni syndrome (sarcomas in children associated with early onset breast cancer in female relatives) and a proportion of these families are associated with germline mutations in the p53 gene on chromosome 17p (Malkin *et al.*, 1990).

Prompted by the observation that A-T homozygotes exhibit an increased risk of cancer,

[1]To whom correspondence should be addressed
[2]Section of Epidemiology, Institute of Cancer Research, 15 Cotswold Road, Sutton, Surrey, SM2 5NG, United Kingdom.
[3]CRC Human Cancer Genetics Research Group, University of Cambridge, Tennis Court Road, Cambridge, CB2 1QP, United Kingdom.

NATO ASI Series, Vol. H 77
Ataxia-Telangiectasia
Edited by R. A. Gatti and R. B. Painter
© Springer-Verlag Berlin Heidelberg 1993

prospective and retrospective epidemiological studies performed by several groups have suggested that heterozygotes for the A-T gene (or genes) also suffer an increased cancer risk (Swift *et al.*, 1976, 1987, 1991; Pippard *et al.*, 1988; Borresen *et al.*, 1990). In particular, the risk for breast cancer appears to be increased five-fold or more over that in the general population. Since A-T heterozygotes may comprise 1% or more of the general population (Swift *et al.*, 1986), this raises the possibility that A-T heterozygotes may account for a significant fraction of breast cancer incidence and of familial cases in particular. We have examined the proposition that heterozygosity for A-T may account for some familial predisposition to breast cancer by performing genetic linkage analysis in breast cancer families using markers in the vicinity of the A-T loci for complementation groups A/C and D on chromosome 11q. Previously this type of analysis has been confounded by the likelihood that several different genes contribute to breast cancer predisposition. However, the problem of genetic heterogeneity in the family set has now been diminished by excluding families with breast and ovarian cancers (most of which are linked to 17q) and families suggestive of the Li-Fraumeni syndrome. Moreover, in the remaining families the LOD scores for linkage to 11q markers have been adjusted to take account of the probability that the family is linked to BRCA1 on 17q.

Materials and Methods
Breast cancer families

Over the last decade we have investigated over 200 breast cancer families, of which sixteen have been included in this study. All these contain at least two affected sisters with breast cancer diagnosed below the age of 45, plus one other relative with breast cancer, or four cases of breast cancer diagnosed below the age of 60. Families containing individuals affected with ovarian cancer in addition to breast cancer were excluded, since the majority of such families appear to be linked to BRCA1 (Easton *et al.*, 1993). Table 1 summarises the basic details of the families that were studied. All families have previously been typed for markers on 17q in the vicinity of BRCA1 (see Linkage Analysis) and most have been examined for p53 mutations by direct sequencing and SSCP analysis (Warren *et al.*, 1992).

<u>Table 1</u> Description of families

Family	Number of breast cancers			Posterior prob. of linkage to 17q[1]	LOD scores at $\theta=0.10$[2]	
	<45*	45+*	Bilateral		D11S35	CD3D
Families inconsistent with linkage to BRCA1[3]						
7	4	7	1	0.08	-0.27	0.12
8	3	0	0	0.18	-0.12	0.00
67	3	1	0	0.11	-0.25	-0.13
78	2	1	0	0.16	0.10	0.07
85	3	4	2	0.17	-0.19	-0.13
135	3	2	2	0.18	-0.21	-0.36
136	3	3	2	0.21	-0.13	0.06
186	3	3	2	0.09	-0.11	0.07
931	3	2	0	0.16	0.00	-0.05
Families consistent with linkage to BRCA1						
17	4	1	3	0.60	-0.27	-0.20
19	2	3	2	0.79	-0.19	-0.26
22	3	1	0	0.52	0.26	0.00
82	3	1	0	0.70	0.00	-0.16
132	0	4	0	0.51	0.04	-0.02
923	2	4	1	0.63	0.00	-0.03

*Age at diagnosis. [1]From a multipoint analysis of D17S588, D17S250 and breast cancer, assuming 45% of families are linked (see Easton *et al.*, 1993). [2]Female recombination fraction. [3]At least one breast cancer case under 60 does not share a 17q haplotype in common with other affected individuals.

Marker Typing and linkage analysis

Five polymorphic microsatellite markers on 11q were typed using the PCR. The following sex-averaged genetic map for these markers has been kindly provided by M. Litt (pers. comm);

cen-D11S35-13-DRD2-12-D11S490-3-CD3D-D11S528-qter

where the distances between the markers are in centimorgans. The A-T locus responsible for families with complementation groups A and C is thought to lie between D11S35 and DRD2 whereas the locus for complementation group D is more distally located and is thought to be close to CD3D.

Two-point LOD scores for linkage of individual markers to breast cancer were computed using the LINKAGE package (Lathrop *et al.*, 1984). Breast cancer susceptibility was assumed to be conferred by an autosomal dominant allele with population frequency 0.005; this is approximately the gene frequency of A-T mutants in the general population assuming that the disease is homogeneous. (The overall prevalence of A-T has been estimated as between 1 in 40,000 and 1 in 100,000 births (Pippard *et al.*, 1988)). However, increasing the gene frequency to 0.02 (which would be a more appropriate estimate if A-T were heterogeneous) made essentially no difference to the results. Estimates of age-specific risks of breast cancer in non-gene carriers were taken from the Cancer and Steroid Hormone Study (Claus *et al.*, 1991). The risk of breast cancer in A-T gene carriers was assumed to be 8 times higher in A-T gene carriers than non-carriers at all ages, this being approximately the average of the relative risk estimates for breast cancer in A-T heterozygotes from published studies (see Appendix). This corresponds to a cumulative breast cancer risk by age 60 of 24% in gene carriers, compared with 2.7% in non-gene carriers. Analyses were also carried out assuming that the breast cancer risk in carriers was the same as given by the model of Claus *et al.*, (1991), which predicts a cumulative risk of 55% by age 60. However, assuming this higher penetrance made little difference to the results.

The female genetic map has been estimated to be 2.72 times longer than the male genetic map over this region (Foroud *et al.*, 1991), and all two-point LOD scores have been calculated on this assumption; results have been summarised according to the female recombination fraction. LOD scores were also calculated allowing for linkage to BRCA1 on chromosome 17q in a proportion of families. Details of these calculations can be obtained on request. In addition to the two-point LOD scores, a multipoint analysis involving D11S35, D11S490 and the disease was also carried out. The A-T locus was assumed to be located 13.7 cM distal to D11S35 on the female map, as suggested by the linkage analysis of Foroud *et al.*, (1991), in which the best estimate for the gene locus was 6.2cM distal to STMY on the female map. STMY, which we have not typed, is 7.5cM distal to D11S35 (M. Litt, pers comm).

To evaluate the evidence for linkage to chromosome 11q without assuming any genetic model, sharing of 11q haplotypes based on the markers D11S35, DRD2 and D11S490 between pairs of relatives both affected below age 60 was also examined. Since DRD2 was often not completely informative and D11S490 is further from the A-T locus than the other two markers, haplotype sharing was determined by the D11S35 genotypes if there was any ambiguity.

Results

Two-point LOD scores for linkage of breast cancer to 11q23 microsatellite markers are given in Table 2. These LOD scores provide no evidence for linkage of breast cancer in these families to 11q23 markers and in particular to the markers D11S35 and D11S490 which flank the major A-T locus. LOD scores after adjusting for the 17q linkage results are similar to or more negative than the unadjusted LOD scores for all markers. There was also no evidence of linkage of breast cancer to the A-T locus in the multipoint analysis involving D11S35, D11S490 and the disease. In this analysis, the multipoint LOD score at the position of the putative major A-T locus was -1.34.

Table 2 Two point LOD scores for linkage of breast cancer to markers on chromosome 11q.

		Female recombination fraction[1]					
		0.001	0.01	0.05	0.1	0.2	0.3
D11S35	Unadjusted[2]	-2.36	-2.24	-1.81	-1.40	-0.85	-0.50
	Adjusted[3]	-2.31	-2.07	-1.82	-1.57	-1.20	-0.95
DRD2	Unadjusted	-0.03	-0.01	0.06	0.09	0.06	.0.00
	Adjusted	-0.53	-0.53	-0.51	-0.52	-0.57	-0.61
D11S490	Unadjusted	-1.50	-1.39	-1.03	-0.75	-0.43	-0.25
	Adjusted	-1.34	-1.30	-1.16	-1.04	-0.89	-0.79
D11S528	Unadjusted	-0.69	-0.66	-0.54	-0.43	-0.28	-0.18
	Adjusted	-0.86	-0.85	-0.81	-0.77	-0.71	-0.68
CD3D	Unadjusted	-1.79	-1.72	-1.40	-1.09	-0.62	-0.31
	Adjusted	-1.35	-1.32	-1.19	-1.05	-0.84	-0.70

[1]Assuming female distance is 2.72 times the male distance. [2]LOD scores assuming homogeneity. [3]LOD scores adjusted for 17q linkage results (see text).

We also assessed linkage to 11q by examining the sharing of 11q haplotypes between pairs of affected relatives. Of thirty pairs of sisters both affected under the age of 60, five shared both 11q haplotypes, 19 shared one haplotype and 6 shared neither haplotype. The expected numbers given no linkage would be 7.5, 15 and 7.5 respectively. Five out of seven pairs of affected second degree relatives shared a haplotype compared with 3.5 expected, and one out of four pairs of third degree relatives shared a haplotype, compared with 1.25 expected. Overall, therefore, there was no evidence of any excess sharing of 11q haplotypes over that expected by chance.

Finally, there is no strong evidence for linkage to any marker in any individual family. The LOD scores with D11S35 and CD3D in each family at female recombination fraction 0.10 are given in Table 1. The more distal markers D11S528 and CD3D are close to the location of an A-T candidate gene responsible for complementation group D. The unadjusted and adjusted LOD scores for these markers are also negative (unadjusted LOD scores at 0=0.1 were -0.43 and -1.09 respectively; see Table 2).

Discussion

We found no evidence of breast cancer linkage in 16 families with 5 microsatellite markers spanning a 26cM region on chromosome 11q. Even after adjusting for the possibility that some families were the result of BRCA1 on chromosome 17q, the LOD scores for all markers were negative.

These results suggest that the A-T gene can be responsible for, at most, a minority of breast cancer families not due to BRCA1. Although this may appear to contradict the epidemiological observations which suggest that A-T heterozygotes suffer a greatly increased risk of breast cancer, this is not necessarily so. The families used have been selected on the basis of multiple cases and are likely to be due to a highly penetrant gene. However the relative risk of 8 for breast cancer in A-T gene carriers implies a risk of breast cancer of 24% by age 60. This contrasts with the risk of 55% previously suggested by the analysis of Claus *et al.*, (1991) based on the Cancer and Steroid Hormone Study. In principle, the breast cancer risks in some A-T heterozygotes could be much higher if the breast cancer risk were restricted to a subset of the complementation groups. Under these circumstances A-T heterozygotes could then generate the type of multiple case family used in this linkage study. The results of this study, however, argue against this possibility.

The epidemiological studies by themselves do not provide a precise estimate of the proportion of familial breast cancer due to A-T. A dominant gene with a population frequency of 0.005 causing an 8-fold increase in risk (the model for breast cancer and A-T assumed here) would result in a risk of breast cancer in the mothers and sisters of breast cancer cases only 1.2 fold increased over that in the general population (Easton and Peto, 1990). This excess familial risk is an order of magnitude lower than the observed familial risk for breast cancer which is two-fold or more (Claus *et al.*, 1991); under this model, therefore, A-T heterozygosity would account for little familial clustering of breast cancer. This conclusion is, however, critically dependent on both the breast cancer risk associated with the A-T genes and its gene frequency. At the other extreme, a 12-fold increased risk (the upper 95% confidence limit for the relative risk from epidemiological studies of A-T heterozygotes, see Appendix) and a gene frequency of 2% (a plausible estimate given heterogeneity) would 'explain' a familial relative risk of more than two-fold in first degree relatives. Under these assumptions, A-T could explain a substantial fraction of the observed familial clustering of breast cancer. Our linkage results tend to exclude these higher estimates of gene frequency and relative risk.

In conclusion, our linkage results suggest that the contribution of A-T to familial breast cancer is likely to be minor, even though A-T heterozygotes may account for a substantial proportion of breast cancer cases. Once the A-T gene(s) has been cloned, it should be possible to determine precisely the risks of breast cancer in A-T heterozygotes, and the contribution of A-T to breast cancer incidence, using population based studies.

Appendix - the relative risk of breast cancer in A-T heterozgotes

The risk of breast cancer in A-T heterozygotes has been examined in a number of studies of A-T families. Here we attempt to obtain a summary estimate of the relative risk. For this purpose, the results from four studies can be combined. The studies by Swift *et al* (1987) and Swift *et al* (1991) estimate the breast relative risks in A-T heterozygotes, compared to spouse controls, to be 6.8 (based on 27 cases in relatives in 3 in spouses) and 5.1 (based on 23 cases in relatives and 3 in spouses) respectively. Crude confidence limits for these estimates can be obtained based on the observed number of breast cancers in blood relatives and spouse controls. Thus if O_1 and O_2 are the number of cases in relatives and controls, and E_1 and E_2 are the expected numbers at national rates, and R is the estimated relative risk of breast cancer in A-T heterozygotes, then:

134

$$O_1/O_2 = (\alpha R + 1 - \alpha)E_1/E_2$$

where α is the proportion of the expected number of breast cancers in relatives E_1 which accrues to A-T carriers. α can be estimated using the above equation. Then:

$$var(R) = var(O_1/O_2)(\alpha E_1/E_2)^2$$
$$= (O_1/O_2)(1/O_1 + 1/O_2)(\alpha E_1/E_2)^2$$

and

$$var(\ln R) = (1/R^2)var(R)$$

Using these formulae, the studies of Swift *et al* (1987) and Swift *et al* (1991) give confidence limits 3.91-11.84 and 2.18-11.93 respectively for the relative risk.

The studies by Pippard *et al* (1988) and Borresen *et al* (1990) can also be included in this analysis. These found, respectively, 2 cases compared with 0.17 expected and 2 cases compared with 0.05 expected in the mothers of A-T cases (i.e. obligate carriers). The remaining studies of A-T heterozygotes do not give results separately for different types of relative, nor do they provide summary estimates of relative risk, so they cannot be combined in this analysis.

The relative risk estimates from these for studies can be combined using a standard inverse variance weighted average of the logarithm of the relative risk. This gives an estimated relative risk of 7.8, with 95% confidence limits 5.2 to 11.9. A relative risk of 8 has therefore been used in the analyses.

Acknowledgements

We would like to thank David Collier, Michael Gill and Michael Litt for providing oligonucleotides, oligonucleotide sequences and linkage maps respectively. We would also like to thank Diane Averill and the families for their help and cooperation. This work was supported by the Cancer Research Campaign.

References

Borresen A-L, Andersen TI, Treti S, Heiberg A and Moller P (1990) Breast Cancer and other Cancers in Norwegian Families with Ataxia-Telangiectasia. *Genes Chrom. Cancer* 2: 339-340

Claus EB, Risch N, Thompson WD (1991) Genetic analysis of breast cancer in the cancer and steroid hormone study. *Am J Hum Genet* 48: 232-241

Easton DF, Bishop DT, Ford D, Crockford GT and the Breast Cancer Linkage Consortium. Genetic linkage analysis in familial breast and ovarian cancer - results from 214 families. (1993) *Am. J. Hum. Genet.* in press.

Easton DF, and Peto J (1990) The contribution of inherited and predisposition to cancer incidence. *Cancer Surveys* 9: 395-416.

Foroud T, Wei S, Ziv Y, Sobel E, Lange E, Chao A, Goradia T, Huo Y, Tolun A, Chessa L, Charmley P, Sanai O, Salman N, Julier C, Concannon P, McConville C, Taylor AMR, Shiloh Y, Lange K, Gatti RA (1991) Localisation of an Ataxia-Telangiectasia locus to a 3 cM interval on chromosome 11q23: Linkage analysis of 111 families by an International Consortium. *Am J Hum Genet* 49: 1263-1279.

Hall JM, Lee MK, Newman B, Morrow J, Anderson L, Huey B and King M-C (1990) Linkage of early-onset familial breast cancer to chromosome 17q21. *Science* 250: 1684-1689.

Lathrop GM, Lalouel JM, Julier C and Ott J (1984) Strategies for multilocus linkage analysis in humans. *Proc Natl Acad Sci USA* 81: 3443-3446

Lynch HT and Hirayama T (1989) Genetic epidemiology of cancer. CRC Press Inc., Boca Raton, Florida.

Malkin D, Li FP, Strong LC, Fraumeni JF, Nelson CE, Kim DH, Kassel J, Gryka MA, Bischoff FZ, Tainsky MA, Friend SH (1990) Germ line p53 mutations in a familial syndrome of breast cancer sarcomas and other neoplasms. *Science*, 250: 1233-1238.

Morrell D, Chase CL and Swift M (1990) Cancer in 44 families with Ataxia-Telangiectasia. *Cancer Genet Cytogenet* 50: 119-123.

Pippard EC, Hall AJ, Barker JP and Bridges BA (1988) Cancer in homozygotes and heterozygotes of Ataxia-Telangiectasia and Xeroderma Pigmentosum in Britain. *Cancer Res* 48: 2929-2932.

Swift M, Sholman L, Perry M and Chase CL (1976) Malignant neoplasms in the families of patients with Ataxia-Telangiectasia. *Cancer Res* 36: 209-215.

Swift M, Morrell D, Cromartie E, Chamberlain AR, Skolnick MH and Bishop DT (1986) The incidence and gene frequency of Ataxia-Telangiectasia in the United States. *Am J Hum Genet* 39: 573-583.

Swift M, Reitnauer PJ, Morrell D and Chase CL (1987) Breast and other cancers in families with Ataxia-Telangiectasia. *New Engl J Med* 316: 1289-1294.

Swift M, Morrell D, Massey RB and Chase CL (1991) Incidence of cancer in 161 families affected by Ataxia-Telangiectasia. *New Engl J Med.* 325: 1831-1836.

Warren W, Eeles RA, Ponder BAJ, Easton DF, Averill D, Ponder MA, Anderson K, deMars R, Love R, Dundas S, Stratton MR, Trowbridge P, Cooper CS and Peto J (1992) No evidence for germline mutations in exons 5-9 of the p53 gene in 25 breast cancer families. *Oncogene* 7: 1043-1046.

Mammography Screening for A-T Heterozygotes

Amos Norman, Ph.D. and
H. Rodney Withers, M.D., D.Sc.
Department of Radiation Oncology
and Jonsson Comprehensive Cancer Center
UCLA Medical Center
Los Angeles, CA   90024-1714
U.S.A.

Swift et al (1992) have shown an increased incidence of breast cancer among A-T heterozygotes who had X-ray examinations five or more years prior to the diagnosis of the disease as compared to the incidence in the A-T heterozygotes who had not received such examinations. They assumed that the examinations were the cause for the increased incidence and suggested, therefore, that mammography screening may not be beneficial for A-T heterozygotes.   We emphatically disagree: mammography screening is particularly beneficial for A-T heterozygotes whose risk for breast cancer is higher than for the general population.

The women in Swift's study were a selected group who had received X-ray examinations for specific medical problems.   The underlying diseases and the therapies for them are likely contributors to the increased cancer incidence.   For example, several of the anesthetic gases used in surgery and many therapeutic agents used in medicine are carcinogenic.   A critical review of the radiobiology of mammography shows that singling out X rays   as the causative agent is unwarranted.

The radiation dose absorbed by each breast during a well conducted mammography screening examination is only 0.15 cGy per film or 0.30 cGy for the standard 2 film examination per breast.   Thus, even an annual examination for 35 years, from ages 40 to 75, where the benefit of mammography screening is well established, will contribute a lifetime radiation dose of 10 cGy.   This is very similar to the lifetime

NATO ASI Series, Vol. H 77
Ataxia-Telangiectasia
Edited by R. A. Gatti and R. B. Painter
© Springer-Verlag Berlin Heidelberg 1993

dose of background radiation received by women living at sea level and less than the lifetime dose received by women living at high elevations, say, in Denver, Colorado. In fact, no association has been found between natural background radiation levels and the incidence of breast cancer in the United States. And no increase in cancer rate at any site has been found in the Japanese populations which absorbed less than 10 cGy in the atomic bombing of Hiroshima and Nagasaki although the presumed elevated risk for cancer among the survivors has lasted now for over 45 years. From these and other studies it has been estimated that the risk of malignant transformation in breast duct epithelium in the total population of women from a radiation dose of 1 cGy is about 1 in 10,000 per year (NRC 1990).

For the general population, the lifetime risk for breast cancer from the annual mammography screening doses is thus about 1.5 in 100 versus the natural lifetime risk of about 1 in 9. The radiation sensitivity of cells in A-T heterozygotes is now estimated to be some 25-30% greater than for normal cells (Cole et al 1988) so that in A-T women the lifetime breast cancer risk from 10 cGy of mammography radiation is perhaps as high as 2 in 100. However, they are also at a much higher natural lifetime risk than the 1 in 9 for the general population. (The exact risk is not yet defined.)

Annual mammography screening examinations in women over 40 has been demonstrated to result in a reduction in mortality of 30% because of early detection of breast cancer. Thus, the small additional risk of inducing breast cancer is more than offset by the reduction in mortality when the cancer is detected early by annual X-ray examinations. In the more radiosensitive heterozygote A-T population, the slightly larger risk of inducing cancer does not alter this calculus significantly. Indeed, the risk-benefit ratio may be even more favorable than for the population at large: at least one study has shown that mammography screening reduces the death rate from breast cancer even more in a group of women with a naturally high incidence of the disease than in a group with a low natural incidence (Rennert 1991).

There is some controversy concerning the benefit of mammography screening for all women in the age group 40 to 50 but it is not relevant to A-T heterozygotes in whom the incidence of cancer peaks in the age group of 45 to 54 (Swift et al 1987). It is important, therefore, to begin screening in this group by age 40.

Certainly mammography is not the ideal screening procedure. Although there is a small increased cancer risk from routine mammography, other problems are of more practical importance, for example false positive and false negative diagnoses, particularly in premenopausal women. But, despite its flaws, it is the only screening method that is proven to save lives. The responsible attitude is to encourage all women to use it and to not make exceptions for A-T heterozygotes.

Acknowledgements

This investigation was supported in part by PHS grant number CA-31612 awarded by the National Cancer Institute, and a Clinical Research Professorship (Dr. Withers) from the American Cancer Society.

The authors thank Eric Hall for useful discussions and Jan Haas for typing the manuscript.

References

Cole J, Arlett CF, Green, MH et al (1988) Comparative human cellular radiosensitivity. II. The survival following gamma irradiation of unstimulated (G_0) T-lymphocytes, T-lymphocyte lines, lympho-blastoid cell lines and fibroblasts from normal donors, from ataxia-telangiectasia patients and from ataxia-telangiectasia heterozygotes. Int J Radiat Biol 54: 929-943

National Research Council (1990)   Health effects of exposure to low levels of ionizing radiation.   BEIR V. National Academy Press, Washington, DC

Rennert G (1991)   The value of mammography in different ethnic groups in Israel-analysis of mortality reduction and costs using CAN*TROL. Cancer Detection and Prevention 15: 477-481

Swift M, Morrell D, Massey, RB, Chase, CL (1992)   Incidence of cancer in 161 families affected by ataxia-telangiectasia.   NEJM 325: 1831-1836

Swift M, Reitnauer PJ, Morrell D, Chase CL (1987) Breast and other cancers in families with ataxia-telangiectasia.   NEJM 316: 1289-1294

IV. Defining the A–T Defect

Lymphoid V(D)J Recombination: Accessibility and Reaction Fidelity in Normal and Ataxia-Telangiectasia Cells

Chih-Lin Hsieh and Michael R. Lieber
Laboratory of Experimental Oncology,
Department of Pathology,
Stanford University School of Medicine, Stanford, CA 94305-5324

INTRODUCTION

The seven antigen receptor loci are targeted for V(D)J recombination at different times, at different developmental stages, and with B or T lineage specificity. The mechanisms remain undefined. The physical basis for the differential accessibility in this site-specific recombination reaction has been a matter of much speculation. Possibilities have included the processes of transcription (Ferrier et al., 1989; Martin et al., 1991; Schlissel et al., 1991) and DNA replication, and the structural features of DNA methylation and chromatin structure (Mather and Perry, 1983; Persiani and Selsing, 1989; Storb and Arp, 1983; Yancopoulos et al., 1986). The relevant order and hierarchy of these parameters in controlling accessibility of the V(D)J recombination activity are poorly understood. Although some studies have raised the possibility that transcription is a requirement for recombination, the temporal resolution of such studies has been limiting. They have not permitted determination of whether transcription and recombination are consequences of a common chromatin change or whether transcription precedes and, thereby, activates recombination.

Recent findings have intensified an interest in locus targeting of V(D)J recombination (Lieber, 1991). First, the length of the essential portions of the recombination signal sequences may not be long enough to stringently specify these sites in the genome. The heptamer can serve as a signal without the nonamer at a reduced, but significant, frequency, potentially allowing cutting at many adventitious sites. Within the heptamer, only 4 base pairs appear to be critical to initiating and completing the reaction (Hesse et al., 1989).

Second, it appears that the V(D)J recombination activity may be able to initiate nucleolytic cuts at a single signal (Lewis et al., 1988; Hendrickson et al.,

NATO ASI Series, Vol. H 77
Ataxia-Telangiectasia
Edited by R. A. Gatti and R. B. Painter
© Springer-Verlag Berlin Heidelberg 1993

1991). These cuts are then reclosed, with some base loss and addition. Hence, the sequence requirements for initiation of the reaction may lie in one rather than two signals. These findings indicate that without some form of locus targeting, V(D)J recombination may catalyze cuts and rearrangements much more frequently than one would expect to be compatible with cell viability. Here we summarize our recent investigations of the role that DNA replication, transcription, CpG methylation and DNA topology have in targeting the V(D)J recombination reaction.

V(D)J Recombination, DNA Replication, and Transcription

We have examined a series of extrachromosomal DNA substrates for V(D)J recombination under replicating and non-replicating conditions (Hsieh et al., 1991). Complete and partial replication were examined by monitoring the loss of prokaryotic-specific adenine methylation at 14 to 22 MboI/DpnI restriction sites (GATC) on the substrates. Some of these sites are within 2 bases of the signal sequence ends. We found that neither coding joint nor signal joint formation requires substrate replication.

After ruling out replication as a substrate requirement, we determined whether replication had any effect on the efficiency of V(D)J recombination. Quantitation of V(D)J recombination efficiency on non-replicating substrates requires some method of monitoring the entry of substrate molecules into the cells. We devised such a method by monitoring DNA repair of substrates into which we had substituted deoxyuridine for 10 to 20% of the thymidine nucleotides in the DNA. The substrates which enter the lymphoid cells are repaired efficiently in vivo by the eukaryotic uracil DNA repair system. Upon plasmid harvest, we distinguish repaired (entered) from unrepaired (not entered) plasmids by cleaving unrepaired molecules with uracil DNA glycoylase and E. coli endonuclease IV in vitro. This method of monitoring DNA entry does not appear to underestimate or overestimate the amount of DNA entry. Using this method, we found no significant quantitative effect of DNA replication on V(D)J recombination efficiency.

It has been shown previously by others that transcription is temporally correlated with the onset of V(D)J recombination at the endogenous antigen receptor loci (Alt et al., 1987). We have been interested in determining whether this temporal correlation indicates a causal connection between these two processes. We have compared V(D)J recombination minichromosome substrates that have transcripts running through the recombination zone with substrates that do not in a transient transfection assay (Hsieh, McCloskey and Lieber, 1992). In this system, the substrates acquire a minichromosome conformation within the first several hours after transfection. We found that the substrates recombine equally well over a 100-fold range in transcriptional variation. In additional studies, we have taken substrates that have low levels of transcription and inhibited them further by methylating the substrate DNA or by treating the cells with a general transcription inhibitor (a-amanitin). Although these treatments decreased the level of expression an additional 10- to 100-fold, there was still no observable effect on V(D)J recombination.

Based on these results, we conclude that transcription is not necessary for the V(D)J reaction mechanism and does not alter substrate structure at the DNA level or at the simplest levels of chromatin structure in a way that affects the reaction.

CpG Methylation and V(D)J Recombination

We used minichromosome substrates to study the role that CpG methylation might play in controlling V(D)J recombination site accessibility (Hsieh and Lieber, 1992). CpG methylation decreased the V(D)J recombination of these substrates more than 100-fold. The decrease correlated with a considerable increase in resistance to endonuclease digestion of the methylated minichromosome DNA. The minichromosomes acquired resistance to both the intracellular V(D)J recombinase and exogenous endonuclease only after DNA replication. Therefore, CpG methylation specifies a chromatin structure that, upon DNA replication, is resistant to eukaryotic site-specific recombination. The implications of these findings to V(D)J recombination as well as to the chromatin assembly of methylated DNA during replication are discussed below.

CpG Methylation, V(D)J Recombination and Accessible Domain Size

CpG methylation on V(D)J recombination substrates results in a striking inhibition of V(D)J recombination. This is clearly not a direct interference of the interaction of the recombination activity with the methylated DNA because no inhibition of recombination is observed in the case of non-replicating substrates. The inhibition due to methylation is only apparent for transfected plasmids that form replicating minichromosomes in the lymphoid cells. This inhibition of site-specific recombination correlates with a degree of restriction endonuclease resistance that is only apparent after substrates have replicated. We infer that replication of methylated DNA results in a chromatin structure that is resistant to lymphoid V(D)J recombination.

Using a V(D)J recombination substrate that is capable of DNA replication in human cells, we found that V(D)J recombination is inhibited more than 200-fold by CpG methylation in a human lymphoid pre-B cell line (unpublished observations). As in the case of the polyoma replicon, CpG methylation did not inhibit origin firing. Therefore, our conclusions regarding the inhibition of V(D)J recombination by CpG methylation are not restricted by species or the choice of replicon. These extents of inhibition are likely to be 10-fold underestimates because what little recombination that does occur happens on the small sub-population of demethylated molecules.

Inaccessibility occurs regardless of the exact placement of the CpG sites relative to the signals, indicating that a regional structure is important rather than a localized interference with the heptamer or nonamer recognition. We find that a CpG gap of 150 bp around one signal and a 91 bp gap around the other signal in one of our substrates (pJH229) still resulted in a 100-fold inhibition of V(D)J recombination. The inhibition does not increase for a substrate with CpG sites located within 4 bp to 8 bp of each signal. It is not clear in any system what length of DNA is critical for the formation of an inaccessible domain. Because the domain of inaccessibility does not appear to be at the length of hundreds of base pairs, one suspects that it is considerably longer.

CpG Methylation and V(D)J Recombination at the Endogenous Antigen Receptor Loci

Analysis of over 50,000 bp of sequence at the endogenous Ig and TCR V, D, and J segments in 8 vertebrate species indicates that they are CpG-rich relative to the bulk genome. In addition, where long stretches of sequence are available at the immunoglobulin loci, the CpG density also appears to be higher than the bulk genome. In a continuous 14,928 bp stretch of the human DH locus that includes twelve DH segments, the CpG density is one in 55 b (Ichihara et al., 1988). With respect to the T-cell receptor loci, analysis of TCR α, β and γ sequences in human and mouse indicate that these sequences are also richer in CpG than the bulk genome (Kabat et al., 1987). Of the Ig and TCR V, D, and J segments in these 8 vertebrate species, only the VH and V_λ genes of mouse are as CpG-deficient as bulk vertebrate DNA, and these recombine with segments that are CpG-rich.

The CpG densities of our substrates are very similar to the observed CpG richness in the endogenous loci. For the substrates, the local CpG densities (within 50 bp) are between one in 15 and one in 48 bp. The regional densities (within 1 to 3 kb) are between one in 19 and one in 37 bp. We see no diminution in the effect of CpG methylation over this range. In fact, we see the highest inhibition on the substrates with the lowest regional and local CpG densities over these ranges. We conclude that the CpG densities studied here are comparable and relevant to the densities at endogenous loci.

Model of the Order of Events Required for Locus Activation for V(D)J Recombination

Based on these functional and structural observations and the structural analyses of others on the endogenous loci, we suggest a model in which targeted demethylation leads to an endonuclease-sensitive chromatin structure that then allows for recombination to occur (Fig. 1). How might the targeted demethylation occur? It is possible that specific sites are recognized by demethylation activities at each locus. Alternatively, binding of transcription factors may target a region for demethylation.

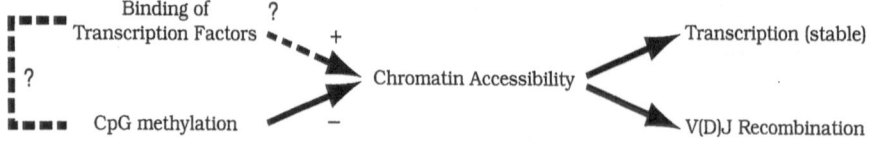

Fig 1: Proposed Order of Events in the Activation
of Antigen Receptor Loci for V(D)J Recombination

CpG Methylation and Genome Stability

Our observations that CpG methylated DNA that has undergone replication is resistant to site-specific endonucleolytic action by the V(D)J recombinase
is of intrinsic significance from a chromatin structure standpoint. If one
considers the V(D)J recombinase as a nuclease, then these studies demonstrate
that the nuclease-resistant chromatin configuration induced by methylation is
present prior to cell fractionation. The relevance of this is two-fold. First, if
methylated DNA is as resistant to recognition by other nucleases as by the V(D)J
recombinase, then CpG methylation may stabilize the genome against the
inadvertent action of the enzymes of DNA metabolism. Second, because 75% of
the CpG sites in the genome are methylated, much of the genome in lymphoid
cells is likely to be protected from rearrangements at adventitious sites that
might otherwise be catalyzed by the V(D)J recombination activity. Given the
minimal requirements for cutting by the V(D)J recombination activity, there may
be as many as 5000 adventitious cut sites for every one signal sequence at a V,
D, or J segment. The chromosomal translocations that occur in childhood
lymphoid leukemia and lymphoma are likely to represent only a fraction of what
would occur if a major portion of the genome were left unprotected. The studies
here suggest that at least a significant portion of the protection against V(D)J
recombination outside of the targeted loci is mediated by CpG methylation.

From an evolutionary standpoint it is interesting to note that, within the
animal kingdom, CpG methylation is used on a genome-wide basis only in the
vertebrates. It is possible that the combination of a longer life span and a more
complex genome made the stability against inadvertent recombination a selec-

tive advantage for retaining some minimal density of methyl-CpG. It is also interesting, in light of the observations here, that the only physiologic, site-directed recombination reaction that has been described in animal cells appears to be restricted to vertebrates, suggesting that the protection provided by methylation might have been a prerequisite for the evolutionary introduction of a site-directed endonuclease.

The V(D)J Recombination Defect in Murine Severe Combined Immune Deficiency

The severe combined immune deficiency (scid) defect in mice manifests as an absence of mature B or T cells. Bosma and colleagues (Schuler et al., 1986) found that these mice were unable to undergo normal antigen receptor gene assembly. Their hypothesis that the scid mutation affected V(D)J recombination was supported by Southern blot analysis of the endogenous loci which showed large deletions at the antigen receptor loci (Schuler et al., 1986). Analysis of the

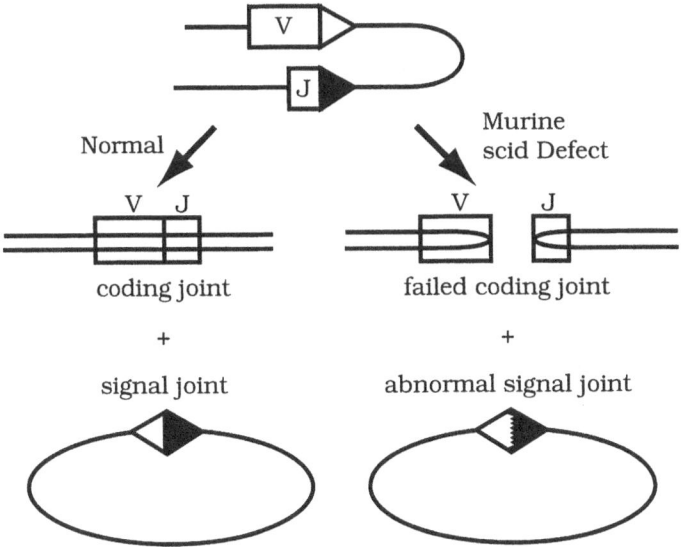

Fig. 2. The Murine Scid Defect. Coding (VJ) joint formation fails to occur despite signal (triangles) joint formation.

details of signal and coding joint formation in scid pre-B and pre-T cells revealed that coding joint formation is depressed relative to signal joint formation at least 1000-fold (Lieber et al., 1988). More recent studies have indicated that approximately one coding joint forms for every 5000 reactions (Harrington et al., 1992). This marked inefficiency in forming coding joints explains the paucity of antigen receptor gene assembly in the B and T cells of these mice (Fig. 2). It is noteworthy that, though signal joints are made, roughly half show loss of the usual precision at the signal ends.

Insofar as the two half-reactions — signal joint and coding joint formation — can be uncoupled in scid mice, it appears that signal ends are able to leave the four-ended intermediate and form signal joints independently of coding ends. Hence, it is not obligatory that signal and coding end resolution occur concurrently.

Coding ends in scid do not appear to be destroyed insofar as they can participate in alternative reactions (Lieber et al., 1988). Coding ends can resolve using long (70-base pair) stretches of homology when present. Why coding ends are unable to join with one another has been unclear but may relate to incompatible end configurations (Harrington et al., 1992). Important information on this point comes from the observation that coding ends from scid primary thymocytes can be found with a sealed (hairpin) configuration (Roth et al., 1992). This blocked configuration fits with the observation that inverted repeats are often found at sites of junctional diversity (Lieber, 1991). Such repeats strongly suggested that a hairpin coding end is a normal intermediate in V(D)J recombination (Lieber, 1992). The Roth et al. (1992) study provides strong physical support for such a model of V(D)J recombination and provides a firm understanding of why the coding ends are failing to join.

As stated above, at a low level, approximately one event in every several thousand, coding ends can join to one another with any of a range of deletion sizes (Malynn et al., 1988; Kim et al., 1988; Okazaki et al., 1988; Hendrickson et al., 1990; Harrington et al., 1992). The short deletions are similar to conventional coding end joints (Hendrickson et al., 1990). Whether these coding end joints are representative of V(D)J recombined coding joints or whether they represent illegitimate recombination is unclear. Regardless of their mechanistic pathway, these coding end joinings may explain part of the leakiness of the scid phenotype; that is, some of the chance normal recombinations of coding ends may give rise to functional antigen receptor chains. The leaky phenotype may be due to more than one process, however. There are other data that suggest that the scid phenotype can revert to normal at some low frequency in rare lymphoid progenitors sometime during the life of each scid mouse (Petrini et al., 1990; Schuler, 1990). These appear to give rise to a few B and T cell clones bearing normal antigen receptors. These revertants may explain most of the leaky phenotype.

The scid mouse has become even more interesting because it may provide a bridge between site-specific and general recombination/repair systems in eukaryotes. Ionizing radiation-induced (Fulop and Phillips, 1990) and drug-induced double-strand breaks are not repaired as efficiently in scid mice or in scid fibroblasts when compared to normal. The ionizing radiation-induced double-strand breaks are repaired at one-half to one-third the normal rate (Biedermann et al., 1991). Gamma radiation-induced single-strand breaks are repaired at the normal rate. The common feature of the V(D)J recombination reaction and the repair of double-stranded breaks is that both involve two free non-specific ends. The scid locus product(s) may be involved in modification, alignment, or ligation of free DNA ends. In the case of the V(D)J recombination reaction, the coding ends may at some point be handled by a factor which also participates in the repair of double-stranded breaks.

V(D)J Recombination in Ataxia-Telangiectasia

Only recently have we been able to analyze V(D)J recombination in human cells (Gauss and Lieber, unpublished). We have begun an analysis of V(D)J recombination in a variety of human immunodeficiency states. It is important to study V(D)J recombination in ataxia-telangiectasia (AT) patients because 80% of malignancies in AT patients are lymphoid malignancies. Possibly one of the site-directed enzymes of the immune system (Peterson and Funkhouser, 1990) contributes to an increased genetic instability, which might explain the predominance of lymphoid malignancy. We are still in the process of examining the fidelity of V(D)J recombination in cells from AT patients. We examined one Group D AT fibroblast cell line for V(D)J recombination by activating its recombination system. We then analyzed the V(D)J recombination reaction by using substrates with which we transfected the cells. Thus far, we have not seen abnormalities in the signal and coding joint formation in this cell line. In additional analyses, we will determine whether accessibility to the V(D)J recombinase is abnormal. We will also determine whether either of the other two site-directed enzyme systems of the immune system—class switch recombination and somatic mutation—is abnormal.

REFERENCES

Alt, F. W., Blackwell, T. K., and Yancopoulos, G. D. (1987). Development of the primary antibody repertoire. Science 238:1079-1087.
Biedermann, K., Sun, J., Giaccia, A., Tosto, L. and Brown, J.M. (1991) The scid mutation in mice confers hypersensitivity to ionizing radiation and a deficiency in DNA double strand break repair. Proc. Natl. Acad. Sci. 88:1394-1397.
Ferrier, P., Covey, L. R., Suh, H., Winoto, A., Hood, L., and Alt, F. W. (1991). T cell receptor DJ but not VDJ rearrangement within a recombination substrate introduced into a pre-B cell line. Int. Immunol. 1:66-74.
Fulop, G.M., and Phillips, R.A. (1990) The scid mutation in mice causes a general defect in DNA repair. Nature 347:479-482.
Harrington, J., Hsieh, C.L., Gerton, J., Bosma, G., Lieber, M. (1992). Analysis of the Defect in DNA End Joining in the Murine scid Mutation. Mol. Cell. Biol. 12:4758-4768.
Hendrickson, E. A., Liu, V. F., and Weaver, D. T. (1991). Strand breaks without DNA rearrangement in V(D)J recombination. Mol. Cell. Biol. 11:3155-3162.
Hendrickson, E.A., Schlissel, M.S., and Weaver, D.T. (1990) Wild-type V(D)J recombination in scid pre-B cells. Mol. Cell. Biol. 10:5397-5407.
Hesse, J. E., Lieber, M. R., Mizuuchi, K., and Gellert, M. (1987). Extrachromosomal DNA substrates in pre-B cells undergo inversion or deletion at immunoglobulin V-(D)-J joining signals. Cell 49:775-783.
Hesse, J. E., Lieber, M. R., Mizuuchi, K., and Gellert, M. (1989). V(D)J recombination: a functional definition of the joining signals. Genes Dev. 3:1053-1061.
Hsieh, C.-L., McCloskey, R. P., Radany, E., and Lieber, M. R. (1991). V(D)J recombination: evidence that a replicative mechanism is not required. Mol. Cell. Biol. 11:3972-3977.
Hsieh, C.-L. and Lieber, M.R. (1992). CpG methylated minichromosomes become inaccessible for V(D)J recombination after undergoing replication. EMBO J. 11:31 5-325.
Hsieh, C.-L., McCloskey, R. P., and Lieber, M. R. (1992). V(D)J recombination is not affected by transcription. J. Biol. Chem. 267 (in press).
Ichihara, Y., Matsuoka, H., and Kurosawa, Y. (1988). Organization of human immunoglobulin heavy chain diversity gene loci. EMBO J. 7:4141-4150.
Kabat, E., Wu, T., Reid-Miller, M., Perry, H., and Gottesman, K. (1987) Sequences of Proteins of Immunological Interest, 4th Ed., U.S. Dept. HHS,

Washington, D.C.

Kim, M.-G., Schuler, W., Bosma, M.J., and Marcu, K.B. (1988) Abnormal recombination of IgH D and J gene segments in transformed pre-B cells of scid mice. J. Immunol. 141:1341-1347.

Lewis, S. M., Hesse, J. E., Mizuuchi, K., and Gellert, M. (1988). Novel strand exchanges in V(D)J recombination. Cell 55:1099-1107.

Lieber, M. R., Hesse, J. E. Mizuuchi, K., and Gellert, M. (1987). Developmental stage specificity of the lymphoid V(D)J recombination activity. Genes Dev. 1:751-761.

Lieber, M.R. (1991) Site-specific recombination in the immune system. FASEB J. 5 (14): 2934-2944.

Lieber, M. R. (1992). The Mechanism of V(D)J Recombination: A Balance of Diversity, Specificity and Stability. Cell 70:873-876.

Malynn, B., Blackwell, T.K., Fulop, G., Rathbun, G., Furley, A., Ferrier, P., Heinke, L.B., Phillips, R., Yancopoulos, G., and Alt, F. (1988) The scid defect affects the final step of the immunoglobulin VDJ recombinase mechanism. Cell 54:453-460.

Martin, D., Huang, R., LeBien, T., and Van Ness R. (1991). Induced rearrangement of k genes in the BLIN-1 human pre-B cell line correlates with germline J-Ck and Vk transcription. J. Exp. Med. 173:639-645.

Mather, E. L., and Perry, R. P. (1983). Methylation status and DNaseI sensitivity of immunoglobulin genes: changes associated with rearrangement. Proc. Natl. Acad. Sci. USA 80:4689-4693.

Okazaki, K., Nishikawa, S., and Sakano, H. (1988) Aberrant immunoglobulin gene rearrangement in scid mouse bone marrow cells. J. Immunol. 141:1348-1352.

Persiani, D. M ., and Selsing, E . (1 989) . DNaseI sensitivity of immunoglobulin light chain genes in Abelson murine leukemia virus transformed pre-B cell lines. Nucl. Acids Res. 17:5339-5348.

Peterson, R. D., and Funkhouser, J.D. (1990). Ataxiatelangiectasia: an important clue. New Engl. J. Med. 322:124-5.

Petrini, J., Carroll, A., Bosma, M. (1990) T-cell receptor gene rearrangements in functional T-cell clones from scid mice: reversion of the scid phenotype in individual lymphocyte progenitors. Proc. Natl. Acad. Sci. 87:3450-3452.

Roth, D. B., J. P. Menetski, P. B. Nakajima, M. J. Bosma, and M. Gellert. 1992. V(D)J recombination: broken DNA molecules with covalently sealed (hairpin) coding ends in scid mouse thymocytes. Cell 70:983-991

Schlissel, M. S., Corcoran, L. M., and Baltimore, D. (1991) Virus-transformed pre-B cells show ordered activation but not inactivation of immunoglobulin gene rearrangement and transcription. J. Exp. Med. 173:711-720.

Schuler, W., Wieler, I., Schuler, A., Phillips, R., Rosenberg, N., Mak, T., Kearny, J., Perry, R ., and Bosma, M. (1986) Rearrangement of antigen receptor genes is defective in mice with severe combined immune deficiency. Cell 46:963-972.

Schuler, W. (1990) The scid mouse mutant: biology and nature of the defect. In Molecular Basis of B Cell Developments. Cytokines, Vol. 3, C. Sorg, ed. (Basel: S. Karger), pp. 132-173 .

Storb, U . and Arp, B. (1983) Methylation patterns of immunoglobulin genes in lymphoid cells: correlation of expression and differentiation with undermethylation. Proc. Natl. Acad. Sci. USA 80:6642-6646.

Yancopoulos, G. D., Blackwell, T. K., Suh, H., Hood, L., and Alt, F. W. (1986). Introduced T cell receptor variable region gene segments recombine in pre-B cells: evidence that B and T cells use a common recombinase. Cell 44:251-259 .

Murine scid cells and human ataxia-telangiectasia cells
complement each other's radiosensitivity.

Kenshi Komatsu
Radiation Biophysics
Atomic Disease Institute
Nagasaki University School of Medicine
Sakamoto-machi, Nagasaki 852, JAPAN.

Introduction

Mice homozygous for the SCID mutation are characterized by
a severe deficiency in both B and T cell immunity. The absence
of B and T lymphocytes results from a failure of V(D)J
recombination activity that normally mediates somatic assembly
of both the immunoglobulin and T-cell receptor gene elements.
Investigation of SCID V(D)J recombination has shown that the
immune gene elements are not correctly rejoined during
rearrangement, because of an aberrant V(D)J recombinase(Lieber
1992). Myeloid cells and fibroblasts from SCID mice also show
a marked increase in radiation sensitivity as measured by cell
killing. Biedermann et al.(1991) and Hendrickson et al.(1991)
have recently demonstrated that this hypersensitivity to ionizing
radiation is due to a defect in rejoining of radiation-induced
DNA double strand breaks. Hence, the site-specific V(D)J DNA
recombination process has been linked to the repair of randomly-
induced double-strand breaks.

An association of immune rearrangement activity with
hypersensitivity to ionizing radiation is also suggested in A-T.
A-T patients show a immunodeficiency of both immune compartments.
Defects in rearrangement of immunoglobulin and T-cell receptor
genes are suggested by studies that show increased frequencies
of interlocus recombination between TCR-γ(V)regions and TCR-
β(J)regions as well as translocations in loci containing the

NATO ASI Series, Vol. H 77
Ataxia-Telangiectasia
Edited by R. A. Gatti and R. B. Painter
© Springer-Verlag Berlin Heidelberg 1993

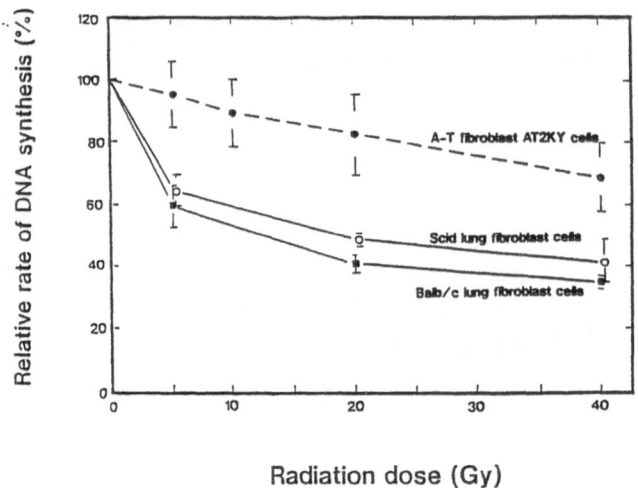

Figure 1. Dose–response curves for inhibition of DNA synthesis
by X–rays

immune genes on chromosomes 7 and 14. Since illegitimate V(D)J
recombination is one of the candidate functions for the basic
defect in A–T(Gatti 1991), comparative studies of murine SCID
mutatnts and A–T were performed.

Post-irradiation DNA synthesis

Hyperradiosensitvitiy as measured by cell lethality and
radioresistant DNA synthesis are two hallmarks of A–T, and both
phenotypes are thought to be strongly associated with the primary
molecular defect in A–T cells(Painter and Young 1980). Primary
cultures of lung fibroblasts from SCID mice(C.P-17/Icr-SCID Jcl)
and SV40 virus-transformed SCID cells(SC3VA2) were used in these
experiments. Figure 1 shows DNA synthesis in AT2KY, SCID and
Balb/c cells. Although A–T cells(AT2KY) maintained a high level
of   DNA   synthesis   throughout   the   range   of   doses
tested(radioresistant DNA synthesis), the SCID cells after
irradiation showed a bi-phasic decrease in DNA synthesis; a steep

decrease, initially followed by a more gradual decline in DNA synthesis at higher doses(Komatsu et al. 1989). This pattern is similar to that of normal Balb/c fibroblast cell DNA synthesis following graded doses of X rays. Transformed SCID cells also showed similar kinetics of DNA synthesis as freshly explanted SCID cells. Thus, SCID cells resembled A-T cells in radiosensitivity but not in DNA synthetic characteristics after irradiation. Our results suggest that the basic defect of the SCID mutation is different from that of the A-T mutation.

Complementation assay by somatic cell fusion

Although radioresistant DNA synthesis is an A-T specific phenotype, this phenotype can be modified under some conditions, such as in (A-T x normal cells) hybrid clones(Komatsu et al. 1989), or in an A-T cell line transfected with a normal gene. In these studies, cell radiosensitivity as measured by survival was restored to levels consistent with normal cells while DNA synthesis behaved like that in A-T. Therefore, we cannot exclude the possibility that the mechanism of hyperradiosensitivity seen in both A-T and SCID cells may have a common basis regardless of their differences in post-irradiation DNA replication. To confirm that different mutations are responsible for SCID and A-T, a cell complementation assay was performed by using somatic cell fusion techniques. AT5BIVA cells, tagged with pSV2neo, were fused with SC3VA2 cells by treatment with polyethylene glycol 1000 and the resulting (A-T X SCID) hybrids were isolated in selection medium containing G418 and ouabain. All hybrid clones obtained from SCID and A-T cell fusions exhibited restoration of radiosensitivity to normal levels as measured by survival. Similarly, Nijmegen Breakage Syndrome(NBS) cells, an A-T variant, were fused with SC3VA2 cells and this same type of complementation was again observed. Thus, the complementation assay indicates that the basic defect of SCID mutations is different from that of A-T and NBS as well. This result substantiates the evidence of post-irradiation DNA synthesis described above.

Mapping of a putative A-T gene by a chromosome transfer technique

In order to identify the human chromosome which carries a mutated gene in cells from a patient with A-T, we performed chromosome transfer experiments via microcell fusion(Komatsu et al. 1990). Monochromosomal hybrid clones of A9 cells, containing a single normal human chromosome 11 or chromosome 12 tagged with the pSV2neo plasmid DNA, were used as donors. After enucleation by cytochalasin B, microcells were collected from donor cells and were fused with AT5BIVA cells(complementation group D) by treatment with polyethylene glycol 1000. Resulting microcell hybrid clones were isolated in medium containing G418. Cytogenetic analysis demonstrated that the microcell hybrid clones obtained by the introduction of a normal chromosome 11 had increased copy numbers of chromsome 11. The hybrid clones in which a chromosome 11 was successfully transfered showed a restoration to wild-type levels of cells death from X-irradiation, whereas all hybrid clones into which a chromosome 12 was introduced(control experiments) remained hyperradiosensitive, like the parental A-T cells. These results indicate that a defective gene in AT-D cells is located on chromosome 11. This is consistent with the results of genetic linkage analysis which has suggested that the defective genes from complementation groups A and C are located on this chromosome.

Mapping of a SCID gene, a human gene homologous to the murine SCID gene

Mapping of the putative SCID gene on a human chromosome region was attempted using the SCID mouse cell line and mouse cell lines to make a hybrid containing a single human chromosome 8; these complemented the hyperradiosensitvity of the SCID mutation (Komatsu et al. 1993). Several radioresistant clones were obtained from somatic cell hybrids between lethally irradiated chomosome 8 donor cells and SC3VA2TG2 recipient cells. Although most of the human chromosome 8 was lost, these new clones contained human chromosomal fragments in a background of mouse chromosomes. Fluorescence in situ hybridization(FISH) using total human DNA as a probe showed that one of these radiation hybrid clones retained a single human DNA fragment. To identify the human DNA fragments retained in the hybrid clones, this human DNA in a hybrid clone was amplified by Alu-PCR with a TC-65 primer. Using these biotinylated Alu-PCR products as probes, chromosomal in situ suppression(CISS) hybridization were utilized for chromosome painting on normal human lymphocyte metaphase cells. These results demonstrated that the SCID gene, a human gene complementing the murine SCID mutation, is localized in a pericentromeric region of human chromosome 8. The XRCC 2 and XRCC 4 genes with defects in the rejoining of double strand breaks have been mapped to human chromosomes 7 and 5, respectively. Ataxia-telangiectasia which is both hyperradiosensitive and immunodeficient was assigned to chromosome 11, as described above(Komatsu et al. 1990). RAG 1 and 2, the controlling genes for V(D)J recombination, and the human ADA-SCID gene are known to be localized on human chromosome 11p and 20q12-13.11, respectively. Therefore, the murine SCID gene does not seem to be the same as any genes already reported and must be different from that of A-T.

Conclusion

Our results indicate that the primary molecular defect of SCID cells is different from that of A-T cells, as exhibited by the evidence of complementation between both mutants and by a different patterns of post-irradiation DNA synthesis. These results were consistent with the studies on the assignment of both mutated genes, i.e., A-T and <u>SCID</u> genes were mapped to human chromsome 11 and 8, respectively. At the molecular level, studies support our results concerning the different mechanisms between the SCID and A-T mutations. V(D)J recombination is a multiple processing event including formation of a hairpin structure at the coding end of the immune gene element. The target of the SCID mutation is presumably an inability to bring two hairpins together during the rearrangement and it gives rise to unrejoined coding sequences(Lieber 1992). Recently, Lipkowitz et al.(1990) demonstrated that A-T cells are catalytically normal in rejoining of V-J hybrid genes between TCR-γ(V)regions and TCR-β (J) regions but the occurrence of this abnormal interlocus recombination is 70-fold higher than in normal individuals. This coincides with cytogenetic studies that show increased frequencies of chromosome 7 inversions in the lymphocytes of A-T patients. The high frequencies of interlocus recombination in A-T cells might be related to the radioresistant DNA synthesis, although the mechanism remains unclear. Thus, A-T cells show a defect in some process of immune rearragement but the target is different from that of the murine SCID gene. Further study of murine SCID in relation to A-T should provide insights into the mechanism involved in the multiple phenotypes expressed in A-T, as well as in immune rearrangements.

References

Biedermann, K. A., Sun, J., Giaccia, A. J., Tosto, L. M., and Brown, J. M.(1991) Scid mutation in mice confers hypersensitivity to ionizing radiation and a deficiency in DNA double-strand break repair. Proc. Natl. Acad. Sci. USA, 88:1394-1397.

Gatti, R. A.(1991) Speculations on the ataxia-telangiectasia defect. Clin. Immunol. Immunopathol., 61:S10-S15.

Hendrickson, E. A., Quin, X. Q., Bump, E. A., Schats, D. G., Oettinger,M., and Weaber, D. T.(1991) a link between double-strand break-related repair and V(D)J recombination: The scid mutation. Proc. Natl. Acad. Sci. USA, 88:4061-4065.

Lieber, M. R.(1992) The mechanism of V(D)J recombination: A balance of diversity, specificity, and stability, Cell, 79:873-876.

Lipkowitz, S., Stern, M. H., and Kirsch, I. R.(1990) Hybrid t cell receptor genes formed by interlocus recombination in normal and ataxia-telangiectasia lymphocytes. J. Expl. Medicine, 172:409-418.

Komatsu, K., Okumura, Y., Kodama, S., Yoshida, M., and Miller, R. C.(1989) Lack of correlation between radiosensitivity and inhibition of DNA synthesis in hybrids(A-T x HeLa). Int. J. Radiat. Biol., 56:863-867.

Komatsu, K., Kodama, S., Okumura, Y., Koi, M. and Oshimura, M.(1990) Restoration of radiation resistance in ataxia telangiectasia cells by the introduction of normal human chromosome 11. Mutation Res., 235:59-63.

Komatsu, K., Yoshida, M. and Okumura, Y.(1993) Murine scid cells complement ataxia telangiectasia cells and show a normal post-irradiation response of DNA synthesis. Int. J. Radiat. Biol., In Press.

Komatsu, K., Ohta, T., Jinno, Y., Niikawa, N. and Okumura, Y.(1993) Functional complementation in mouse-human radiation hybrids assigns the putative murine scid gene to human chromosome 8. Submitted to Human Molecular Genetics.

Painter, R. B., and Young, B. R.(1980) Radiosensitivity in ataxia-telangiectasia: a new explanation. Proc. Natl. Acad. Sci. USA., 77:7315-7317.

ATAXIA-TELANGIECTASIA: DEFECTIVE IN A P53-DEPENDENT SIGNAL TRANSDUCTION PATHWAY

Michael B. Kastan
Department of Oncology
Johns Hopkins University School of Medicine
600 N. Wolfe St.
Baltimore, Md. 21287
USA

Damage to DNA in proliferating cells results in alterations of progression through the cell cycle (e.g. Tolmach et al, 1977; Painter and Young, 1980; Lau and Pardee, 1982; Weinert and Hartwell, 1988; Kaufmann et al, 1991; O'Connor et al, 1992). Such cell cycle "checkpoints" appear to be active cellular responses which permit optimal repair of DNA damage so that the cell will not replicate a damaged DNA template (G_1 arrest) nor segregate damaged chromosomes (G_2 arrest). Defects in these checkpoints are thought to contribute to decreased cell survival and increased propagatable genetic abnormalities following DNA damage (Hartwell and Weinert, 1989). One consequence of failing to repair DNA damage prior to replicative DNA synthesis is that mutagenic lesions could be fixed and propagated and could thus contribute to the genomic changes which result in neoplastic transformation. Abnormalities in the RAD9 gene in yeast result in a defect in the G_2 arrest following ionizing irradiation - such mutant yeast exhibit increased sensitivity and increased genetic abnormalities following exposure to ionizing radiation (Weinert and Hartwell, 1988; Hartwell and Weinert, 1989). However, little has been clarified about the molecular and genetic controls of these checkpoints in mammalian cells.

We recently began to investigate some of the molecular mechanisms which control cell cycle progression following DNA damage in mammalian cells. In agreement with observations from many other laboratories, we found that ionizing

NATO ASI Series, Vol. H 77
Ataxia-Telangiectasia
Edited by R. A. Gatti and R. B. Painter
© Springer-Verlag Berlin Heidelberg 1993

radiation (IR) can block cells at both G_1 and G_2 checkpoints. In addition, we observed that levels of the "tumor suppressor" nuclear protein, p53, increase in temporal association with the decrease in replicative DNA synthesis (Kastan et al., 1991). Levels of p53 mRNA did not change following IR and increases in p53 protein occurred despite the use of actinomycin D (at transcription-inhibiting doses) as the damaging agent; these observations demonstrated that the increase in p53 protein following irradiation was due to post-transcriptional changes. This made teleologic sense - transcription utilizing a damaged DNA template would be almost as undesirable as replication using a damaged template. Since p53 is the most commonly mutated gene in human malignancies (Vogelstein, 1990; Hollstein et al., 1991) and since environmental DNA damaging agents have been implicated in the development of up to 80% of human cancers (Doll and Peto, 1982), linking p53 function to the cellular response to DNA damage had significant implications in terms of understanding mechanisms of human carcinogenesis.

A functional role for the p53 gene product in the cellular response to certain types of DNA damage was strongly suggested by the observation that cells with wild-type p53 genes arrested in G_1 following IR, while cells with abnormal p53 genes lacked this checkpoint (Kastan et al., 1991; Kuerbitz et al., 1992). Since all cells evaluated, irrespective of p53 status, retained the G_2 arrest checkpoint, it appeared that p53 protein was involved in the G_1, but not in the G_2, arrest following ionizing radiation. A cause and effect relationship between p53 function and the arrest in G_1 following IR was then established by demonstrating: 1) acquisition of the G_1 arrest after ionizing radiation following transfection of wild-type p53 genes into cells lacking endogenous p53 genes (Kuerbitz et al., 1992); 2) loss of the G_1 arrest after irradiation following transfection of mutant p53 genes into cells with wild-type endogenous p53 genes (Kuerbitz et al., 1992); and 3) loss of the G_1 arrest in normal cells obtained from mice in which both p53 alleles were disrupted by homologous recombination (Kastan et al., 1992).

Exposure of cells to caffeine potentiates the cytotoxicity of DNA damaging agents (Tolmach et al, 1977). The mechanism of this potentiation appears to be at least partially due to inhibition of the cell cycle arrests (Walters et al, 1974; Lau and Pardee, 1982). We observed that both the G_1 and G_2 arrests following ionizing irradiation were abrogated by the presence of caffeine and that the increase in p53 protein levels were also blocked (Kastan et al., 1991). Inhibition of protein synthesis by cycloheximide treatment blocked the G_1, but not the G_2, arrest and also abrogated the increase in p53 protein levels following IR. These results with caffeine and cycloheximide demonstrated that the G_1 arrest after IR is an active physiologic response to the DNA damage and does not result simply from a structural blockage of DNA synthesis. Thus, it appears that the cell "senses" abnormalities in the DNA, initiates a signal transduction pathway which results in a post-transcriptional increase in the levels of p53 protein, which subsequently causes cells to arrest in the G_1 phase of the cell cycle. The arrest in G_2 may result from the same signal in the DNA, but is independent of p53 function.

Characterization of the molecular mechanisms of the induction of p53 protein and the mechanism by which this induction causes the G_1 arrest following IR are intense areas of investigation at this time. The inhibition of the p53 induction by caffeine provides one insight into these mechanisms - perhaps a cyclic nucleotide-dependent process is required for p53 induction following IR. Poly(ADP-ribose) synthesis following strand breaks has been implicated as a critical participant in the DNA repair process (e.g. Satoh and Lindahl, 1992). However, prior reports suggested that 3-aminobenzamide, an inhibitor of poly(ADP-ribos)ylation, does not affect the radiation-induced inhibition of DNA synthesis in human cells (James and Lehmann, 1982; Painter, 1985). In agreement with this observation, we observed no alterations in cell cycle checkpoints or in p53 induction following IR when cells were treated with 3-aminobenzamide (Kastan and Plunkett, unpublished observations).

Ataxia-telangiectasia (A-T) is a human autosomal recessive disorder with many phenotypic characteristics, including: 1) hypersensitivity to ionizing radiation; 2) "radioresistant" DNA synthesis; and 3) a markedly increased incidence of cancer (for reviews, see McKinnon, 1987 and Gatti et al, 1991). Painter and Young (1980) were the first to report an abnormality in the ability of A-T cells to cease replicative DNA synthesis following ionizing radiation. Several other laboratories reproduced this observation - interestingly, the cell cycle checkpoint defect in A-T cells (Rudolph and Latt, 1989) was virtually identical to the abnormality we were observing in cells with defective p53 function (Kastan et al, 1991; Kuerbitz et al, 1992) (see Figure 1). Therefore, a link between the defect in A-T and the signal

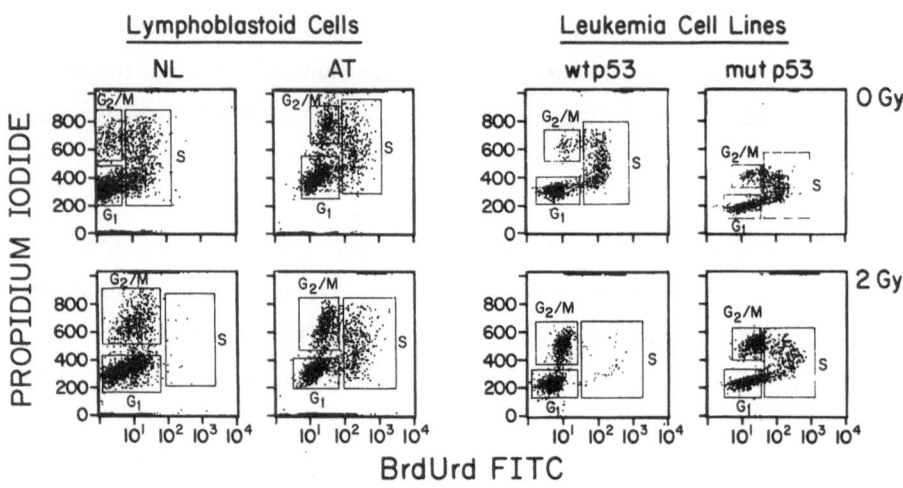

Figure 1. Cell cycle status of cells following ionizing radiation as a function of the status of p53 and A-T genes. Cells were pulsed for 4 hours with bromodeoxyuridine 17 hours (lymphoblastoid cells) or 24 hours (leukemia cells lines) after exposure to 0 Gy (upper row) or 2 Gy (lower row) ionizing radiation. Following harvest, staining with fluorescein-conjugated anti-BrdUrd antibodies and counterstaining with propidium iodide, the cells were analyzed by flow cytometry - all procedures were done as previously described (Kastan et al, 1991, 1992 and Kuerbitz et al., 1992). Lymphoblastoid cells from normal (NL; 2184 cells) and A-T patients (BMA cells; complementation group C) are shown in the left pair of panels and leukemia cells with wild-type (WT; ML-1 cells) and mutant (MUT; Raji cells) p53 are shown in the right pair of panels. (Refer to Kastan et al., 1991 and 1992 for prior characterizations of these cell lines.) Cell populations representing the G_1, S and G_2/M phases of the cells cycle are depicted in the boxes in each panel. This figure demonstrates the phenotypic similarity resulting from mutations in the p53 gene and in an A-T gene - normal cells and leukemia cells with wild-type p53 genes cease entering S-phase following IR, while A-T cells and cells with mutant p53 genes continue to enter S-phase despite the DNA damage.

transduction pathway which utilizes p53 in causing the G_1 arrest following IR was investigated. We reasoned that if this A-T phenotypic characteristic were due to a defect proximal to p53 in this response pathway, A-T cells would lack the induction of p53 protein that is seen in normal cells following irradiation.

Therefore, the ability of a number of cell lines from A-T patients to increase p53 protein levels following IR was evaluated. Assessments of p53 protein levels by immunoprecipitation, immunoblot, and flow cytometry all clearly demonstrated a lack of induction of p53 protein levels in cells from A-T patients (Kastan et al., 1992). This defect was noted in both EBV-immortalized lymphocytes and in normal diploid fibroblasts from A-T patients. Though the complementation groups of some of the A-T cell lines utilized in these studies was not known, cell lines from patients which had been previously characterized as group A and group C were tested and were defective in the induction of p53 protein following IR. There was a suggestion, however, that the defect in cells from group C patients may not be as quantitatively severe as that seen in cells from group A patients. Since 83% of all A-T patients fall into complementation groups A or C (Jaspers et al., 1988), it appears that the vast majority of A-T patients are defective in this p53-dependent response to IR.

A gene distal to p53 in this signal transduction response pathway has also been identified - transcription of the *GADD45* gene (a growth arrest and DNA damage-inducible gene) is enhanced by IR only in cells with wild-type p53 function (Kastan et al., 1992). A binding site for p53 was identified in the *GADD45* gene and wild-type, but not mutant, p53 protein binds to this site. This binding site can also activate transcription of a reporter CAT gene in the presence of wild-type, but not mutant, p53. Consistent with the observation mentioned above that A-T cells are defective in the induction of p53 protein following IR, Fornace and collaborators had previously shown that A-T cells are defective in their ability to induce *GADD45* transcription following IR (Papathanasiou et al., 1991). These experiments thus suggest the following steps in a signal transduction pathway which controls the arrest of cells at the G_1/S border following ionizing irradiation: following IR-type damage, the cell "recognizes" this damage and increases p53 protein levels via a post-transcriptional mechanism; this induction of p53 protein is dependent on the A-T gene product(s) at some step. Subsequently, this increased/altered p53 protein functions as a transcription factor to up-regulate the expression of *GADD45* and possibly other effector genes, which triggers the arrest. Further characterization of the various steps in this pathway, including elucidation of the signal in the DNA which initiates this pathway, is currently underway.

Linkage of p53 and the A-T gene(s) in this pathway suggest that some previous observations about p53 and A-T and the development of human tumors are more than just coincidence. Lymphoid malignancies are the most common (or the first) tumors seen in both A-T patients (Morrell et al., 1986; Hecht and Hecht, 1990) and mice in which both p53 alleles have been disrupted (Donehower et al., 1992; Jacks and Weinberg, unpublished observations) - these are both situations in which the gene defect is **homozygous**. In contrast, the risk of breast (and other non-lymphoid) tumors is markedly increased in situations in which individuals inherit defects in **only one allele** of either the p53 gene or the A-T gene(s) - Li-Fraumeni patients inherit an abnormality of one p53 allele and have an increased risk of breast, brain, lymphoid and other tumors (Malkin et al., 1991; Srivasta et al., 1991) and A-T heterozygotes appear to have a significantly increased risk of developing breast cancers (Swift et al., 1987, 1991). Interestingly, the increased incidence of breast cancer in A-T heterozygotes has been suggested to be related to exposure to low doses of IR (Swift et al., 1991). The reasons for the development of these particular tumors with these particular gene defects remain to be elucidated.

As mentioned above, one predicted physiologic consequence of losing cell cycle checkpoints is the increased risk of developing genetic abnormalities following exposure to DNA damaging agents. Thus, defects at any step in this p53-dependent signal transduction pathway is likely to increase the chance that daughter cells will develop heritable genetic abnormalities. Such increases in genetic instability following IR have been observed in yeast with RAD9 mutations, which lack a G_2 checkpoint (Hartwell and Weinert, 1989; Weinert and Hartwell, 1990). The observations that cells from A-T patients have increases in genetic abnormalities following IR (e.g. Zampetti-Bossler and Scott, 1981; Nagasawa et al, 1985) are consistent with these concepts and provide a direct example of genetic instability resulting from defects in this pathway. This model thus suggests that the high frequency with which tumor cells exhibit both p53 gene abnormalities (e.g. Hollstein et al., 1991) and gross chromosomal changes (Solomon et al, 1991) is causally related through abnormalities in this response pathway to DNA damage.

Though abnormalities in this pathway are likely to be significant contributors to the development of malignancies, the issue of whether defects in this G_1 checkpoint lead to increased sensitivity to ionizing radiation is far from resolved. The observations that the G_1 arrest can be dissociated from the radiosensitivity of A-T cells during genetic manipulations (Lehman et al, 1986; Kapp and Painter, 1989) suggest that the radiosensitivity of AT cells is not dependent on loss of this checkpoint and may be due to some other manifestation of the deficiency in A-T. In light of the link established between p53 and the A-T gene product(s), the observation that SV40-transformed cells from normal individuals (which should have nonfunctional p53 gene products due to binding of SV40 T antigen to p53 protein) continue to be more radioresistant than SV40-transformed cells from A-T patients (e.g. Lambert et al, 1991; Sullivan and Lyne, 1990), would further support the notion of a dissociation between the G_1 checkpoint and cellular sensitivity to ionizing radiation since normal p53 function is required for the G_1 arrest. Finally, the observation that the failure to block replicon initiation in **S-phase** cells following irradiation also contributes to the radioresistant DNA synthesis in A-T cells provides another difference between A-T cells and cells with mutant p53 genes.

Thus, it is feasible that the A-T genes function at a relatively "proximal" step in the cellular response to ionizing irradiation and leads to p53 induction and the G_1 arrest by one pathway (which predisposes cells to genetic instability and tumor development when abnormal) and leads to increased cell death (i.e. "radiosensitivity") by a separate pathway when abnormal. Preliminary observations in our laboratory that: 1) abnormal p53 gene function by itself does not result in increased sensitivity to IR; and 2) and that there appears to be a good correlation between the types of DNA damage which increase p53 protein levels by this pathway and the agents to which A-T cells exhibit hypersensitivity, are consistent with these concepts. Further studies of the functions of these gene products and the physiologic ramifications of defects in their functions should continue to provide useful insights into mechanisms of human carcinogenesis and cellular sensitivity to DNA damaging agents.

ACKNOWLEDGEMENTS

This work was supported in part by grants from the NIH (ES 05777) and the Council for Tobacco Research.

References

Doll, R. and Peto, R. (1981). The causes of cancer in the United States today. J.N.C.I. *66*, 1192-1308.

Donehower, L.A., Harvey, M., Slagle, B.L., McArthur, M.J., Montgomery C.A., Butel, J.S., and Bradley, A. (1992). Mice deficient for p53 are developmentally normal but susceptible to spontaneous tumours. Nature *356*, 215-221.

Gatti, R.A., Boder, E., Vinters, H.V., Sparkes, R.S., Norman, A., and Lange, K. (1991). Ataxia-telangiectasia: an interdisciplinary approach to pathogenesis. Medicine *70*, 99-117.

Hartwell, L.H. and Weinert, T.A. (1989) Checkpoints: Controls that ensure the order of cell cycle events. Science *246*, 629-634.

Hecht, F. and Hecht, B.K. (1990). Cancer in Ataxia-telangiectasia patients. Cancer Genet. Cytogenet. *46*, 9-19.

Hollstein, M., Sidransky, D., Vogelstein, B., and Harris, C.C. (1991). p53 mutations in human cancers. Science *253*, 49-53.

James, M.R. and Lehmann, A.R. (1982). Role of poly(adenosine diphosphate ribose) in deoxyribonucleic acid repair in human fibroblasts. Biochemistry *21*, 4007-4013.

Jaspers, N.G.J., Gatti, R.A., Baan, C., Linssen, P.C.M.L., and Bootsma, D. (1988). Genetic complementation analysis of ataxia telangiectasia and Nijmegen breakage syndrome: a survey of 50 patients. Cytogenet. Cell. Genet. *49*, 259 -263.

Kapp, L.N., and Painter, R.B. (1989). Stable radioresistance in ataxia-telangiectasia cells containing DNA from normal human cells. Int. J. Radiat. Biol. *56*, 667 -675.

Kastan, M. B., Onyekwere, O., Sidransky, D., Vogelstein, B., and Craig, R. W. (1991). Participation of p53 protein in the cellular response to DNA damage. Cancer Res *51*, 6304-6311.

Kastan, M.B., Zhan, Q., El-Deiry, W.S., Carrier, F., Jacks, T., Walsh, W.V., Plunkett, B.S., Vogelstein, B., and Fornace, A.J., Jr. (1992). A mammalian cell cycle checkpoint pathway utilizing p53 and *GADD45* is defective in ataxia telangiectasia. Cell *71*, 587-597.

Kaufmann, W.K., Boyer, J.C., Estabrooks, L.L., and Wilson, S.J. (1991). Inhibition of replicon initiation in human cells following stabilization of topoisomerase -DNA cleavable complexes. Mol. Cell. Biol. *11*, 3711-3718.

Kuerbitz, S. J., Plunkett, B. S., Walsh, W. V., and Kastan, M. B. (1992). Wild-type p53 is a cell cycle checkpoint determinant following irradiation. Proc. Natl. Acad. Sci. USA *89*, 7491-7495.

Lambert, C., Schultz, R.A., Smith, M., Wagner-McPherson, C., McDaniel, D., Donlon, T., Stanbridge, E.J., and Friedberg, E.C. (1991). Functional complementation of ataxia-telangiectasia group D (AT-D) cells by microcell -mediated chromosome transfer and mapping of the AT-D locus to the region 11q22-23. Proc. Natl. Acad. Sci. USA 88, 5907-5911.

Lau, C.C. and Pardee, A.B. (1982). Mechanism by which caffeine potentiates lethality of nitrogen mustard. Proc. Natl. Acad. Sci. 79, 2942-2946.

Lehman, A.R., Arlett, C.F., Burke, J.F., Green, M.H.L., James, M.R., and Lowe, J.E. (1986). A derivative of an ataxia-telangiectasia (A-T) cell line with normal radiosensitivity but A-T-like inhibition of DNA synthesis. Int, J. Radiat. Biol. 49, 639-643.

Malkin, D., Li, F.P., Strong, L.C., Fraumeni, J.F.,Jr., Nelson, C.E., Kim, D.H., Kassel, J., Gryka, M.A., Bischoff, F.Z., Tainsky, M.A., and Friend, S.H. (1990). Germ line p53 mutations in a familial syndrome of breast cancer, sarcomas, and other neoplasms. Science 250, 1233-1238.

McKinnon, P.J. (1987). Ataxia-telangiectasia: an inherited disorder of ionizing -radiation sensitivity in man. Hum. Genet. 75, 197-208.

Morrell, D., Cromartie, E., and Swift, M. (1986). Mortality and cancer incidence in 263 patients with ataxia-telangiectasia. J. Natl. Cancer Inst. 77, 89-92.

Nagasawa, H., Latt, S.A., Lalande, M.E., and Little, J.B. (1985). Effects of x-irradiation on cell-cycle progression, induction of chromosomal aberrations and cell killing in ataxia telangiectasia (AT) fibroblasts. Mut. Res. 148, 71 -82.

O'Connor. P.M., Ferris, D.K., White, G.A., Pines, J., Hunter, T., Longo, D.L., and Kohn, K.W. (1992). Relationships between cdc2 kinase , DNA cross-linking, and cell cycle perturbations induced by nitrogen mustard. Cell Growth and Diff. 3, 43-52.

Painter, R.B. and Young, B.R. (1980). Radiosensitivity in ataxia-telangiectasia: a new explanation. Proc. Natl. Acad. Sci. USA. 77, 7315-7317.

Painter, R.B. (1985). 3-Aminobenzamide does not affect radiation-induced inhibition of DNA synthesis in human cells. Mut. Res. 143, 113-115.

Papathanasiou, M. A., Kerr, N. C., Robbins, J. H., McBride, O. W., Alamo, I. J., Barrett, S. F., Hickson, I. D., and Fornace, A. J. Jr. (1991). Induction by ionizing radiation of the gadd45 gene in cultured human cells: lack of mediation by protein kinase C. Mol Cell Biol 11, 1009-1016.

Rudolph, N.S. and Latt, S.A. (1989). Flow cytometric analysis of x-ray sensitivity in ataxia-telangiectasia. Mut. Res. 211, 31-41.

Satoh, M.S. and Lindahl, T. (1992). Role of poly(ADP-ribose) formation in DNA repair. Nature 356, 356-358.

Solomon, E., Borrow, J., and Goddard, A.D. (1991). Chromosome aberrations and cancer. 254, 1153-1160.

Srivasta, S., Zou, Z., Pirollo, K., Blattner, W., and Chang, E.H. (1990). Germ-line transmission of a mutated p53 gene in a cancer-prone family with Li -Fraumeni syndrome. Nature 348, 747-749.

Sullivan, N. and Lyne, L. (1990). Sensitivity of fibroblasts derived from ataxia -telangiectasia patients to calicheamicin γ_1. Mut. Res. 245, 171-175.

Swift, M., Reitnauer, P.J., Morrell, D., and Chase, C.L. (1987). Breast and other cancers in families with ataxia-telangiectasia. N. Engl. J. Med. 316, 1289 -1294.

Swift, M., Morrell, D., Massey, R.B., and Chase, C.L. (1991). Incidence of cancer in 161 families affected by ataxia-telangiectasia. N. Engl. J. Med. *325*, 1831 -1836.

Tolmach, L.J., Jones, R.W., and Busse, P.M. (1977). The action of caffeine on X -irradiated HeLa cells. I. Delayed inhibition of DNA synthesis. Rad. Res. *71*, 653-665.

Vogelstein, B. (1990). A deadly inheritance. Nature *348*, 681-682.

Walters, R.A., Gurley, L.R., and Tobey, R.A. (1974). Effects of caffeine on radiation-induced phenomena associated with cell-cycle traverse of mammalian cells. Biophys. J. *14*, 99-118.

Weinert, T.A. and Hartwell, L.H. (1988). The RAD9 gene controls the cell cycle response to DNA damage in saccharomyces cerevisiae. Science *241*. 317 -322.

Weinert, T.A. and Hartwell, L.H. (1990). Characterization of RAD9 of saccharomyces cerevisiae and evidence that its function acts posttranslationally in cell cycle arrest after DNA damage. Mol. Cell. Biol. *10*, 6554-6564.

Zampetti-Bosseler, F. and Scott, D. (1981). Cell death, chromosome damage and mitotic delay in normal human, ataxia telangiectasia and retinoblastoma fibroblasts after X-irradiation. Int. J. Radiat. Biol. *39*, 547-558.

DNA Recombination in the Transgenic Mouse Brain

Linda Kingsbury and Hitoshi Sakano
Division of Immunology
Department of Molecular and Cell Biology
University of California
Berkeley, California 94720

Ataxia-telangiectasia   has been associated with abnormalities in the DNA recombination process that occurs in lymphocytes.   This chapter will discuss the possibility that somatic DNA recombination may also occur in the brain (Matsuoka, et al., 1991).

Parallels have long been observed between the immune system and the nervous system (Jerne, 1967).   First, both systems have the ability to "recognize" and "remember" signals from the outside.   Second, an increasing number of cell surface molecules (many of them members of the immunoglobulin superfamily) have been found to be expressed on both lymphocytes and brain cells (Parnes and Hunkapiller, 1987).   Finally, the discovery that the V-(D)-J recombination activating gene RAG-1 is transcribed in the brain led some to speculate that DNA recombination may also occur in the brain (Oettinger, et al., 1990; Chun, et al., 1991; Alt, et al., 1991).

To address this question, we constructed a recombination reporter gene (Figure 1) consisting of two V-(D)-J recombination signal sequences (RSS's) flanking the bacterial lacZ gene, which is situated in an inverse orientation with respect to the β-actin promoter-enhancer complex (Matsuoka, et al., 1991).   Due to the tandem orientation of the RSS's, DNA rearrangement results in inversion of the intervening DNA, such that the lacZ gene is relocated in the correct transcriptional orientation with respect to the promoter.   The chicken β-actin promoter-enhancer complex, which is believed to function fairly ubiquitously, was chosen to allow detection of recombination in whatever tissues we wished to examine.

If recombination in another tissue were less precise in site-specificity than V-(D)-J recombination (as switch recombination is), then the DNA cleavage event might take place anywhere within a few kilobases.

NATO ASI Series, Vol. H 77
Ataxia-Telangiectasia
Edited by R. A. Gatti and R. B. Painter
© Springer-Verlag Berlin Heidelberg 1993

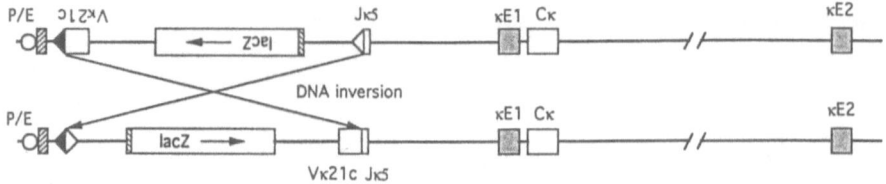

Figure 1. The recombination reporter transgene. $V_{\kappa 21c}$ and $J_{\kappa 5}$ are immunoglobulin κ chain gene segments, shown with their adjacent recombination signal sequences (triangles, not to scale). After inversion recombination, the lacZ gene is placed in the correct transcriptional orientation with respect to the chicken β-actin promoter-enhancer complex (P/E). Hatched boxes represent RNA splice sites.

To allow for such "flexibility" in recombination, we left several kb of DNA in front of the lacZ gene. To compensate for this extra DNA, we introduced splice donor and acceptor sites to allow for proper processing of the RNA transcript.

The substrate DNA was injected into fertilized oocytes to produce transgenic mice. To confirm that the reporter gene was working properly as a detector of V-(D)-J recombination in lymphocytes, we isolated spleen cells from the transgenic mouse and stained them with X-gal, a chromogenic substrate for β-galactosidase. Blue-stained lymphocytes were present, indicating that the reporter gene had undergone rearrangement in those cells.

In most other tissues examined, there was no difference in staining between transgenic and nontransgenic animals. Most tissues were unstained in both animals, while some tissues, such as artery, were stained in both the transgenic and the nontransgenic mouse, reflecting the existence of endogenous β-galactosidase activity in those tissues. In the brain, however, we found blue staining that was unique to the transgenic animal. Strikingly, the staining was confined to certain regions of the brain, including the cerebral cortex, cerebellum, hippocampus, and amygdala.

It was important to rule out several potential causes of staining in the absence of recombination activity. For example, blue staining might be caused by endogenous β-galactosidase activity, as it was in artery. Indeed, when nontransgenic brains were stained for over 24 hours, they did develop blue color; therefore, we always stained the brains for less than 6 hours, and a nontransgenic control was always included for comparison. In addition, we incubated brain sections with antibodies against <u>bacterial</u> β-galactosidase and found that only the transgenic brain was positive.

Another possibility was that <u>lacZ</u> expression might have been caused by a mechanism other than DNA recombination (Matsuoka, et al., 1992). For example, the <u>lacZ</u> gene in one copy of the transgene could be activated by the promoter in a neighboring copy. There are two situations in which this might occur. The first is when two copies of the transgene are integrated in a tail-to-tail fashion. Normal transcription starting at the promoter in one copy could activate the <u>lacZ</u> gene in the other copy, and vice versa. However, such transcription would generate a very long transcript (over 30 kb), which is unlikely because there are (presumably) three transcriptional terminators between the promoter and the <u>lacZ</u> gene. Furthermore, if this occurred, one would expect to see staining in all tissues, not just in the brain and in lymphocytes.

A second situation exists when the transgenes are integrated in tandem. Transcription might be initiated in an unusual backwards direction from the promoter in the second copy, leading to expression of the <u>lacZ</u> gene in the first copy (Abeliovich, et al., 1992). Here, the transcript would be a little over 10 kb, and one would have to hypothesize the existence of a cryptic RNA splice donor site near the promoter. We are now working on isolating the RNA transcripts and sequencing the cDNA to address this question.

Finally, another possibility is that integration of the transgene next to an endogenous promoter or splice site could result in tissue-specific expression of <u>lacZ</u>. (These phenomena are known as "promoter traps" and "gene traps," respectively.) To rule out this possibility it is important to examine two or more independent transgenic founders. Numerous areas in the brain of the second founder were also stained, indicating that it is unlikely that <u>lacZ</u> expression could be due to integration of the transgene near an endogenous tissue-specific promoter.*

To determine more directly whether the transgene was actually undergoing rearrangement in the brain, we used PCR to amplify DNA from the signal joint. (No DNA was amplified from the unrearranged transgene, due to the tandem orientation of the primers and the large distance between them.) The amplified DNA was analyzed by Southern blotting using the region upstream of $J_{\kappa 5}$ as a probe. DNA amplified from spleen

---

* The staining was not identical in the two founders, however. In general the staining was lighter in the second founder, probably because it contained fewer copies of the transgene. But in addition, staining was not always found in exactly the same regions within the brain. The integration site of the transgene may affect its accessibility to the recombination machinery in different cells. We are now constructing additional transgenic founders to further investigate this matter.

and thymus cells gave a band of the size expected for normal V-(D)-J type rearrangement, while the tail and kidney contained no rearranged DNA. The liver sample contained a small band of the same size as found in spleen and thymus, probably due to contaminating lymphocytes. The brain samples, however, contained rearranged DNA of many sizes, each different from the size expected for normal V-(D)-J type recombination.

The amplified DNA was cloned and sequenced, and we found that spleen and thymus cells contained DNA rearranged in the manner normally expected for V-(D)-J recombination, with the heptamers joined in a head-to-head fashion. In the brain, however, we found that DNA rearrangement took place in a much less precise manner. Recombination sometimes occurred near the RSS's, but other times it occurred as much as 700 bp away. At this point, we do not know whether the V-(D)-J recombination signal sequences in the substrate are recognized by the brain recombination machinery; our substrate may not contain all the proper signals for recombination in the brain.

The next question was whether recombination was happening in neurons as opposed to glia. In 1 micron plastic-embedded sections, the blue staining is usually located in a membrane-bound compartment within neuronal cell bodies; however, sometimes it is clearly located outside of cell bodies -- possibly in axons or dendrites, possibly in glia. Thus recombination occurred in neurons; it may have also occurred in glia.

We also wanted to determine at what point in development recombination occurred. Blue staining first appears shortly before birth and progresses through adulthood. In areas which are largely unstained in the 2-week-old brain, there are a few stained cells, and the number increases as the mouse grows; blue color does not appear "all at once" in a region. However, there may be a "lag time" between the point at which the substrate rearranges and the point at which sufficient β-galactosidase has accumulated that it can be detected by X-gal staining. Thus the first appearance of blue color may not coincide with the time of recombination activity. In newborns descended from the first founder, the only area stained to any great extent is the granule cell layer of the cerebellum. This staining first appears around embryonic day 16 in the mouse.

What role could DNA recombination play in the brain? There are at least three possibilities. First, DNA recombination could be used to activate a gene by bringing its promoter and enhancer elements (or its promoter-enhancer and its coding region) into close proximity. Second, it could be used to diversify gene sequences, as in antigen receptor genes.

Finally, it could be used to switch biological effector functions of a molecule, as immunoglobulin class switching does.

In summary, we now believe that DNA recombination, or a similar event, may occur in the brain, although its function is still unclear. Hopefully, identification of the rearranging genes and their functions will help to answer this question.

It is not yet clear whether the DNA rearrangement we observed in the brain plays a role in A-T. Since A-T is associated with some abnormalities in antigen receptor gene rearrangement, it could potentially have an effect on DNA recombination in the brain. If abnormalities in DNA recombination could be linked to the neuropathological effects of A-T, a more coherant understanding of the etiology of A-T could be developed.

References

Abeliovich A, Gerber D, Tanaka O, Katsuki M, Graybiel A M and Tonegawa S (1992) On somatic recombination in the central nervous system of transgenic mice (letter). Science 257: 404-408.

Alt F W, Rathbun G and Yancopoulos G D (1991) DNA recombination in the brain? Current Biology 1: 3-5.

Chun J J M, Schatz D G, Oettinger M A, Jaenisch R and Baltimore D (1991) The recombination activating gene-1 (RAG-1) transcript is present in the murine central nervous system. Cell 64: 189-200.

Jerne N K (1967) Antibodies and learning: selection versus instruction. In The Neurosciences (edited by G C Quarton, T Melnechuk, and F O Schmitt), Rockefeller University Press, New York, pp. 200-205.

Matsuoka M, Nagawa F, Okazaki K, Kingsbury L, Yoshida K, Mueller U, Larue D T, Winer J A and Sakano H (1991) Detection of somatic DNA recombination in the transgenic mouse brain. Science 254: 81-86.

Matsuoka M, Nagawa F, Kingsbury L and Sakano H (1992) On somatic recombination in the central nervous system of transgenic mice (response). Science 257: 408-410.

Oettinger M A, Schatz D G, Gorka C and Baltimore D (1990) RAG-1 and RAG-2, adjacent genes that synergistically activate V(D)J recombination. Science 248: 1517-1523.

Parnes J R and Hunkapiller T (1987) L3T4 and the immunoglobulin gene superfamily: new relationships between the immune system and the nervous system. Immunological Reviews 100: 109-127.

V. A–T Variants

Clinical Variants of Ataxia-Telangiectasia

O.Sanal[1], A.I. Berkel[1], F. Ersoy[1], I.Tezcan[1], H. Topaloglu[2]
Division of Pediatric [1]Immunology and [2]Neurology
Hacettepe University Medical School
Ankara
Turkey

Although ataxia-telangiectasia (A-T) can be diagnosed on purely clinical grounds and often on inspection, a number of case reports have shown clinical variability that makes diagnosis difficult without laboratory assistance such as determination of serum alpha-fetoprotein (AFP), demonstration of chromosomal aberrations or cellular radiosensitivity studies (Curry et al., 1989; Fiorilli et al., 1985; Sedgwick and Boder, 1991; Stankler and Bennet, 1988; Taylor et al., 1987; Terenty et al., 1978; Tsukahara et al., 1986; Ying and Decoteau, 1981). While some of the variants are characterized by a complete phenotype with additional features, others lack early onset of ataxia, telangiectasia or normal intelligence. Patients without clinical features of A-T but with the characteristic cellular radiosensitivity or chromosomal instability have also been reported (Conley et al., 1986; Weemaes et al., 1981; Wegner et al., 1988).

In our division, we have seen about 30 patients who have variant or presumed A-T in addition to 220 typical A-T patients. In this report, we describe 14 of the above 30 patients from 7 families whose diagnoses were based on the presence of one or more major parameters (progressive ataxia, telangiectasia, high serum AFP level, cerebellar atrophy in CT or MRI). They all showed some differences from typical A-T. The cellular radiosensitivity studies that are needed for a definite diagnosis in some of these patients are still in progress.

CASE REPORTS

Family 1. Five branches of this family had seven affected children (one by history) (Fig. 1). The affecteds of branches A, B, and C had clinical markers diagnostic for A-T, however, their serum AFP levels were normal except for one

NATO ASI Series, Vol. H 77
Ataxia-Telangiectasia
Edited by R. A. Gatti and R. B. Painter
© Springer-Verlag Berlin Heidelberg 1993

which was slightly high (25.7 ng/ml) and that individual was mentally retarded as the other patients in this family (Table 1). In branches D and E. the predominant features were mental and motor retardation.

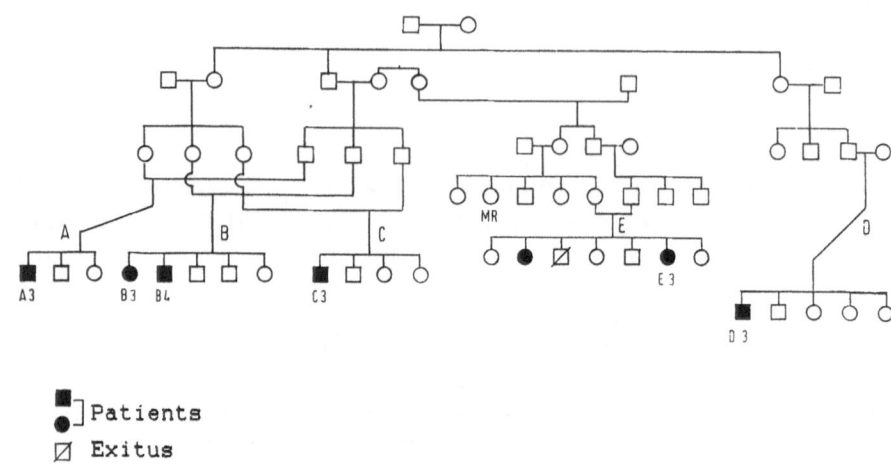

■
●] Patients
▨ Exitus

Fig. 1. The Pedigree of Family 1

Family 2. The patient presented clinically as immunodeficiency with hyperIgM at the age of 26 months and developed ataxia and telangiectasia at age of 4-5 years (Table 2). The serum AFP was high at age of 5. Of special interest for this patient is that an older brother who died at the age of 16 months with infection also had hypogammaglobulinemia (IgG was 150 mg/dl, IgA undetectable, IgM 27 mg/dl) and showed normal cerebellum (Bielschowsky staining and micro-scopic examination kindly performed by R.A. Gatti) and severe lymphoid depletion on postmorten histopathological examination. His serum AFP was unknown.

Family 3. This family had three affected children (one by history). Upon examination the older patient had mild ataxia and minimal telangiectasia; however, he also had mental retardation. The younger patient had only mild ataxia. Serum AFP and Ig levels were normal in both siblings (Table 2). Although without documentation of chromosomal aberration and/or cellular radiosensi-tivity the diagnosis is open to question, this family shows linkage to 11q22-23.

Table 1. Features of Patients in Family 1.

Patient	A3	B3	B4	C3	D3	E3
Age (Yrs), Sex	19 (M)	26 (F)	25 (M)	9 (M)	18 (M)	10 (F)
Ataxia	+	+	+	+	Unsteadiness	Unsteadiness
Telangiectasia	+	Minimal	Minimal	Minimal	–	–
Frequent Infections	–	–	–	–	–	+
Characteristic Facies	+	?	?	–	–	–
Growth Retardation	–	?	?	+	+	+
Mental Retardation	Delayed speech (4-5 years)	Delayed speech	Delayed speech	Delayed speech (5 years)	Delayed speech (5 years)	Delayed speech (6-7 years)
Head Circumference	N	N	N	N	N	?
Serum Afp (Ng/Ml)	8.0	8.1	25.7	1.9	0.5	0.1
Serum Ig's	N	N	N	N	N	N
Other Features	–	–	–	–	Nystagmus, Poor fine motor coordination	Poor fine motor coordination

186

Table 2. Clinical Features of A-T Variants.

	FAMILY 2	FAMILY 3		FAMILY 4	FAMILY 5	FAMILY 6		FAMILY 7
Age (Yrs), Sex	9 (M)	12 (M)	11 (F)	16 (M)	7 (M)	5 (M)	4 (F)	7 (F)
Ataxia	+	Mild	Mild	Widened base gait	+	+	+	+
Telangiectasia	+	Minimal	–	+	+/–	Minimal	Minimal	Minimal
Frequent Infections	+	–	–	–	–	–	–	+ (Skin?)
Mental Retardation	–	+	+	–	–	+	+	+
Growth Retardation	+	–	–	+	–	+	+	+
Typical Facies	+	–	–	–	–	–	–	–
Head Circumference	N	N	N	<5%	N	<5%	<5%	<5%
Consanguinity of Parents	+ (First degree)	+ (First degree)		–	–	+ (Third degree)		–
Serum AFP (ng/Ml)	43.2	4.7	4.8	147	5.0	0	?	2.1
Serum Ig's (mg/dl)	IgG 110, IgA 0 IgM 290	N	N	IgA <21	N	N	?	N
Other Features	Sibling history (see text)	Links to 11q22-23		An older brother has similar complaints	Cerebellar atrophy (CT, MRI)	Cerebellar atrophy (CT) An older brother has bulbar telangiectasia without ataxia		Cerebellar-cortical atrophy (CT) Hodgkin's lymphoma

Family 4. The propositus was first seen in our department at the age of 16 years because of low serum IgA level found during the evaluation of growth retardation. On physical examination he had microcephaly without mental retardation, bulbar telangiectasia, nystagmus and widened base gait without remarkable ataxia. Motor coordination was normal and serum AFP level was high (Table 2). An older brother with similar complaints has yet to be examined.

Family 5. A 7-year-old boy whose parents are unrelated had progressive ataxia beginning at the age of 3.5 years. He had questionable telangiectasia and no frequent infections. Somatic growth was within normal limits as were the serum AFP and Ig levels. MRI and CT scan showed cerebellar atrophy.

Family 6. Patients DFT and FT are 5-year-old (male) and 4 year-old (female) siblings, whose parents are third degree relatives; both developed ataxia rather rapidly at the ages of 2.5 and 3 years, respectively. Both had microcephaly, mental retardation and minimal bulbar telangiectasia. CT scan performed in the older patient showed cerebellar atrophy and his serum AFP and Ig values were normal. An 8-year-old brother who had neither ataxia nor microcephaly had bulbar telangiectasia with normal serum AFP and Ig levels.

Family 7. The patient was referred to Hacettepe Childrens' Hospital at the age of 7 years for evaluation of cervical lymphadenopathy and unstable gait. She began to walk at age of 18 months and developed unsteadiness rather rapidly at the age of 3, which progressed slowly during the following years. Recently,she was unable to walk without assistance. She did not have any febrile disorder suggestive of central nervous system infection. She had marked ataxia. minimal bulbar telangiectasia, mental retardation, and cerebellar and cortical athrophy on CT. A lymph node biopsy at age 7 revealed Hodgkin's lymphoma. The serum AFP and Ig levels have been within normal ranges.

DISCUSSION

Numerous reports have been published describing clinical variants of A-T. All these variations strongly suggest genetic heterogeneity. Examples of these clinical variants include absence of telangiectasia, presence of peripheral neuropathy as the prominent clinical picture, presence of generalized skin pigmentation, presence of microcephaly and mental retardation and presence of bird-like face in addition to microcephaly and mental retardation (Curry et al., 1989; Fiorilli et al., 1985; Sedgwick and Boder, 1991; Stankler and Bennett, 1988; Taylor et al., 1987; Terenty et al., 1978; Tsukahara et al., 1986; Ying and Decoteau, 1981).

In addition to these clinical variants, patients have been described with different levels of cellular radiosensitivity (Fiorilli et al., 1985; Taylor et al., 1987; Ying and Decoteau, 1981). Elevated serum AFP, a rather consistent marker of A-T, is not invariably high in all patients.

Additional laboratory studies are needed on most of these patients (i.e. demonstration of chromosomal aberrations and/or cellular radiosensitivity) both to confirm the diagnosis and to demonstrate whether they show any correlated pattern with respect to the radiosensitivity. Following the first positive report of genetic linkage of A-T to chromosome 11q22-23 (Gatti et al., 1988) there has been some more progress in the localization of A-T gene, but characterization of A-T variants probably will have to await the cloning and sequencing of the common A-T gene(s).

REFERENCES

Conley ME, Spinner NB, Emanuel BS, Nowell PC, Nichols WW (1986) A chromosomal breakage syndrome with profound immunodeficiency. Blood 67:1251-1256.

Curry CJR, Tsai J, Hutchinson HT, Jaspers NGJ, Wara D, Gatti RA (1989) AT Fresno: A phenotype linking ataxia-telangiectasia with the Niimegen Breakage Syndrome. Am J Hum Genet 45:270-275.

Fiorilli M, Antonelli A, Russo G, Crescenzi M, Carbonary M, Petrinelli P (1985) Variant of ataxia-telangiectasia with low level radiosensitivity. Hum Genet 70:274-277.

Gatti RA, Berkel I, Boder E, Braedt G, Charmley P, Concannon P, Ersoy F, Foroud T, Jaspers NGJ, Lange K, Lathrop GM, Leppert M, Nakamura Y, O'Connell P, Paterson M, Salser W, Sanal O, Silver J, Sparkes R, Susi E, Weeks DE, Wei S, White R, Yoder F (1988) Localization of an ataxia-telangiectasia gene to chromosome 11q22-23. Nature (London) 336:577-580.

Sedgwick RP, Boder E (1991) Ataxia-telangiectasia. In Handbook of Clinical Neurology, Chap. 26: Hereditary Neuropathies and Spinocebellar Atrophies (de Jong JMBV ed), Elsevier Science Publishers B.V. , Amsterdam pp 347-423.

Stankler L, Bennett FM (1988) Ataxia telangiectasia. Case report of a benign variant with telangiectasia, recurrent infection and low IgA. Brit J Dermatol 88:187-189.

Taylor AMR, Flude E, Laher B, Stacey M, McKay E, Waat J, Green SH, Harding AE (1987) Variant forms of ataxia telangiectasia. J Med Genet 24:669-677.

Terenty TA, Robson P, Walton JH (1978) Presumed ataxia-telangiectasia in a man. Brit J Med ii,802.

Tsukahara M, Masuda M, Ohshiro K, Kobayashi K, Kajii T, Ejima YJ, Sasaki SS (1986) Ataxia telangiectasia with generalized skin pigmentation and early death. Eur J Pediatr 145:121-124.

Weemaes CMR, Hustinx TWJ, Scheres JMJC, van Munster PJJ, Bakkeren JAJM, Taalman RDFM (1981) A new chromosomal instability disorder: The Nijmegen breakage syndrome. Acta Pediatr Scand 70:557-564.

Wegner RD, Metzger M, Hanefeld F, Jaspers NGJ, Baan C, Magdorf K, Kunze J, Sperling K (1988) A new chromosomal instability disorder confirmed by complementation studies. Clin Genet 33:20-32.

Ying KL. Decoteau WE (1981) Cytogenetic anomalies in a patient with ataxia, immune deficiency and high alphafetoprotein in the absence of telangiectasia. Cancer Genet Cytogenet 4:311-317.

Epidemiology of Ataxia-Telangiectasia in Italy

L. Chessa*, M. Fiorilli#
*Dipartimento di Medicina Sperimentale, and #Istituto di Clini-
ca Medica III, Universita' "La Sapienza", Viale Regina Elena
324, 00161 Roma, Italy.

A cohort study of Ataxia-Telangiectasia (A-T) families has
been followed in Italy since 1986 through a Registry sent to
clinicians and geneticists working in the Universities or in
public hospitals (Chessa et al., 1987). The Registry asks for
informations on the probands, such as clinical data and laboratory values (IgA, AFP, cytogenetics and radiobiology), and on
their family (parents, grandparents, siblings and relatives).
An accurate pedigree is requested. The purpose of the Registry
is to collect data on: 1) the frequency and the prevalence of
A-T in Italy; 2) the clinical heterogeneity of the disease, and
3) the causes of death among the patients and their relatives.

The families collected in the Registry originate from a
variety of places around Italy, with two large highly inbred
pedigrees, one from Calabria and the other from Sardinia (Fig.
1). At this moment, information regarding 58 families has been
received; for two of them the data were not sufficient for
analysis.

Consanguinity is reported in 8 families, denied in 42, unknown in 8. The consanguineous parents are first cousins in 4
cases, first cousins once removed in two, second cousins in one
and third cousins in another one. The mean rate of consanguinity in this group, whose marriages were celebrated between 1945
and 1985, is 0.0063. Moroni and Zei (unpublished data), on the
basis of the Catholic Church registries established until 1964
for all Italian provinces, fixed the consanguinity rates from
1945 to 1964 as 0.0005 for northern Italy, 0.0008 for central
Italy and 0.0017 for southern Italy.

NATO ASI Series, Vol. H 77
Ataxia-Telangiectasia
Edited by R. A. Gatti and R. B. Painter
© Springer-Verlag Berlin Heidelberg 1993

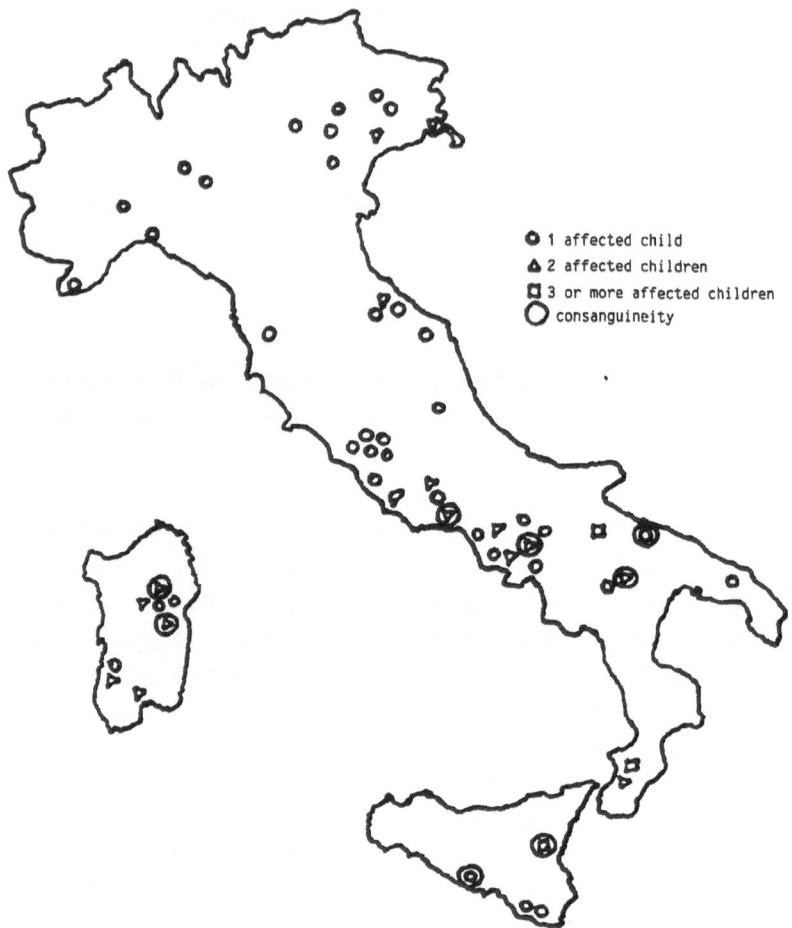

⊙	1 affected child
▲	2 affected children
⊡	3 or more affected children
◯	consanguineity

Figure 1 - Geographic distribution of A-T in Italy

Interestingly enough, the mean consanguinity rate for Italy from 1964 to 1980 decreased from 0.0010 to 0.0008 (Zei, personal communication), indicating a trend away from consanguineous marriages, a trend common throghout the occidental world.

A preliminary analysis of consanguinity data confirms the autosomal recessive inheritance of the disease in Italy, indicated by the exceedingly high rate of consanguineous marriages

193

in A-T families compared to region/5 year-matched control families. This is at variance with the data reported by Woods et al. (1990), who found a low consanguinity rate among A-T families from West Midlands and suggested, therefore, a non-recessive mode of inheritance.

An analysis of the composition of A-T families showed that in 6 families the proband is the only child, while 29 families have an affected child and one or more non-A-T siblings, 16 have two affected children, 1 three and 2 four. The number of unaffected sibs is 98. 1246 ancestors and relatives are reported; for three of them, dead in their infancy, A-T was suspected. Twenty-six families were informative for the presence of cancer (Table I). Interestingly, the most frequent neoplasia noticed in these families was gastric carcinoma (11/61). Breast carcinoma, the most frequent cancer in A-T relatives (Swift et al., 1983) was noted only in 3 out of 61 cancers. A high number of unspecified tumors (25/61) is reported. Diabetes was noted in 12 ascendents/relatives from 6 families.

Table I - Frequency and sites of malignancies in A-T families

site of tumor	patient	parents	grandparents	sibs	aunts/uncles	others
blood (leukemia)	2			1		1
blood (lymphoma)	3				1	1
stomach		7	1		1	2
lung		1	1			
colon		1				
uterus	1	2				1
breast		1			2	
other	2	1			1	1
unspecified	1	7			9	7

Eighty-one patients (50 males, 31 females) from 56 families were recorded. It is noteworthy that two of them are adopted sons. The oldest patient was born in 1949, the youngest in 1989 (Fig. 2).

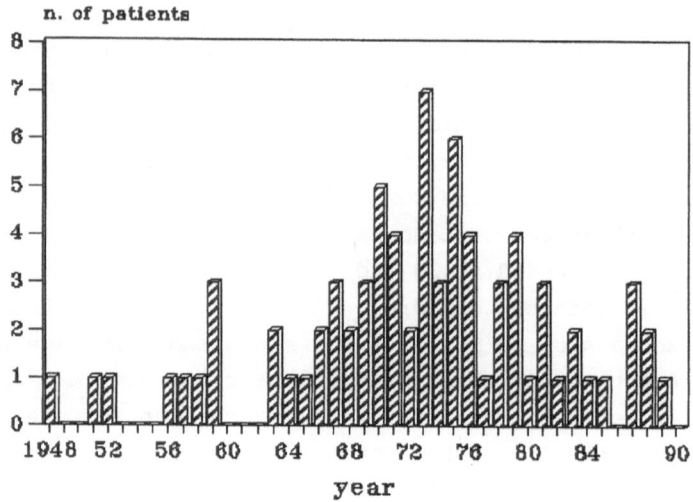

Figure 2 – Date of birth of A–T patients

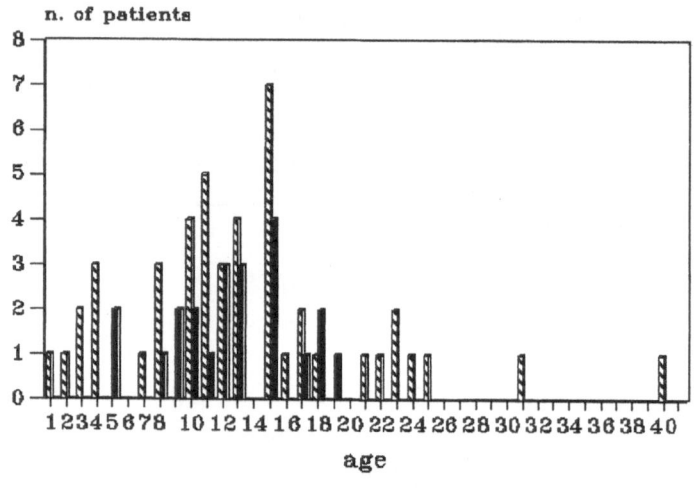

Figure 3 – Survival in A–T patients

The patients' survivals, i.e. the last time they were seen by the referring clinician, varied from 1 to 40 years (Fig. 3). Forty-six affecteds are still alive, 22 died; no data on the other 15 are obtained.

The reported causes of death were: sinopulmonary disease in 18 cases, lymphoma in three, leukemia in two, rhinopharyngeal carcinoma in one, osseous sarcoma in one.

The age of onset of ataxia for 64 patients ranged from 7 months to 12 years. The age of onset of telangiectasia, for 32 patients, ranged from 18 months to 8 years. AFP was increased in 34 cases, normal in 4. Serum IgA was decreased or absent in 42 patients, normal in 21. Recurrent infections were noted in 57 patients, while in two "no infections" were noted. Many other features were of normal frequency in A-T subjects; it is noteworthy that, among them, juvenile diabetes was described in one patient, and cafè-au-lait spots in 9. A three-year-old girl with A-T has been diagnosed as having a Castleman's lymphoma (not listed in Table I) accompanied by marked hyper-IgM (>4,000 mg/dl). Clinical remission of the lymphoma was achieved by low-dose corticosteroids and the patient remains in relatively good clinical condition one year after diagnosis.

Contemporaneously with the Registry compilation blood samples from the patients and their relatives were taken whenever possible. Lymphoblastoid cell lines were established and used for linkage analysis to localize the A-T region to 11q22.3-23.1 (Foroud et al., 1991; Sobel et al., 1992). At this moment our A-T Cell Repository includes 162 lymphoblastoid cell lines, 41 of which are from A-T patients, 52 from their parents (obligate heterozygotes) and 69 from their relatives.

Eleven A-T patients, six males and five females, ranging from 2 to 22 years of age, were evaluated by clinical examination, by M-mode and by two-dimensional echocardiography color Doppler (Bastianon et al., in press). ECGs were normal in all the patients. Five of them presented with echocardiographic anomalies. Mitral valve prolapse was found in four patients; in three of them mild mitral valve regurgitation was also present. One patient presented with aortic root dilation. These results suggest a high incidence of cardiac anomalies in the A-T syndrome, a finding previously not observed.

We performed cellular radiosensitivity tests and evaluated radioresistant DNA synthesis (RDS) on twelve A-T patients displaying the typical clinical manifestations and the immunological deficiences characteristic of classical A-T (Chessa et al.,

1986; Chessa et al., 1992). Radiosensitivity was evaluated by means of gamma-survival and chromosomal breakage induced by bleomycin. In three patients (two sibs and one unrelated case), radiosensitivity was at an intermediate level between classical A-T and normal cells, and RDS ranged from normal to intermediate values. Our data and a literature review of the low radiosensitivity A-T cases (LR-AT) suggest that RDS, cellular radiosensitivity, and the clinical hallmarks behave independently.

We tried to focus on some precocious clinical signs suggestive of the disease by examining three early onset cases of A-T (Leuzzi et al., in press). Case 1 and 2 were observed a few months after the onset of the disease. Case 3 is the younger sister of a patient affected by A-T and was examined at 9 months of age, when "asymptomatic". The earliest clinical sign was the truncal ataxia; in all these patients it was present at the first clinical observation. During the second year of life the patients exhibited extrapiramidal disorders such as dystonic postures and movements. A second clinical sign, appearing before the age of 3, was a subtle disorder of eye movements, i.e. a spontaneous blinking before gaze changing or an increase in the latency and hypometry of horizontal saccades . Anomalous head posture (tilted laterally) was observed in cases 1 and 3 at the age of 42 and 21 months respectively. All movement disorders seemed to be amplified by fatigue and stress.

The analysis of the current data on A-T in Italy confirm: a) the autosomal recessive inheritance of the disease; b) the existence of radiobiological variants (with intermediate radiosensitivity); c) the increased frequency of neoplasia both in patients and in heterozygotes; and d) an unusual frequency of cardiovalvular anomalies in homozygotes. The increased occurrence of gastric carcinoma in A-T families has also been noted in Costa Rica (Porras et al., this volume). Further progress on the epidemiological aspects of the disease is warranted by the steady increase of new Italian A-T families referred to the Registry.

ACKNOWLEDGEMENTS
This work was supported in part by grants Consiglio Nazionale
Ricerche Progetto Finalizzato A.C.R.O. n. 92.02160.PF39 and
Associazione Italiana Ricerca sul Cancro.

BIBLIOGRAPHY

Bastianon V, Fiorilli M, Giglioni E, Businco L, Chessa L Car-
    diac anomalies in Ataxia-Telangiectasia. Am J Dis Child (in
    press)
Chessa L, Federico A, Arlett C, Harcourt S, Cole J, Palmieri S,
    Guazzi GC, Gandini E (1986) Is the Ataxia-Telangiectasia ge-
    ne for radiosensitivity in Italy different from the classi-
    cal one? 7th ICHG, Berlin.
Chessa L, Terracini B, Gandini E (1987) Italian Registry for
    Ataxia-Telangiectasia: purpose for a collaborative study.
    International Congress on DNA Damage and Repair, Roma.
Chessa L, Petrinelli P, Antonelli A, Fiorilli M, Elli R, Mar-
    cucci L, Federico A, Gandini E (1992) Heterogeneity in Ata-
    xia Telengiectasia: classical phenotype associated with low
    cellular radiosensitivity. Am J Med Genet 42: 741-746
Foroud T, Wei S, Ziv Y, Sobel E, Lange E, Chao A, Goradia T,
    Huo Y, Tolun A, Chessa L, Charmley P, Sanal O, Salman N,
    Julier C, Concannon P, McConville C, Taylor M, Shiloh Y,
    Lange K, Gatti RA (1991) Localization of an ataxia-telan-
    giectasia locus to a 3-cM interval on chromosome 11q23:
    linkage analysis of 111 families by an international con-
    sortium. Am J Hum Genet 49: 1263-1279
Leuzzi V, Elli R, Antonelli A, Chessa L, Cardona F, Marcucci L,
    Petrinelli P Neurological and cytogenetic study in early
    onset Ataxia-Telangiectasia (AT) patients. Eur J Pediatr
    (in press)
Sobel E, Lange E, Jaspers NGJ, Chessa L, Sanal O, Shiloh Y,
    Taylor AMR, Weemas CMA, Lange K, Gatti RA (1992) Ataxia-
    Telangiectasia: Linkage evidence for genetic heterogeneity.
    Am J Hum Genet 50: 1343-1348
Swift M, Chase C (1983) Cancer and cardiac deaths in obligatory
    ataxia-telangiectasia heterozygotes. Lancet i: 1049-1050
Woods CG, Bundey SE, Taylor AMR (1990) Unusual features in the
    inheritance of Ataxia Telangiectasia. Hum Genet 84: 555-562

Epidemiology of Ataxia-Telangiectasia in Costa Rica

O. Porras, O. Arguedas, M. Arata, M. Barrantes, L. González and E. Sáenz
Departments of Immunology and Oncology
National Children's Hospital
Apartado 1654 1000 San José
Costa Rica

INTRODUCTION

Costa Rica is around 50,000 square Km with 3 million people, a third of them below 19 years of age. In 1985, a primary immunodeficiency (PID) registry was begun. Children with recurrent infections or PID from the whole country were admitted to one clinic at the Children's Hospital in San José. Ataxia Telangiectasia (A-T) was registered as the most frequent PID (34%). A-T was more frequent than symptomatic Selective IgA deficiency. The prevalence was higher than SCID and Endocrine Congenital Defects, but 5-fold lower than Down Syndrome (Porras et al 1991).

A-T was first noted (8 cases) in Costa Rica by Faingezicht and Mohs in 1970 (unpublished). Campos and Loria (unpublished) in 1989 reviewed 14 cases that were attending a pediatric neurology clinic.

A-T registry began in 1986 at the Immunology Department. Since then forty-five cases among 39 families have been identified. The present report describes the clinical and immunological findings of the A-T group followed in Costa Rica.

MATERIALS AND METHODS

A-T diagnosis was based on clinical features (Sedgwick et al 1991 and Gatti et al 1991) associated with a T cell defect, demonstrated by a low response to PHA. T cells numbers were measured by rosetting with sheep erythrocytes

NATO ASI Series, Vol. H 77
Ataxia-Telangiectasia
Edited by R. A. Gatti and R. B. Painter
© Springer-Verlag Berlin Heidelberg 1993

(SRBC). Lymphocyte stimulation was done with a PHA final concentration of 6.25 ug/ml (González et al 1986).

Immunoglobulin (Ig) levels were measured using radial gel immunodiffusion. Alpha-feto-protein (AFP) was measured by double antibody competitive RIA in which ^{125}I-labeled AFP competes with AFP in the patient sample for antibody-binding sites (DPC, L.A., Ca). The standards were human sera having AFP values ranging from 3 to 300 IU/ml. The assay has been standardized against the WHO international standard for AFP #72/225. The normal level was 24. 2 ng/ml.

Handicap grading was done as follows: children capable of doing all the usual tasks expected for age while at home and school were graded I. The patient was graded II if aid was needed to walk. Grade III included the severe handicapped, those unable to walk, in need of a wheelchair or been oxygen dependent.

RESULTS

The study group included 39 families consisting of 21 girls and 24 boys, with a female:male ratio of 0.9. Parental consanguinity was 17.8% (n=8); within families the occurrence was 21.6% (8 cases). Patients' average age was 10.2 years with a range between 3.7 and 18.4 years. Thirty—two patients (71.1%) were school children and nine adolescents. A-T was diagnosed at an average age of 4.8 years with a range between 1.6 and 14 years. Fifty-one percent of the cases were diagnosed before 4 years of age (Fig. 1).

An estimated prevalence of 2.87 per 100,000 was obtained by relating the number of A-T children in Costa Rica to the country population between 0-19 years. Cases were detected in all the geographic areas except the Atlantic coast, no cases were registered among the black population living there. An average of three new A-T cases were detected every year in Costa Rica; however, seven or more cases per year were registered in 1989, 1990 and 1992.

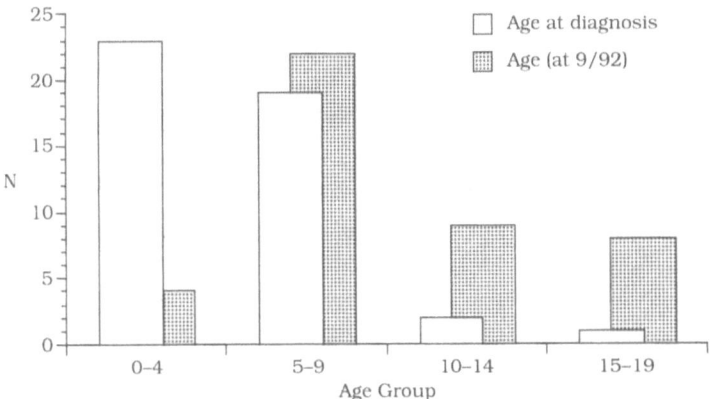

Fig. 1. Age distribution in children with A-T

Clinical features

The frequency of the A-T classical features are shown in Fig. 2. All had cerebellar ataxia and oculo-cutaneous telangiectasia. Ninety-one percent had apraxia of eye movements, dysarthric speech and the characteristic facies. Recurrent respiratory tract infections were identified in 87% of the cases. Motor problems or abnormal movements were the main complaint during the first visit to the hospital (59.4%). Fig. 3 displays the chronic disease features found in the group. Fifty percent were handicapped, with a third using wheelchairs (n=15) and 9% being oxygen dependent (n=4). Clubbing of the fingertips (Fig. 4), a clinical feature not previously described in A-T, was found in one-third of the cases and chronic lung disease was diagnosed in 15 cases. The most frequent infections were pulmonary, skin and upper respiratory tract, with 60% having otitis media and 7.8 % chronic otitis.

Malignancy

Three children (6.7%) had neoplasias, histologically defined as two non-Hodgkin lymphomas and one hepatoblastoma. We registered 12 cancer cases among parents and grandparents (n=64) in 16 families; half of them were gastric cancer.

Mortality

Five A-T patients (11.1%) died during the follow-up period. The cause of death was chronic lung disease in four of them, and a hepatoblastoma in the other.

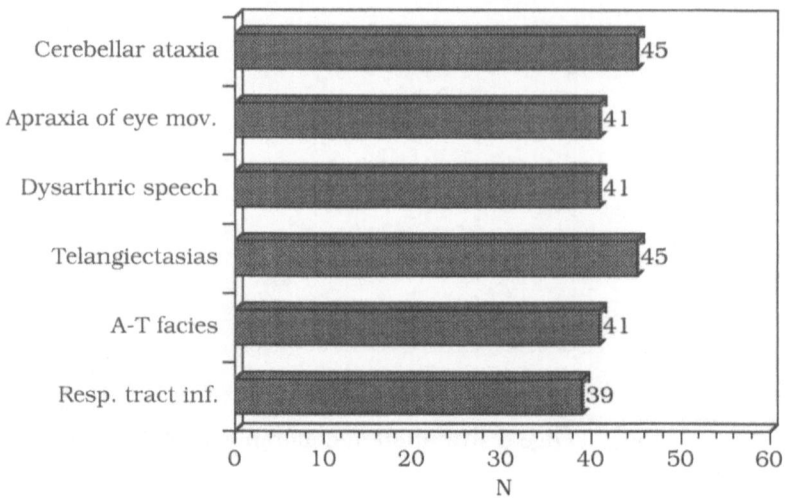

Fig. 2. Classical A-T clinical features

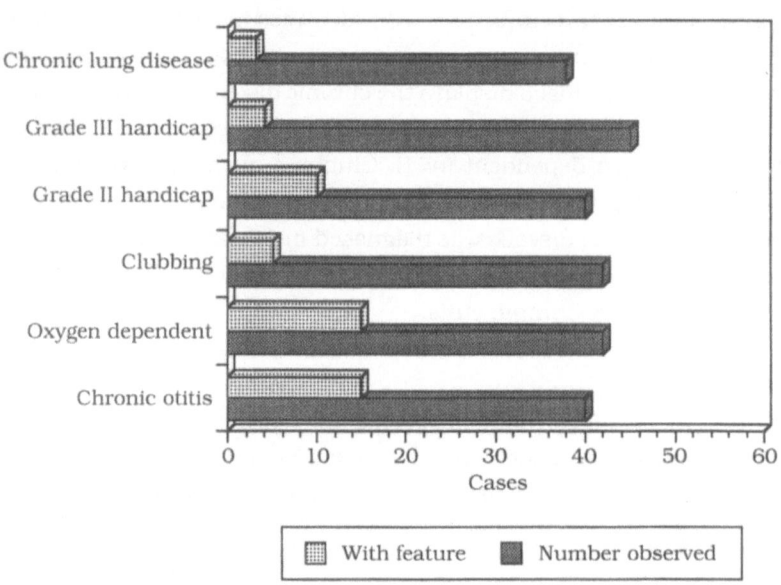

Fig. 3. Chronic disease features in A-T Children

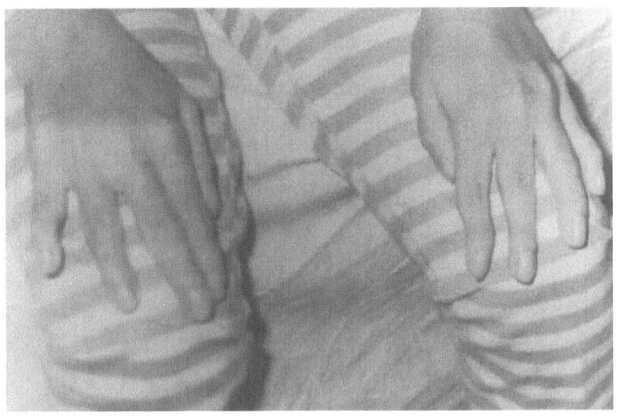

Fig. 4. Clubbing of the fingertips in an A-T girl
Photograph by R. Gatti

Immunology

Ninety-one percent of the children had a T cell defect demonstrated by a deficient response to mitogen (PHA). Only four cases had a normal *in vitro* lymphocyte response to PHA (Fig. 5).

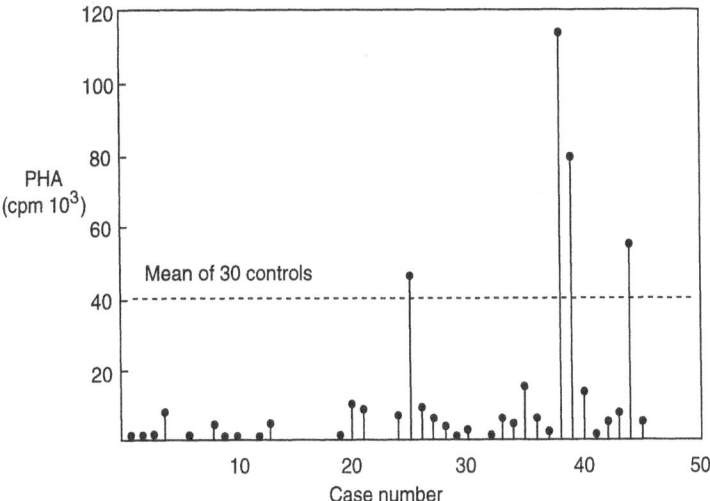

Fig. 5. PHA lymphocyte stimulation in A-T patients

A humoral immune status was heterogeneous, with absent (>0.05 g/L) or low levels (> mean -2SD of the normal age level) of IgA in 21 of 37 cases (56.8%) (Fig. 6). IgG2 deficiency (IgG2D) was found in 26.7% of the patients (n=8/30), associated with IgA deficiency in 10% and as a selective IgG2D in 10% (Fig. 7).

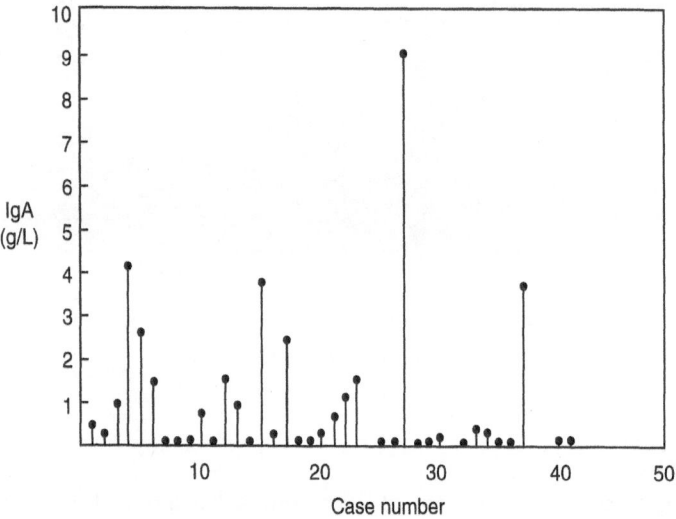

Fig. 6. Immunoglobulin A (g/L) levels in A-T children

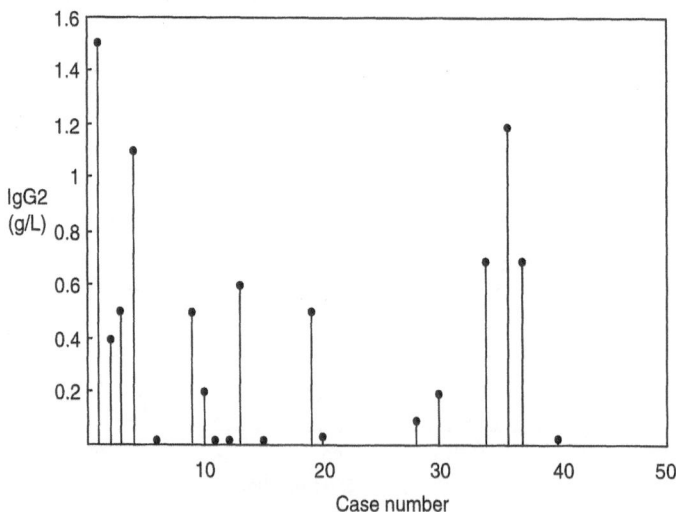

Fig. 7. Immunoglobulin G2 (g/L) levels in A-T children

Alpha-fetoprotein

Data on the AFP levels were available in 21 children. Only one child had a normal AFP level. Age and AFT level had a linear correlation (Fig. 8).

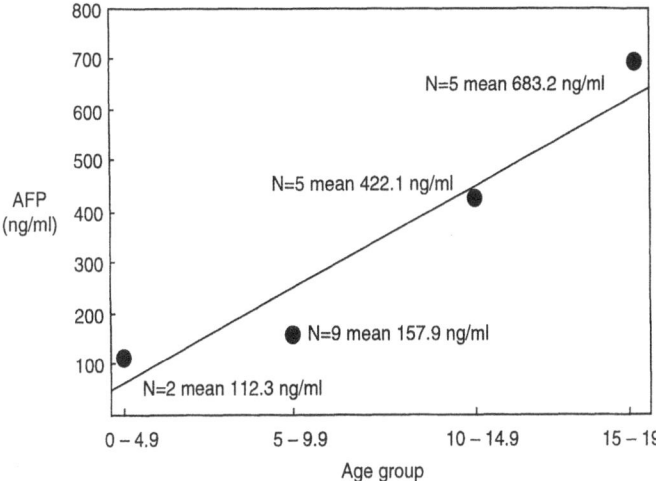

Fig. 8. Alpha-fetoprotein levels (ng/ml) in A-T age groups

DISCUSSION

A-T is defined as an autosomal recessive multisystem disease with progressive cerebellar ataxia, oculocutaneous telangiectasia and chronic lung disease (Sedgwick et al 1991 and Gatti et al 1991). Based on clinical features, immunological defect and increased AFP, a group of 45 A-T cases were registered in Costa Rica.

A-T was the most frequent PID reported in Costa Rica, as it was in Kuwait (20%) (White et al 1988). Other PID registries report A-T as a rare disease with frequencies between 1.4% in Sweden (Fasth 1984) and 7.3% in Japan (Hayakawa et al 1981). Costa Rican people are mainly a mixture between Spaniards and Amerindians. They are characterized by heavy inbreeding, a consequence of isolated founding groups. Because of the numerous cases detected in a relatively small population, we expect a high frequency of heterozygotes in Costa Ricans.

Cancer develops in A-T patients at a rate 100 times higher than a control population (Swift et al 1991), 80% are lymphoid malignancies (Peterson et al

1992). Heterozygotes for the A-T gene have a cancer risk of 3.8 in men and 3.5 in women, when compared with non carriers. There is an even higher risk for breast cancer in female carriers (Swift et al 1991). Eighteen percent of immediate relatives had cancer, mainly gastric, an association that needs further study in Costa Rica, a country where gastric cancer has a high frequency. Three non-Hodgkin lymphomas had been documented among A-T cases in our country before 1986 (Barrantes M. personal communication).

A study of 160 Turkish cases noted a higher malignancy rate than that reported in Costa Rica (Ersoy et al 1991). AFP levels showed no association with malignancy, but were correlated to age.

Mortality was most frequently related to chronic lung disease with terminal oxygen dependence. This may reflect the relatively high altitude of most of Costa Rica. Early antibiotic treatment in febrile children, intravenous immunoglobulins in IgG or IgG2 deficiency, and infection prophylaxis gives a better quality of life and survival.

Further research is needed in some aspects of the Costa Rican A-T group, like the relatives association with gastric cancer and the evidence of early severe lung disease as shown by the frequent finding of clubbing. It is possible that the somewhat different Costa Rica phenotype of A-T may represent a unique mutation in the A-T gene.

ACKNOWLEDGMENTS

This study was supported by a grant from The A-T Medical Research Foundation. Dr. González and Dr. Sáenz work at INCIENSA.

REFERENCES

Ersoy F, Berkel AJ, et al (1991) Twenty-year follow-up of 160 patients with Ataxia-Telangiectasia. Turk J Pediatr 33:205-215.

Fasth A (1984) Immunodeficiency in children in Sweden 1974-1983. In: Griscelli C, Vossen J (eds) Progress in Immunodeficiency Research and Therapy I, pp 461-467. Elsevier Amsterdam.

Gatti RA, Boder E, et al (1991) Ataxia-Telangiectasia: An interdisciplinary approach to pathogenesis. Medicine 79:99-117.

González L, Frajman M, et al (1986) Effect of tinidazole on the cellular immune response. J Antimic Chemoth 18:499-502.

Hayakawa H, Tsutomo I, et al (1981) Primary immunodeficiency syndrome in Japan. J Clin Immunol 1:31-39.

Peterson RD, Funkhouser JD, et al (1992) Cancer susceptibility in Ataxia-Telangiectasia. Leukemia 6(Sl):8-13.

Porras 0, Arguedas 0, et al (l991). Primary immunodeficiencies in Costa Rica. Report from a hospital-based Registry. In: Chapel HM, Levinsky RJ, Webster ADB (eds) Progress in Immunodeficiency III p 102. Royal Society of Medicine, London.

Sedgwick RP, Boder E (1991). Ataxia-Telangiectasia (208900; 208910; 208920). In: de Jong JMBV (ed) Handbook of Clinical Neurology: Hereditary Neuropathies and Spinocerebellar Atrophies pp 347-424. Elsevier Amsterdam.

Swift M, Morrell D, et al (1991) Incidence of cancer in 161 families affected by Ataxia-Telangiectasia. N Engl J Med 325: 1831-1836.

White AG, Raju KT, et al (1988) A six year experience with recurrent infection and immunodeficiency in children in Kuwait. J Clin Lab Immunol 26:97-101.

Clinical and cellular heterogeneity in ataxia-telangiectasia

A.M.R. Taylor, C.M. McConville, C.G. Woods*,
P.J. Byrd and D. Hernandez
CRC Department of Cancer Studies,
The Medical School,
University of Birmingham,
Edgbaston,
Birmingham B15 2TT, U.K.

Ataxia-telangiectasia (A-T) is a progressive neurological disorder with a birth frequency of about 1 in 300,000 (Swift et al., 1986; Woods et al., 1990). The major neurological features include progressive cerebellar ataxia presenting in infancy, oculomotor dyspraxia, and dysarthria (Sedgwick and Boder, 1991). About 10% of all A-T homozygotes develop a malignancy in childhood or early adulthood. A minority of tumours are epithelial cell cancers but with an unusually high predisposition to stomach carcinoma and smaller excesses of liver, uterine and ovarian tumours (Spector et al., 1982). The vast majority of tumours are however lymphoid in origin. All the leukaemias reported by Spector et al. (1982) were lymphoid with no myeloid tumours. A 70-fold and 250-fold excess of leukaemias and lymphomas respectively was reported by Morell et al. (1976).

Ataxia-telangiectasia would appear to be a fairly homogeneous disorder clinically in terms of the range of clinical features present but the degree to which some symptoms are present can be very variable. There is a more clearcut heterogeneity observed at the genetic or cellular levels. The purpose of this review is to tabulate evidence for heterogeneity at all levels and question its significance for our understanding of the disorder.

There would appear to be some fairly objective means by

---

*Department of Clinical Genetics, Churchill Hospital,
Headington, Oxford OX3 7LJ, U.K.

NATO ASI Series, Vol. H 77
Ataxia-Telangiectasia
Edited by R. A. Gatti and R. B. Painter
© Springer-Verlag Berlin Heidelberg 1993

which particular patients with this disorder can be grouped. One of these is by allocation to a genetic complementation group.

Genetic Heterogeneity

Genetic heterogeneity in A-T was first observed following investigation of genetic complementation in cultured A-T fibroblasts. Complementation groups were established by the analysis of rates of DNA synthesis in γ-irradiated heterodikaryons obtained from fusions between different A-T fibroblast cell strains. By producing different combinations of fusions four different complementation groups were defined. There are designated group A (55% of patients), group C (28% of patients), group D (14% of patients) and group E (3% of patients) (Murnane and Painter, 1982; Jaspers et al., 1982, 1988). Table 1 shows some clinical and cellular features of one or two Birmingham patients from each complementation group. Some basic features appear to be common to all complementation groups. Firstly the clinical features involving cerebellar degeneration are indistinguishable between groups. Susceptibility to infections appears to be shared by at least two complementation groups (A and D), although the siblings in group D appear to be differentially affected by infections. Secondly, at the cellular level there is increased radiosensitivity chromosomally and by colony forming assays in all groups. There is no easily discernable quantitative difference in colony forming ability between the groups although at the chromosomal level there may be more induced aberrations associated with the two group E siblings. Thirdly, spontaneous chromosome abnormalities are similar in type across the groups; in four individuals in these complementation groups there is evidence of a large clonal T cell population with an unusual chromosomal translocation. In two of the groups (D and E) patients have developed T cell prolymphocytic leukaemias and died (Taylor and Butterworth, 1986; Taylor et al., 1992). Heterogeneity in the patients in Table 1 is therefore not very obvious apart from the index of complementation groups. In the

Table 1: Clinical and cellular features of patients in different complementation groups

Patient	Comp. groups	Age	Sex	Telang.	Speech	Eye move.	Infect.	Spont. chrom.	Radiosen. surv.	Radiosen. chrom.	RDS	Tumour
AT3BI	A	15	M	2	3	2	1	+	++++	++++	ND	−
AT4BI	C	25	M	1	1	1	1	+*	++++	+++	ND	−
AT5BI	D	27	M	2	3	1	0	+*	++++	++++	++++	T-PLL
AT6BI		34	F	2	3	2	3	+	++++	++++	ND	−
AT2BI	E	36	F	2	2	1	0	+*	++++	++++	++++	−
AT8BI		43	F	2	1	1	0	+*	++++	++++	++++	T-PLL

All patients showed severe cerebellar ataxia and an immobile or impassive facies.

AT5BI and AT6BI are sibs; AT2BI and AT8BI are sibs;

*All stimulated T cells were clonal: AT4BI complex t(14;14)
 AT5BI inv(14)(q11q32)   (Taylor and Butterworth, 1986)
 AT2BI t(14;14)(q11;q32)
 AT8BI t(X;14)(q28;q11)   (Taylor et al., 1992)

Comp. groups = complementation group; Telang - conjunctional telangiectasia, 1 - mild or find vessels, 2 - moderate, 3 - prominent; Speech, 1 - mild slurring, 2 - dysarthria, 3 - difficult to interpret without time and effort. Eye movements, 1 - full movement but difficult, 2 - sacchades difficult, 3 - forward vision only; Infections, 0 - none, 1 - possible increase in infections, 2 - definite increased number or 1 severe infection, 3 - severe infections; Radio-sensitivity measured by colony survival or chromosomally; RDS - radioresistant DNA synthesis.

literature cells from relatively few patients have been allocated to complementation groups and no detailed clinical data are easily available to correlate with this information.

Although generally believed to be an autosomal recessive disorder, there is some evidence that this is not the case for all families. There is a well founded relationship between the birth frequency of an autosomal recessive disorder and the proportion of parents of patients who are consanguineous. This relationship holds true as long as the recessive disorder consists of a single entity. The expected level of parental consanguinity in ataxia-telangiectasia with a birth frequency of 1 in 300,000 is 10%. In a study of 47 families in the UK, a low parental consanguinity rate was observed (0/47 families). This was also confirmed from information in the literature (see Woods et al., 1990). There are only 5 reports of parents being first cousins or more closely related, in a total of 383 families. An explanation for the deficit of consanguineous parents is that A-T is not always an autosomal recessive disorder. One possibility is that some patients have a new dominant mutation. This would give a high risk of transmission of the gene to the patients offspring, but no examples have been described of classical A-T patients having a child. The family of Terenty et al. (1978) however did show dominant transmission of the gene. The explanation that A-T is not always a strictly homozygous recessive disorder, but possibly a result of compound heterozygosity is supported by the observation of parents of mixed race having children with A-T, together with the presence of the gene in different races.

The A-T gene has been mapped to chromosome 11q22-23 (Gatti et al., 1988; McConville et al., 1990a, b; Foroud et al., 1991). In view of the four complementation groups there may be a number of genes in this segment. The alternative possibility that the complementation studies indicate genes at different loci is unlikely firstly because in this case parental consanguinity rates would need to be higher, and secondly because all the linkage/recombination evidence points to a single chromosome segment. It is now clear that the A-T locus for patients in groups A and C is at 11q22-23 (Gatti et al., 1988; Ziv et al., 1991) and both genes may be between NCAM/DRD2 and

STMY/D11S385. Fibroblasts from a group D patient have been complemented by chromosome 11 microcell fusions (Komatsu et al., 1989). Kapp et al. (1992) have recently reported the cloning of a candidate group D gene and have shown this maps about 20 cM distal to the A/C locus, and telomeric to THY1. There are no families among the 50 studied in Birmingham in which the chromosome segment between NCAM/DRD2 and STMY/D11S385 can be excluded as a possible A-T locus. Since however group D families are only 14% of all families it is possible that there are insufficient group D families in the Birmingham study to give appropriate recombinations. There is some linkage evidence in support of a second A-T locus distal to THY1 from an international study of 111 families (Sobel et al., 1992). While it seems certain that complementation groups A and C map to 11q22-23 it is not yet clear whether these represent separate loci. One group E family we have studied did not provide any support for the existence of this A-T locus outside the 11q22-23 region.

In one additional family in which two first cousins presented with clinical features of ataxia telangiectasia, and the typical cellular features of increased radiosensitivity and spontaneous chromosome abnormalities, there was no clear evidence that the gene for A-T in this family was on 11q22-23. The affected individuals did show some clinical differences compared with most A-T patients. In general the clinical course was milder. Both patients are still ambulatory at ages 25 and 20 years respectively. The proband was short (>-2SD for age) and had no ocular telangiectasia. AFP and IgA levels were normal. She was unsteady from age of 3-4 years, had vertical nystagmus, slow saccadic eye movement, slight choreiform movements of arms, intention tremors, absent ankle reflexes and flexor plantars. Dysarthria was also present. Her male cousin presented at 3-4 years with ataxia gait and constant drooling. At age 20 years, he showed normal stature, had progressive unsteadiness in walking, dysarthria, drooling, vertical mystagmus and loss of pursuit movements, choreiform movement of the hands, moderate peripheral ataxia, dysdiadochokinesis, absent ankle reflexes, flexor plantars, decreased sensation to vibration and pinprick and pes cavus. There was no cutaneous telan-

giectasia and AFP and immunoglobulin levels were normal. The
proband showed an identical chromosome 11q22-23 haplotype as an
unaffected sibling using 21 markers. The two affected cousins
showed very little haplotype similarity and the proband did not
inherit the chromosome which in her cousin appears to contribute to A-T. A possible explanation is that she is homozygous
for a gene at a different locus and therefore the extended
family may be carrying more than one mutation for A-T. If two
separate loci were responsible for the A-T seen in this family,
then phenotypic differences might be expected between cousins.
Minor differences do exist e.g. height and drooling, but the
similarities appear stronger, especially the cellular radiosensitivity.

Heterogeneity at the clinical level

Evidence for heterogeneity can be analysed in a different
way based on clinical features but with the emphasis on details
such as age of onset of cerebellar symptoms, the rate of progress of symptoms, and the range of severity of symptoms. This
approach is more subjective but has the advantage of providing
a more complete clinical description with which some correla-
tions may be attempted however imperfect.

Table 2 shows the clinical features in which variation has
been observed. The age of onset of ataxia symptoms, infancy
versus childhood can be relatively easily distinguished. At
the extreme we are aware of two brothers one of whom developed
the first symptom of A-T in infancy and the other at age 10
years. Regarding the rate of progress of the ataxia, most
children are usually confined to a wheelchair early in teenage,
and find it impossible to move around the house on foot. Other
patients are still ambulatory in teenage or later however
poorly (see above).

In a study of 70 A-T individuals from 62 families the age
of onset of abnormal symptoms as judged by parents was under 1
year in 13/66 patients, under 2 years in 43/66 patients and
under 4 years of age in 56/66 patients. Abnormalities of
balance and gait were the first abnormalities noted by parents

215

Table 2: <u>Clinical and cellular features showing variations in</u>
<u>presentation</u>

1.   Cerebellar ataxia – age at onset.
                       rate of progress.
                       severity.

2.   Other cerebellar effects – speech.
                               Oculomotor dyspraxia.

3.   Telangiectasia – severity on bulbar conjunctivae.
                      presence elsewhere.

4.   Degree of humoral and cellular immunity.

5.   Suceptibility to infection.

6.   Cellular abormalities – variations in chromosomal radio-
                             sensitivity.
                             variations in colony forming
                             ability following exposure to
                             γ-rays.
                             variations in radioresistant DNA
                             synthesis.

Table 3:   <u>Simultaneous irradiation of blood cultures at G_2 from</u>
           <u>normal and A-T patients</u>

	No. cells	r	dic	f	ctg	ctb	csg	tri	qr
Following exposure to 1.0 Gray at G_2									
AT5BI	50	22*	1	9	84	53	0	5	2
AT19BI	50	1	0	3	16	10	0	1	0
Con 1584	50	0	0	3	9	5	0	2	1
Con 1585	50	0	0	1	8	6	1	0	0

* High level of rings in AT5BI are due to the presence of a
ring containing clone.

in 61 cases. Eight individuals who were symptomatic after age
4 years had a slower disease progression (Woods and Taylor,
1992).

According to Sedgwick and Boder (1991), the diagnostic
sine qua non remains early onset progressive cerebellar ataxia
with later onset oculocutaneous telangiectasia. They also
suggest that rates of progress of the disorder and its severity
may vary considerably from one patient to another. It has
become evident that milder forms of the disorder exist, with
respect to the cerebellar ataxia. Some patients with early
onset ataxia are still ambulatory at age 20 years or more
(Hernandez et al., 1992). Sedgwick and Boder (1991) described
two brothers in whom the disease had a slower course. The
younger brother although definitely ataxic was able to walk
unaided at age 18 years. The older brother was more markedly
ataxic but did not require a wheelchair until aged 21 years.
However, now in their 20s and 30s they present with classical
A-T.

The cerebellar ataxia is initially truncal but within 5
years peripheral co-ordination also becomes involved. Dystonia
and athetosis are seen in the majority of patients. All patients show apraxia of horizontal and vertical sacchadic eye
movements. Speech is dysarthric in all patients. The face is
impassive and relaxed.

One of the most striking variations in A-T patients is the
degree of ocular telangiectasia. In 70 patients, all but one
showed this feature (Woods and Taylor, 1992). The median age
at which telangiectasia was first noted was 6 years. In 15
cases, telangiectases were very marked causing cosmetic dis-
tress, and 6 patients had marked telangiectasia on the butter-
fly area of the face. Even within a family two affected
siblings can have striking differences in the degree of telangiectasia (Sedgwick and Boder, 1991). It is possible therefore
that heterogeneity in the degree of telangiectasia is influenced by other genes and not a purely allelic feature.
Sedgwick and Boder (1991) concede that it is conceivable that
ataxia-telangiectasia may exist without telangiectasia. This
may be true in rare cases as one extreme of the range of variation in this feature.

Aicardi et al. (1988) and Maserati et al. (1988) reported patients with ataxia without telangiectasia. It seems unlikely, however, that all these patients fall into a homogeneous grouping outside A-T, and it is possible that some represent true A-T patients with variations in presenting features. Interestingly, the two siblings described by Maserati et al. also have the spontaneous chromosomal abnormalities typical of A-T together with the early onset ataxia, but with normal IgA and serum AFP levels. Radiosensitivity studies were not undertaken in either study.

Heterogeneity of immunological abnormalities and susceptibility to infection

A-T patients display a variable dysgammaglobulinaemia with a characteristic selective deficiency of serum IgA, and serum IgE in association with normal or elevated levels of IgM. Total IgG levels can be low as can levels of IgG_2 and IgG_4. The thymus shows agenesis or may be absent, reflecting the defect in cellular immunity seen in all patients. The immunodeficiencies are very variable, even between affected individuals within a single family. Frequent sinopulmonary infection is a prominent feature in A-T patients but a low incidence of recurrent respiratory infection has been reported in some A-T patients (Roifman and Gelfand, 1985). Affected siblings may show a quite different susceptibility to recurrent infections.

Heterogeneity in the type of spontaneous chromosome abnormalities seen in A-T patients

The types and frequencies of spontaneously occurring chromosome abnormalities seen in A-T patients is remarkably consistent between patients. These consist almost entirely of lymphocyte translocations involving chromosomes 7 and 14. The translocations include inv(7)(p13q35), t(7;7)(p13;q35), t(7;14)(p13;q11), t(7;14)(q35;q11), t(14;14)(q11;q32),

inv(14)(q11q32) and t(X;14)(q28;q11). Most of these translocations occur at a low frequency in lymphocytes of non A-T patients. In A-T patients the frequency may be 50 times higher,
making these a useful aid in the diagnosis of the disorder.
Typically 10-15% of lymphocytes from an A-T patient may contain
a single translocation or inversion. Different translocations
may be represented in different cells or alternatively the same
translocation may be present possibly inferring clonal evolution. There appears to be little variation in the presentation
of these translocations, although as few as 2% of cells may
contain them.

Unusual families with ataxia-telangiectasia

These rare families display unusual features either in the
inheritance of the disorder or in the presenting clinical features, sufficient to make us question some established facts
concerning ataxia-telangiectasia. Some families, however,
clearly do not have ataxia-telangiectasia.

The first unusual family was described by Ying and
Decoteau in 1981. The proband was a Saskatchewan Mennonite in
whom a neurological disturbance was noted at age 10 years. At
age 44 years a diagnosis was made of spinocerebellar degeneration in association with choreiform movement. No telangiectasia was noted. At 52 years of age he was still walking, had
absent serum IgA, low serum IgE and increased serum levels of
AFP. His lymphocytes showed the typical chromosome translocations associated with A-T. He died of lymphoma at age 57
years. His sister was diagnosed with spinocerebellar degeneration and choreiform movement at age 46 years but again with no
telangiectasia. His niece developed ataxia at 12 months of age
and by 15 years was confined to a wheelchair. She also showed
bulbar telangiectasia and had severe sinopulmonary infections,
and died at 20 years of age from pneumonia.

The proband was clearly not a typical A-T patient, having
a mild ataxia and no telangiectasia, but with other features of
the disorder. His niece does appear to have been a typical A-T
patient.

Explanations for the occurrence of these similar disorders in two generations of the family are difficult to provide. Multiple allelism may be a possibility with the niece inheriting a different allele from her mother, although this seems unlikely. Consanguinity was not completely ruled out which might imply some form of anticipation (increasing severity with successive generations) if these are the same gene. The presence or absence of telangiectasia in this family may be of little significance as it is clear that this feature can be variable even between siblings.

Swift et al. (1986) show pedigrees of four unusual families with homozygotes in more than one sibship. In family A in particular, without evidence of consanguinity, A-T patients were apparently documented in four sibships.

Byrne et al. (1984) reported a family with three cases of ataxia without telangiectasia but with IgE deficiency. The patients were also unusual in showing very slow progression of the ataxia, dementia in all three cases, a normal serum level of AFP and no evidence of t(7;14) translocations in lymphocytes. There must be some doubt as to whether these were bona fide ataxia-telangiectasia patients.

Similarly the family of Terenty et al. (1978) showed apparent dominant inheritance of ataxia-telangiectasia. Although telangiectasia was present, IgA was low and AFP raised, the onset of the neurological disorder was clearly different from A-T. There was a predominant peripheral neuropathy. Evidence of cerebellar dysfunction was slight, making it more likely to be a hereditary axonal neuropathy.

Heterogeneity in radiosensitivity in ataxia-telangiectasia patients

The increased sensitivity of A-T cells to ionising radiation is well established using both chromosomal methods (Rary et al., 1975; Taylor et al., 1976) and by cell survival (Taylor et al., 1975). Chromosomal radiosensitivity is best observed following exposure during the G_2 phase of the cell cycle, since at this stage the differential between A-T and normal

cells is greatest. Chromatid type damage is the major form of
aberration observed at this stage. An interesting feature of
the increased chromosomal radiosensitivity of A-T cells is the
high level of chromatid type damage observed following exposure
of A-T cells to ionising radiation during the G_0 phase of the
cell cycle (Taylor et al., 1976). Over recent years it has
become clear that some A-T patients show a lower degree of
cellular radiosensitivity compared with others, as assessed by
either chromosomal radiosensitivity or by cell survival (Cox et
al., 1978; Fiorilli et al., 1985; Taylor et al., 1987; Chessa
et al., 1992).

When lymphocytes from a large group of A-T patients are
irradiated it can be seen that the level of induced damage is
very variable between patients, possibly indicating a heterogeneous response to the effects of ionising radiation. This
apparent range of chromosomal radiosensitivity may in part be
the result of dosimetric differences at different times, or the
result of irradiating different samples at different stages of
the cell cycle. When blood samples from patients are irradiated simultaneously, however, a variable response can again be
observed between patients indicating a truly heterogeneous
response (Taylor et al., 1987) (Table 3). When the colony
forming ability of fibroblasts from these patients is analysed,
no difference in survival is observed in cells from patients in
different complementation groups.

It is not clear if there is any relationship between the
level of chromosomal radiosensitivity and different complementation groups. Taylor et al. (1987) tentatively ranked into
groups patients who showed a different lymphocyte chromosomal
radiosensitivity even though their fibroblasts showed the same
level of colony forming ability. Three possible groups were
described; group 1 consisted of siblings AT2BI and AT8BI (complementation group E), with the highest level of induced
chromosome aberrations. Group 2 consisted of unrelated
patients AT5BI and AT17BI (complementation group D) and group 3
consisted of only patient AT7BI with a lower radiosensitivity.
The complementation group of this patient is not known. Repeat
samples of blood gave broadly the same levels of radiosensitivity for these individuals. More careful work on a variety of

samples from patients of known complementation groups would need to be undertaken in order to be sure that different complementation groups reflected different levels of chromosomal radiosensitivity.

In addition to heterogeneity of radiosensitivity within what might be called classical A-T patients there appears to be another group of patients showing a much lower level of chromosomal radiosensitivity. Some of these patients are particularly striking because in the presence of all the typical clinical features together with the spontaneous translocations involving chromosomes 7 and 14, there is no increased chromosomal radiosensitivity over normal. It is important to stress that there is no doubt about the clinical diagnosis of these A-T patients. Repeat blood samples from the same individuals show the same low/normal level of chromosomal radiosensitivity and affected siblings in these families are concordant for low induced levels of damage (unpublished results). We have now observed low chromosomal radiosensitivity in 15 patients in 12 families which is about 15% of all A-T families we have analysed. Interestingly the low chromosomal radiosensitivity in these individuals is reflected in a higher survival of fibroblasts exposed to γ-rays. The D_0 for fibroblasts for 'classical' A-T patients falls in the range 0.490-0.601 Gray (Taylor et al., 1987; Cox et al., 1978; Arlett et al., 1980; Weichselbaum et al., 1980) (Fig. 1). The D_0 value for the two radiosensitivity variants described by Taylor et al. (1987) were 0.809 and 0.756 Gray respectively. These are very similar to values of 0.80 and 0.78 Gray reported by Cox et al. (1978) for fibroblasts from two probable A-T patients, one of which we have confirmed chromosomally and by cell survival to have low radiosensitivity (AT1LO). There appears therefore firstly to be a genuine group of low radiosensitivity A-T patients, and secondly there is a general correlation between decreased lymphocyte chromosomal radiosensitivity and increased fibroblast survival in these patients. Jaspers et al. (1988) also reported two patients with a very mild form of A-T one of whose fibroblast cultures showed a D_0 = 0.98 only slightly lower than their normal range. Both Ziv et al. (1989) and Chessa et al. (1992) have also described

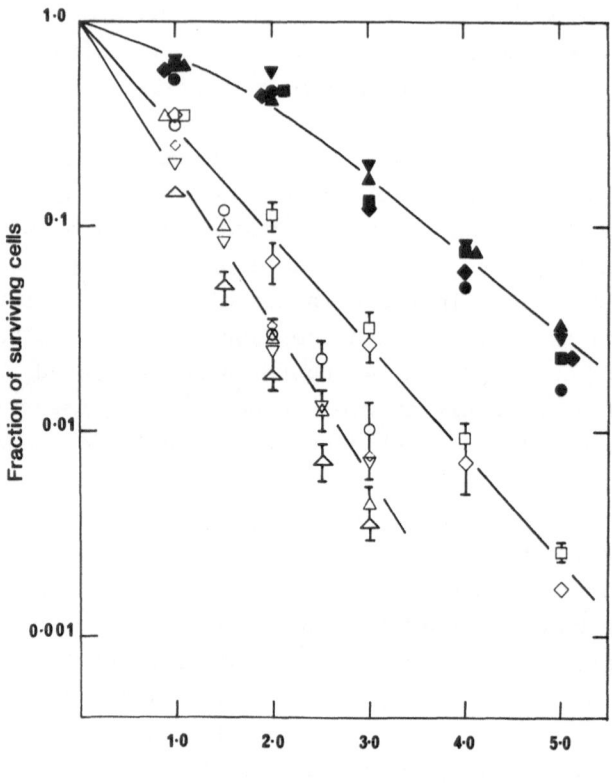

Dose of gamma rays(Gray)

<u>Figure 1</u>: Colony forming ability of normal and A-T fibroblast
strains following exposure of cells to γ-ray doses of 1-5Gy.
Four normal strains Con Bak, ▼ , Con Bri, ▲ , Con Bro, ■ ,
Con Cra, ◆ , gave a mean Do value of 1.273Gy. Five classical
A-T patients AT2BI, △ , AT3BI, ▽ , AT4BI, ◇ , AT5BI, ○ ,
and AT7BI, △ , gave a Do range of 0.490-0.601Gy. Do values
of the two intermediate radiosensitivity patients AT1AB, □ ,
and AT19BI, ◇ , gave Do values of 0.809 and 0.756Gy respectively. An unusual patient AT38BI, ● , gave a Do value in the
normal range (from Taylor <u>et al</u>., 1987, with permission).

strains of A-T fibroblasts showing a higher D_0 value following exposure to γ-rays although neither reported the levels of
ionising radiation-induced chromosome breaks in their fibroblast strains.

There appears to be some heterogeneity of response of DNA synthesis in these radiosensitivity variants following exposure of their cells to ionising radiation. In some variants the radioresistant DNA synthesis (RDS) response is the same as classical A-T patients (Taylor et al., 1987) (Fig. 2) but in other patients RDS has a normal response (Fiorilli et al., 1985; Jaspers et al., 1988; Ziv et al., 1989; Chessa et al., 1992), or possible intermediate response (Fiorilli et al., 1985; Chessa et al., 1992).

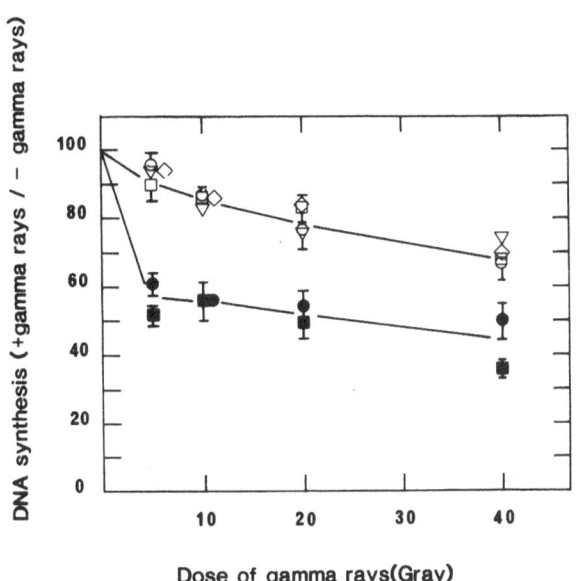

Dose of gamma rays(Gray)

Figure 2: The effect of increasing γ-ray dose on DNA synthesis in normal and A-T fibroblast strains. The normal strains Con Jon, ● , and Con Bro, ■ , are compared with two classical A-T patients AT3BI, ▽ , and AT5BI, △ , and two intermediate radiosensitivity patients AT1AB, □ , and AT19BI, ◇ . The classical and intermediate radiosensitivity patients show the same radioresistant DNA synthesis (from Taylor et al., 1987, with permission).

Ataxia-telangiectasia and Nijmegen Breakage Syndrome

It is intriguing that there is a second disorder which shows quite different clinical features compared with ataxia

telangiectasia, but an almost identical cellular phenotype.
This is the Nijmegen Breakage syndrome. Patients show microcephaly, short stature, a "bird-like" face, immunodeficiency,
café au lait spots and a predisposition to lymphoid tumours
(Hustinx et al., 1979; Weemaes et al., 1981; Taalman et al.,
1989). There appears to be some heterogeneity in the presentation of the disorder, but there is no cerebellar abnormality
(Hustinx et al., 1979; Weemaes et al., 1981; Taalman et al.,
1983; Conley et al., 1986; Jaspers et al., 1978; Seemanova
et al., 1985; Curry et al., 1989).

Translocations occur in T lymphocytes between chromosomes
7 and 14 at the same breakpoints as seen in A-T, giving for
example the t(7;14)(q35;q11) translocation or inv(7)(p14q35)
inversion. No inv(14)(q11q32) inversions have been observed in
NBS patients and t(14;14)(q11;q32) translocations are infreq-
uent (Taalman et al., 1989). The frequency of the 7/14 translocations in NBS patients is 20-25% which appears to be higher
than the average for A-T patients (10-15% of cells). There are
no reports of very large translocation clones in NBS patients
although far fewer patients have been examined compared with
A-T. An increased chromosomal sensitivity to X-rays and bleomycin has been reported as for A-T patients (Taalman et al.,
1983; Conley et al., 1986). Increased radiosensitivity is also
seen by fibroblast survival where again D_0 values are similar
to A-T fibroblasts (Jaspers et al., 1988). There is a lack of
inhibition of DNA synthesis in NBS cells following exposure of
cells to either γ-rays or bleomcyin (Taalman et al., 1983;
Jaspers et al., 1988). The cellular phenotypes of A-T and NBS
are clearly very similar.

NBS patients have been allocated to one of two complementation groups, V1 or V2, again using RDS as an indication of
complementation. Cell strains from all NBS patients will complement A-T cell strains suggesting these are quite different
mutations (Jaspers et al., 1988). Twins were described by
Curry et al. (1989) with features of both ataxia-telangiectasia
and NBS, A-T$_{FRESNO}$. They showed microcephaly,
mental retardation, progressive truncal ataxia, apraxic eye
movements, elevated serum AFP levels, increased chromosomal
breakage and increased cellular radiosensitivity. Partial

genetic complementation was observed with cells from A-T groups A, C and E as well as NBS group V2 cells, but not with complementation group V1. This suggests that the genetic effects of both disorders are related through a common pathway or perhaps involve the same gene. It is possible that different mutations in the same gene could give rise to different clinical phenotypes. A-T and NBS may be part of a spectrum of disorders and may not be entirely distant entities. It is possible therefore that additional clinical phenotypes may eventually be recognised which reflect further mutations in this region of the genome.

Conclusions

Patients with the classical form of A-T can be segregated according to complementation groups but as Table 1 suggests there are as yet no clinical or cellular features unique to any one complementation group. It is not known whether the low radiosensitivity variant individuals can also be segregated into some system of complementation groups. It is interesting, however, that the evidence suggests that the A-T gene in these patients may also map to chromosome 11q22-23.

At the clinical level, differences between A-T patients can be observed by symptoms resulting from cerebellar degeneration, particularly ataxia. In addition, difference in the degree of telangiectasia, immunodeficiency and frequency of upper respiratory tract infections are common. At the cellular level, clear differences in the level of radiosensitivity between individuals can be very striking. Between affected sib pairs, however, there is good concordance for the degree of cerebellar ataxia and also for cellular radiosensitivity. Other features including telangiectasia, the level of immunodeficiency and susceptibility to infections can be more variable between siblings. It seems likely therefore that the A-T mutation(s) has a more direct affect on cerebellar function and on cellular radiosensitivity and other features may be more easily influenced by additional genes.

Immunodeficiency and susceptibility to infections appears

Table 4: Groupings of ataxia telangiectasia and Nijmegen Breakage Syndrome in patients

Patient group	Ataxia	RDS (comple. group)	Gene Location	Radiosen. surv.	chrom.	Freq. (all A-T)	Comments
1.Classical A-T. (early onset ataxia. Telang. infect. immunodef. variable,RS & RDS)	++++	++++ (A)	11q22-23	++++	++++	85%	Gatti et al 1988 for gene location. Ziv et al 1989 for gene location. Kapp et al 1992 for gene location.
	++++	++++ (C)	11q22-23	++++	++++		
	++++	++++ (D)	11q22-23	++++	++++		
	++++	++++ (E)	?11q22-23	++++	++++		
2.Radiosensitivity variants of A-T. (later age of onset, poss. slow rate of progress).	++	++++ (?)	11q22-23	++	+	15%	Recombination events consistent with A-T gene being at 11q22-23 (unpublished). RDS may also be wild type or intermediate.
3.Ataxia variant of A-T	++	?	?	++++	++++	rare	Hernandez et al 1993
4.Nijmegen B.S.	-	++++ (V1)	?	++++	++++	rare	Jaspers et al 1988a,b. Taalman et al 1983. Conley et al 1986, Wegner et al 1988.
	-	++++ (V2)	?	++++	NK		
5.AT FRESNO	++	++++ (V1)	?	NK	NK	rare	Curry et al 1989, Jaspers et al 1988b.

RS - radiosensitivity; RDS - radioresistant DNA synthesis.

to be a more consistent feature of NBS, although the frequency of infections again appears to be episodic. In A-T patients, T cell tumours occur at a much higher frequency compared with the normal population, but it is not clear whether NBS patients are also more like to develop T cell tumours. A-T and NBS are distinct genes as shown by the ability of cells to complement each other, yet A-T$_{FRESNO}$ has the features of both disorders but is in NBS complementation group V1. This might imply that a mutation can occur at a step in a biochemical pathway common to both NBS and A-T. The similarity of the cellular responses to ionising radiation in NBS and A-T is very striking, but this cellular similarity does not preclude a quite different underlying molecular mechanism for each disorder.

The A-T patients and NBS patients can be grouped into one of five groupings given in Table 4. These are classical A-T patients (85% of total), radiosensitivity variants (15% of total) as well as the much rarer ataxia variants of A-T, NBS patients and AT FRESNO like patients.

Our understanding of the genetic groupings will obviously become much clearer once the mutations are identified. There are, meanwhile, several problems. Firstly, the evidence that not all A-T patients inherit the gene in an autosomal recessive fashion is quite compelling; on the other hand, the linkage evidence, based on a recessive model, gives very convincing evidence that the A-T gene(s) is on chromosome 11q22-23. Secondly, there appear to be rare A-T families in which the gene may not be on 11q22-23. Thirdly, there are clearly are families where the level of chromosomal radiosensitivity is no different from normal. As the chromosomal response to ionising radiation is one of the first screening tests for confirmation of the A-T diagnosis, there is perhaps a need in these patients to give extra weight to the presence of 7;14 translocations in the absence of increased chromosomal radiosensitivity, and assaying for survival using skin fibroblasts is indicated. The variation in radiosensitivity in A-T patients is now quite clear and forms part of the overall heterogeneity which is becoming more evident in this disorder.

References

Aicardi, J., Barbosa, C., Andermann, E., Andermann,. F., Morcos, R., Ghanem, Q., Fukuyama, Y., Awaya, Y., Moe, P. (1988) Ataxia-ocular motor apraxia: A syndrome mimicking ataxia telangiectasia. Ann. Neurol. 24:497-502

Arlett, C.F., Harcourt, S.A. (1980) Survey of radiosensitivity in a variety of human cell strains. Cancer Res. 40:926-932

Byrne, E., Hallpike, J.F., Manson, J.F., Sutherland, G.R., Thong, Y.H. (1984) Ataxia without telangiectasia. Progressive multisystem degeneration with IgE deficiency and chromosome instability. J. Neurol. Sci. 66:307-314

Chessa, L., Petrinelli, P., Antonelli, A., Fiorilli, R., Elli, R., Marcucci, L., Federico, A., Gandini, E. (1992) Heterogeneity in ataxia telangiectasia: classical phenotype associated with intermediate cellular radiosensitivity. Am. J. Med. Genet. 42:741-746

Conley, M.E., Spinner, M.B., Emanuel, B.S., Nowell, P.C., Nicholls, W.W. (1986) A chromosome breakage syndrome with profound immunodeficiency. Blood 67:1251-1256

Cox, R., Hosking, P., Wilson, J. (1978) Ataxia telangiectasia, evaluation of radiosensitivity in cultured skin fibroblasts as a diagnostic test. Arch. Dis. Child. 53:386-390

Curry, C.J.R., Tsai, J., Hutchinson, H.T., Jaspers, N.J.G., Wara, D., Gatti, R.A. (1989) AT FRESNO: A phenotype linking ataxia telangiectasia with the Nijmegen breakage syndrome. Am. J. Hum. Genet. 45:270-275

Foroud, T., Wei, S., Ziv, Y., Sobel, E., Lange, E., Chao, A., Goradia, T., Huo, Y., Tolun, A., Chessa, L., Charmley, P., Sanal, O., Salman, N., Julier, C., Concannon, P., McConville, C.M., Taylor, A.M.R., Shiloh, Y., Lange, K, Gatti, R.A. (1991) Localisation of an ataxia telangiectasia locus to a 3cM interval in chromosome 11q22-23: linkage analysis of 111 families of an international consortium. Am. J. Hum. Genet. 49:1263-1279

Fiorilli, M., Businco, L., Pandolfi, F., Paganelli, R., Russo, G., Aiuti, F. (1982) Heterogeneity of immunological abnormalities in ataxia telangiectasia. J. Clin. Immunol. 3:135-141

Fiorilli, M., Antonelli, A., Russo, G., Crescendi, M., Carbonari, M., Petrinelli, P. (1985) Variant of ataxia telangiectasia with low level radiosensitivity. Hum. Genet. 70:274-277

Gatti, R.A., Berkel, I., Boder, E., et al. (1989) Localisation of an ataxia telangiectasia gene to chromosome 11q22-23. Nature 336:577-580

Hustinx, T.W.J., Scheres, J.M.J.C., Weemaes, C.M.R., ter Haar, B.G.A., Janssen, A.H. (1979) Karyotype instability with multiple 7/14 and 7/7 rearrangements. Hum. Genet. 49:199-208

Hernandez, D., McConville, C.M., Stacey, M., Woods, C.G., Brown, M.M., Shutt, P., Rysiecki, G., Taylor, A.M.R. (1993) A family showing no evidence of linkage between the ataxia telangiectasiaa gene and chromosome 11q22-23. J. Med. Genet. (in press)

Jaspers, N.G.J., Bootsma, D. (1982) Genetic heterogeneity in ataxia telangiectasia studied by cell fusion. Proc. Natl.

Acad. Sci. (USA) 79:2641-2644

Jaspers, N.G.J., Gatti, R.A., Baan, C., Linssen, P.C.M.L., Bootsma, D. (1988a) Genetic complementation analysis of ataxia telangiectasiaa and Nijmegen Breakage Syndrome: a survey of 50 patients. Cytogenet. Cell. Genet. 49:259-263

Jaspers, N.G.J., Taalman, R.D.F.M., Baan, C. (1988b) Patients with an inherited syndrome characterised by immunodeficiency, microcephaly, and chromosomal instability: genetic relationship to ataxia telangiectasia. Am. J. Hum. Genet. 42:66-73

Kapp, L.N., Painter, R.B, Yu, L-C., van Loon, N., Richard, C.W., James, M.R., Cox, D.R., Murnane, J.P. (1992) Cloning of a candidate gene for ataxia telangiectasia group D. Am. J. Hum. Genet. 51:45-54

Komatsu, K., Kodama, S., Okumura, Y., Koi, M., Oshimura, M. (1989) Restoration of radiation resistance in ataxia telangiectasia cells by the introduction of normal human chromosome 11. Mutation Res. 235:59-63

Maserati, E., Ottolini, A., Veggiotti, P., Lanzi, G., Pasquali, F. (1988) Ataxia - without telangiectasia in two sisters with rearrangements of chromosomes 7 and 14. Clin. Genet. 34:283-287

McConville, C.M., Woods, C.G., Farrall, M., Metcalfe, J.A., Taylor, A.M.R., (1990a) Analysis of 7 polymorphic markers at chromosome 11q22-23 in 35 ataxia telangiectasia families: further evidence of linkage. Hum. Genet. 85:215-220

McConville, C.M., Formstone, C.J., Hernandez, D., Thick, J., Taylor, A.M.R. (1990b) Fine mapping of the chromosome 11q22-23 region using PFGE, linkage and haplotype analysis: localisation of the gene for ataxia telangiectasia to a 5cM region flanked by NCAM/DRD2 and STMY/CJ52.75/φ2.22. Nucleic Acids Res. 11:4335-4343

Morell, D., Cromartie, E. and Swift, M. (1986) Mortality and cancer incidence in 263 patients with ataxia telangiectasia. J. Natl. Cancer Inst. 77:89-92

Murnane, J.P., Painter, R.B. (1982) Complementation of the defects in DNA synthesis in irradiated and unirradiated ataxia telangiectasia cells. Proc. Natl. Acad. Sci. (USA) 79:1960-1963

Rary, J.M., Bender, M.A., Kelly, T.E. (1974) Cytogenetic status of ataxia telangiectasia. Am. J. Hum. Genet. 26:70A

Roifmann, C.M., Gelfand, E.W. Heterogeneity of the immunological deficiency in ataxia telangiectasia: absence of a clinical pathological correlation. In: Gatti, R.A. and Swift, M. (eds). Ataxia telangiectasiaa, New York, Alan R. Liss Inc. 1985 pp3-87

Sedgwick, R.P., Boder, E. Ataxia telangiectasia. In: J.M.B.V. de Jong (ed). Handbook of Clinical Neurology. Hereditary Neuropathies and Spinocerebellar Atrophies. Vol. 16, pp 347-423. Amsterdam: Elsevier Science Publishers BV (1991)

Seemanova, E.E., Passarge, E., Beneskova, D., Houstek, J., Kasel, P., Sevcikova, M. (1985) Familial microcephaly with normal intelligence, immunodeficiency and risk for lymphoreticular malignancies. Am. J. Med. Genet. 20:639-648

Sobel, E., Lange, E., Jaspers, N.E.J., Chessa, L., Sanal, O., Shiloh, Y., Taylor, A.M.R., Weemaes, C.M.A., Lange, K., Gatti, R.A. (1992) Ataxia-telangiectasia: linkage evidence for genetic heterogeneity. Am. J. Hum. Genet. 20:1343-1348

Spector, B.D., Filipovich, A.H., Perry, G.S., Kersey, J.H. (1982) Epidemiology of cancer in ataxia telangiectasia. In: Bridges B.A., Harnden, D.G. (eds). Ataxia telangiectasia - a cellular and molecular link between cancer neuropathology and immune deficiency. John Wiley, Chichester, p103-138

Swift, M., Morell, D., Cromartie, E., Chamberlin, A.R., Skolnick, M.H., Bishop, D.H. (1986) The indicence and gene frequency of ataxia telangiectasia in the United States. Am. J. Hum. Genet. 39:573-583

Taalman, R.D.F.M., Jaspers, N.G.J., Scheres, J.M.J.C., de Wit, J., Hustinx, T.W.J. (1983) Hypersensitivity to ionising radiation in vitro in a new chromosome breakage disorder, the Nijmegen breakage syndrome. Mutation Res. 112:23-32

Taalman, R.D.F.M., Hustinx, T.W.J., Weemaes, C.M.R., Seemanova, E., Schmidt, A., Passarge, E., Scheres, J.M.J.C. (1985) Further delineation of the Nijmegen breakage syndrome. Am. J. Med. Genet. 32:425-431

Taylor, A.M.R., Harnden, D.G., Arlett, C.F., Harcourt, S.A., Lehmann, A.R., Stevens, S., Bridges, B.A. (1975) Ataxia telangiectasia: a human mutation with abnormal radiation sensitivity. Nature 258:427-429

Taylor, A.M.R., Metcalfe, J.A., Oxford, J.M., Harnden, D.G. (1976) Is chromatid type damage in ataxia telangiectasia after irradiation at Go a consequence of defective repair? Nature 260:441-443

Taylor, A.M.R., Butterworth, S.V. (1986) Clonal evolution of T cell chronic lymphocytic leukaemia in a patient with ataxia telangiectasia. Int. J. Cancer 37:511-516

Taylor, A.M.R., Flude, E., Laher, B., Stacey, M., McKay, E., Watt, J., Green, S.H., Harding, A.E. (1987) Variant forms of ataxia telangiectasia. J. Med. Genet. 24:669-677

Taylor, A.M.R., Lowe, P.A., Stacey, M., Thick, J., Campbell, L., Beatty, D., Biggs, P., Formstone, C.J. (1992) Development of T cell leukaemia in an ataxia telangiectasia patient following clonal selection in t(X;14) containing cells. Leukaemia 6:961-966

Terenty, T.R., Robson, P., Walton, J.N. (1978) Presumed ataxia telangiectasia in a man. Brit. Med. J. 2:802

Woods, C.G., Bundey, S.E., Taylor, A.M.R. (1990) Unusual features in the inheritance of ataxia telangiectasia. Hum. Genet. 84:555-562

Woods, C.G., Taylor, A.M.R. (1992) Ataxia telangiectasia in the British Isles. The clinical and laboratory features of 70 affected individuals. Quart. J. Med. New Series 82 No. 298 pp169-179

Weemaes, C.M.R., Hustinx, J.W.J., Scheres, J.M.J.G., van Munster, P.J.J., Bakkeren, J.A.J.M., Taalman, R.D.F.M. (1981) A new chromosomal instability disorder. The Nijmegen breakage syndrome. Acta Paed. Scand. 70:557-564

Wegner, R.D., Metzger, M., Hanefield, F., Jaspers, N.G.J., Baan, C., Magdorf, K., Kunze, J. (1988) A new chromosomal instability disorder confirmed by complementation studies. Clin. Genet. 33:20-32

Weichselbaum, R.R., Nove, J. Little, J.B. (1980) X-ray sensitivity of fifty-three human diploid fibroblast cell strains

from patients with characterised genetic disorders. Cancer
Res. 40:920-925

Ying, K.L., Decoteau, W.E. (1981) Cytogenetic anomalies in a
patient with ataxia, immune deficiency and high alpha-feoto-
protein in the absence of telangiectasiaa. Cancer Genet.
Cytogenet. 4:311-317

Ziv, Y., Amiel, A., Jaspers, N.G.J., Berkel, A.I., Shiloh, Y.
(1989) Ataxia telangiectasia: a variant with altered in
vitro phenotype of fibroblast cells. Mutation Res.
210:211-219

Ziv., Rotman, G., Frydman, M., Dagan, J., Cohen, T., Foroud,
T., Gatti, R.A., Shiloh, Y. (1991) The ATC (ataxia telan-
giectasia group C) locus localises to chromosome 11q22-23.
Genomics 9:373-375

Acknowledgements

We thank the Cancer Research Campaign (U.K.), the Ataxia
Telangiectasia Society, the Thomas Appeal (A-T Medical Research
Trust U.K.) and the Medical Research Council for continued
support.

VI. Overviews

Biochemical Defects in Ataxia-Telangiectasia

Martin F. Lavin

Queensland Cancer Fund Research Unit

Queensland Institute of Medical Research

The Bancroft Centre

300 Herston Road,

Brisbane QLD 4029

Australia

Ever since it was established by Thieffry et al (1961) that a deficiency in serum IgA existed in ataxia-telangiectasia (A-T), considerable effort has been expended in attempting to determine the biochemical defect in this disease. While there are several cellular and molecular abnormalities associated with A-T, a description of the actual defect at a molecular level remains elusive. The existence of up to 5 complementation groups adds to the difficulty of describing a single biochemical abnormality.

The description of cellular hypersensitivity to ionizing radiation by Taylor et al (1975) largely shaped the emphasis of research into the nature of this defect over the past 18 years. This observation, together with the description of chromosome instability and a propensity to develop tumours, paved the way for a variety of studies designed to investigate possible abnormalities in chromatin structure, defective DNA processing as well as gene mapping and cloning.

Hypersensitivity to radiation, an important hallmark, could not be explained by reduced excision of damaged sites in DNA, reduced capacity to repair strand breaks or by reduced activity of enzymes involved in oxygen radical metabolism. Attempts to associate the increased sensitivity with cellular levels of thiol

NATO ASI Series, Vol. H 77
Ataxia-Telangiectasia
Edited by R. A. Gatti and R. B. Painter
© Springer-Verlag Berlin Heidelberg 1993

compounds and other radical scavengers have produced mixed results. Radio-resistant DNA synthesis was shown to be a universal trait in A-T as was abnormality in cell cycle traverse post-irradiation. DNA topoisomerase II, an enzyme involved in altering DNA supercoiling, was demonstrated to be either reduced or increased in A-T cells. More recently an abnormality in the cellular distribution of a specific DNA-binding protein has been described. This protein is translocated from the cytoplasm/perinuclear region to the nucleus in response to radiation damage in control cells but is constitutively present in the nucleus in A-T cells. At this stage a unifying model to fit these various anomalies to the A-T phenotype remains unresolved. In this chapter studies on the various biochemical parameters investigated in A-T will be reviewed and an attempt will be made to relate some of the abnormalities described.

General

A review of the literature over the last 20 years reveals a variety of biochemical studies aimed at delineating the basic defect in this syndrome. Most of these studies have been based on the major characteristics of the disease that include immunodeficiency, developmental abnormalities, sensitivity to ionizing radiation, chromosome instability, defective DNA processing and predisposition to cancer (Sedgwick and Boder 1991). A comprehensive list of molecular and cellular changes observed in A-T cells with or without response to ionizing radiation appears in Table 1. At first glance the list appears to reflect the apparent unrelatedness of the major progressive components of this disease, such as oculocultaneous telangiectasia, cerebellar ataxia and sinopulmonary infection (Boder 1985). This list can be somewhat simplified by regrouping the various abnormalities under 10 areas varying from radiosensitivity to altered cell receptor binding capacity (Table 2). In this article, I will review the evidence for some of these abnormalities and attempt to produce a unifying hypothesis to explain the divergent observations. Without knowledge of the basic defect(s) in A-T this, of course, becomes a difficult task.

Table 1

BIOCHEMICAL/CELLULAR ABNORMALITIES IN A-T

IgA, IgE ↓	DNA-PROTEIN BINDING
IgG SUBCLASS IMBALANCE	DIFFUSIBLE FACTOR
LOW MOLECULAR WEIGHT IgM ↑	CLASTOGENIC FACTOR
AFP ↑	CATALASE ↓
CEA ↑	dRp MODIFICATION
FIBRONECTIN EXPRESSION	HEPATIC DYSFUNCTION
MEMBRANE PROTEINS	GLUCOSE INTOLERANCE
ACTIN DEGRADATION	INSULIN RESISTANCE
RADIOSENSITIVITY	INSULIN RECEPTORS
RADIOMIMETIC AGENTS	GROWTH RETARDATION
LONGER S PHASE	DEFECTIVE T CELL FUNCTION
REDUCED G1 PHASE DELAY	INAPPROPRIATE TCR EXPRESSION
PROLONGED G2 PHASE DELAY (G1 + S PHASE CELLS)	α/β - γ/δ IMBALANCE
RADIORESISTANT DNA SYNTHESIS	TELANGIECTASIA FACTOR
RADIORESISTANT DNA SYNTHESIS FACTOR	DHFR AMPLIFICATION
CHROMOSOME BREAKS	SV40 - T ANTIGEN - RADIORESISTANCE
CHROMOSOME REARRANGEMENTS	ABNORMAL TRANSCRIPTION
RECOMBINASE DEFECT	POLY ADP-RIBOSE SYNTHESIS
INACCURATE BREAK REJOINING	NUCLEOMEGALY
RESIDUAL STRAND BREAKS	ABNORMAL DEVELOPMENT
DNA REPAIR DEFECT	MUTATION FREQUENCY ↓
ALKALI STABLE ADDUCTS	CANCER PREDISPOSITION
HCR OF ADENOVIRUS 2	
POTENTIALLY LETHAL DAMAGE REPAIR (PLDR) ABSENT	
CHROMATIN ACCESSIBILITY	
TOPOISOMERASE II	
ETOPOSIDE SENSITIVITY	

The description of chromosomal instability in A-T shaped the way for a variety of studies on the DNA repair capability of cells from these individuals (Paterson et al 1976; Vincent et al 1975; Lavin and Davidson 1981; Cornforth and Bedford 1985; Mirzayans et al 1989). While this seemed a logical approach, given the correlation between UV sensitivity and defective DNA repair in xeroderma pigmentosum (Cleaver 1968), in the case of A-T it is much more complex, possibly involving a defect in DNA processing (Hanawalt and Painter 1985). However, it is possible that the chromosomal instability could be explained by a defect at one of the many stages involved in the transmission of a particular stimulus from the level of the plasma membrane to chromatin.

Table 2

CHARACTERISTICS OF A-T

RADIOSENSITIVITY
CELL CYCLE BEHAVIOUR
IMPAIRED GLUTATHIONE BIOSYNTHESIS
ALTERED GENE EXPRESSION
ACTIN ABNORMALITIES
GROWTH RETARDATION
Ig SUPERFAMILY REGULATION
DEVELOPMENTAL ABNORMALITIES
ALTERED SURFACE PROTEINS/RECEPTORS
DISTRIBUTION OF DNA-BINDING PROTEIN

Cell surface and membrane studies

A cardinal clinical feature of A-T is recurrent sinopulmonary infection which probably reflects defects in both B and T cells (Waldmann 1982). It seems likely that a defect in tissue differentiation could account for the immune dysfunction and indeed some of the other features of A-T. The immune disorders and the propensity to develop lymphoid malignancies might be explained by abnormalities in cellular interactions leading to self regulation by cells of the immunological system (Waldmann 1982).

There exists some evidence for aberrations in membrane proteins/receptors in A-T. This includes reduced responses of cells to growth factors (Shiloh et al 1982), altered cell morphology and microfilament array (McKinnon 1987), failure to express immunoglobulin isotypes for genes located most distantly 3^l to IgH variable genes and abnormal ratios of γ/δ to α/β - bearing T cells (Carbonari et al 1990), enhanced expression of procollagenase (Aggeler and Murnane 1990), aberrations in plasma membrane potential; increased CD3 expression (Boutin et al 1987), abnormalities in number and affinity of insulin receptors, loss of a major lymphocyte cell surface protein (Ozer et al 1985), altered synthesis of surface proteins (Murnane and Painter 1983; Lavin and Seymour 1984), presence of heat stable E-receptors in A-T leukaemia blasts (Dussault et al 1977), reduced concanavalin A capping (Gatti et al 1982) and abnormalities in DNA - induced blastogenesis (O'Connor and Scott-Linthicum 1980).

While there is some evidence for an actual defect at the level of the membrane, the results of O'Connor and Scott-Linthicum (1980) suggest that PHA binding to the membrane is normal but a defect of cytoplasmic-nuclear interaction could account for failure to induce blastogenesis, perhaps as a result of a failure to generate a cytoplasm to nucleus signal or an inability of the nucleus to respond. Paterson (1991) has also suggested that a defect may exist in the circuitry of a mitogenic signal transduction pathway in A-T cells. (this volume)

All of these surface changes could be explained by a defect in a gene regulating the expression of a number of genes.

240

Cytoskeletal abnormalities

McKinnon and Burgoyne (1985a) reported an unusual decrease in levels of actin in A-T lymphoblastoid cells. As actin decreased, an increase in a 37 kD protein was observed, which was shown to be actin-like from peptide analysis. It seems likely that actin is proteolytically cleaved to the 37 kD sized molecule in A-T lymphoblastoid cells. This degradation of actin was not evident in A-T fibroblasts. Immunofluorescence studies also showed that actin-containing microfilaments were altered in their arrangement in A-T cells and, after disruption by agents such as DMSO, recovery was slower (McKinnon and Burgoyne 1985b). Other studies using anti-actin fluorescent antibodies have shown that A-T cells possess fewer actin "cables" that are shorter in length and more dispersed compared to the pattern in normal cells (Becker 1986). In view of these findings, McKinnon (1987) postulated that the anomaly in A-T may exist at the level of the actin cytoskeleton, which could account for several of the seemingly diverse facets of the syndrome. Since there are several actin-binding proteins in the cell and since these interactions are influenced by physiological stimuli such as $[Ca^{2+}]$ (Vandorckhove, 1990), it is conceivable that a defect in actin or one of these proteins could have wide-ranging effects similar to those seen in A-T. For example, actin appears to have an involvement in control of gene expression (Scheer et al 1984), in chromatin condensation (Jamil 1984) and in the organisation of the structure of chromatin (Ashall and Puck 1984). In addition, interference with cytoskeletal function appears to be linked to genome instability (Lechner et al 1985); it would also help to explain the concanavalin A capping abnormality described by Gatti et al (1982).

Metabolic abnormalities

A great deal of emphasis has been placed on investigating possible defects in the ability of cells to cope with radiation damage to DNA. As will be discussed in a later section, it is unlikely that the radiosensitivity observed in A-T cells is due to a defect in excision repair of radiation damage (McKinnon 1987). Since A-T cells are particularly sensitive to oxidative damage, it has been suggested that reduced detoxification of active oxygen species might account for the sensitivity. Glutathione peroxidase is capable of detoxifying hydrogen peroxide, a byproduct of radiation damage. Given the failure to describe a repair defect in A-T cells, it seemed likely that some impairment in gluthatione metabolism might account for the increased sensitivity to radiation. Indeed, increased sensitivity to such agents as adriamycin and hydrogen peroxide support this contention (Shiloh et al 1985). Meredith and Dodson (1987) demonstrated that A-T fibroblasts and lymphoblasts failed to resynthesize glutathione after depletion of this compound. This could be explained by a reduced ability to accumulate cysteine, a limiting substrate for glutathione biosynthesis. Transport of both cysteine and cystine was shown to be 8- and 5- fold slower, respectively, in A-T cells than in controls. While a reduced ability to resynthesize glutathione seemed to be an attractive explanation for the defect in A-T cells, it later became apparent that this was not generally observed. Dean et al (1988) demonstrated that this was not a consistent feature of A-T cells, regardless of complementation group.

With the exception of the studies on glutathione biosynthesis, there is remarkably little information on other metabolic abnormalities in this syndrome. A consistent feature of A-T is reduced levels of serum IgA and IgE, as well as imbalances in IgG subclasses (Rivat-Peran et al 1981; Gatti et al 1982; Oxelius et al 1982; Waldmann 1982). Partial defects in both B- and T-cell function contribute to impaired antibody response in A-T. While the B cell defect can be explained in part by a helper T cell deficiency, it is also apparent that the basic defect in A-T must account for some of the dysfunction. At this stage most of the evidence would seem to preclude a biochemical defect in Ig synthesis or turnover but rather point to a defect in some aspect of isotype switching (Waldmann et al 1982; Davis et al 1985).

Radiosensitivity

Of all the characteristics described for A-T cells, radiosensitivity has played the most important role in determining the emphasis of research into the biochemical basis of this disease over the past 15 years. *In vivo* sensitivity of A-T patients to radiation was first demonstrated by Gotoff et al (1967) and Morgan et al (1968); Taylor et al (1975) were the first to describe hypersensitivity of A-T cells in culture. A number of other reports confirmed this observation in other cell types (Chen et al 1978; Paterson et al 1979; Cole et al 1988). It is not surprising that considerable effort was made to equate the radiation hypersensitivity in A-T cells with a reduced capacity to remove radiation damage from DNA, as had been described previously for xeroderma pigmentosum in cell lines where increased UV sensitivity could be explained by reduced or absent excision repair (Cleaver and Kraemer 1989, Robbins 1989). One report observed a repair defect in two A-T cell lines exposed to radiation damage (Paterson et al 1977). In all other lines it was not possible to detect a deficit in excision repair of radiation damage. However, more recent data by Mirzayans et al (1989) provide evidence that faulty execution of the excision repair process operating on alkali-stable 4NQO adducts occurs in three A-T cell lines. Since A-T cells show additional anomalies to radiosensitivity, including radioresistant DNA synthesis (Houldsworth and Lavin 1980, Painter and Young 1980) and abnormal chromosomal rearrangements involving hot spots for genetic recombination (Davis et al 1985), the phrase "DNA processing defect" has been suggested to describe the defect in this syndrome (Hanawalt and Painter 1985; Hanawalt and Sarasin 1986).

Over the years a number of attempts have been made to describe a defect at the level of chromatin structure or in the recognition of that structure as a means of explaining chromosomal instability and other abnormalities in A-T (Lavin and Davidson 1981; Painter 1982; Smith 1984). The various observations made with A-T cells that can be related to a defect at the level of chromatin are depicted in Figure 1. One report by Smith (1984), using the DNA ligand bis-benzimidazole, demonstrated increased sensitivity in A-T cells, increased ligand-induced breaks, and an enhanced accessibility to chromatin. More recently, Pandita and Hittleman (1992a) showed that A-T cells had nearly two-fold higher initial levels of chromosome damage than normal cells in both G1 and G2 phases of the cell cycle. They suggested that this may be due to a higher rate of conversion of DNA double-strand breaks into chromosome breaks in A-T cells, perhaps as a consequence of difference in chromatin organization or stability. Other studies have failed to find any anomalies in chromatin structure in A-T cells.

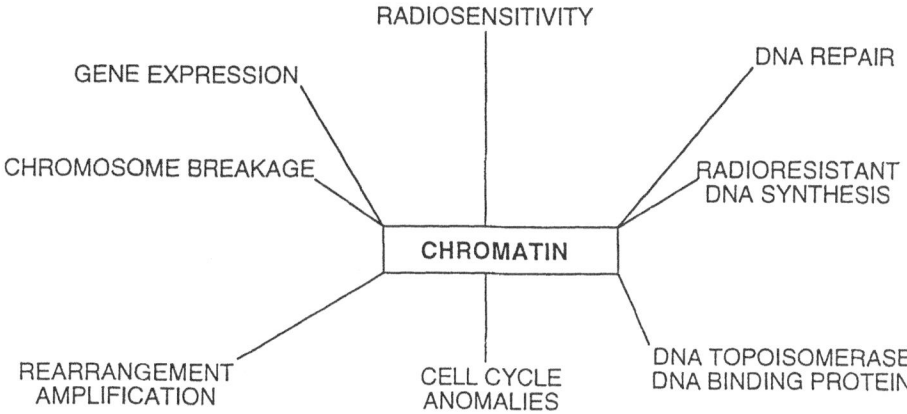

Figure 1: Chromatin structure/function anomalies in A-T

A variety of enzymes associated with the processing of DNA in normal and damaged cells are present at normal levels in A-T cells. However, some reports had pointed to defects in DNA toposomerase II (Mohamed et al 1987; Singh et al 1988) and in an activity that modifies deoxyribose-phosphate residues (dRp) present in A-T cell extracts (Karam et al 1990). Reduced activity of DNA topoisomerase II, assayed by unknotting of P4 phage DNA, was demonstrated in partially purified extracts from five A-T lymphoblastoid cell lines. The reduction in activity was greater than 10-fold in four of the cell lines (Singh et al 1988). On the other hand, later northern and western blot analyses failed to reveal any changes in expression of the topoisomerase II gene or in the size or amount of the protein produced (Singh and Lavin 1989). In contrast to the results described for A-T lymphoblastoid cells, Davies et al (1989) described elevated topoisomerase II activity in transformed and untransformed A-T fibroblasts compared to controls. The increased activity was also reflected in a several-fold higher level of topoisomerase II protein. Taken together, these apparently conflicting results suggest that the central defect in A-T cells does not reside in the topoisomerase II *per se*. In addition, the three most common A-T genes have been localized to 11q (Gatti et al 1988; McConville et al 1990; Foroud et al 1991; Komatsu et al 1991) whereas topoisomerase II is localized to chromosome 17 (Tsai-Pflugfelder et al 1988). However, the changes in topoisomerase II activity could be accounted for by aberrations in an associated protein as part of a DNA repair complex or replisome (see below).

Another hallmark of A-T is an increased level of chromosome aberrations, which is most marked in cells exposed to ionizing radiation (Taylor 1982). Extensive studies have failed to reveal a reduced capacity of A-T cells to repair single strand breaks in DNA, and only one report points to an abnormality in the repair of double strand breaks (Pandita and Hittleman 1992b). Cornforth and Bedford (1985) have also shown that a higher fraction of unrejoined prematurely condensed chrosomes (DCCs) is found in A-T cells after irradiation. In an investigation into the fate of 5' terminal base-free deoxyribose-phosphate (dRp) at strand interruptions in DNA, Karam et al (1990) observed that A-T lymphoblastoid cell extracts produced a covalent modification of dRp whereas control extracts failed to do so. This activity was present in control extracts but was inhibited by a heat-stable low molecular weight component. The inhibitor appears to be absent in A-T cells. To date the structure of the modified form of dRp has not been determined and the significance of this finding to the biochemical defect in A-T remains unresolved.

Protein activation and gene induction

Stress-causing agents cause the preferential transcription of some genes and in other cases the activation of pre-existing proteins (Angel et al 1986, Boothman et al 1989; Kramer et al 1990; Singh and Lavin 1990). Exposure of cells to ionizing radiation leads to increased expression of EGRI, c-jun and gadd45 (Hallahan et al 1991; Papathanisiou et al 1991; Kasten et al, this volume). We have recently described the "activation" of a DNA-binding protein in human cells exposed to ionizing radiation (Singh and Lavin 1990). This factor is normally present in the cytoplasm of unirradiated cells and appears to be translocated to the nucleus in response to damage by ionizing radiation and radiomimetic agents. Translocation is transient, reaching a maximum in the nucleus at 1 hr post-irradiation and disappearing from the nucleus after 7 hr. This protein was first detected using the SV40 enhancer as a substrate and the binding site was localized to nucleotides 247-249 in the 5^{l} flanking sequence of the distal repeat, between the AP-3 and AP-5 binding sites (Singh and Lavin 1990). More recently we have shown that the enhancer of the immunoglobulin K chain gene contains such a binding site, and multiple sites exist in human genomic DNA (Hobson et al 1991). Purification of this activity revealed the presence of three DNA-binding species and the factor with highest binding affinity had an approximate molecular weight of 70 kDa (Teale et al 1992). Binding activity was found to be dependent on phosphorylation.

The DNA-binding activity found in normal cell nuclei post-irradiation was constitutively present in nuclei from A-T cells (unpublished results). Activity was present in unirradiated nuclear extracts from three A-T cell lines, was not detected in two control lines and was present only at a low level in two other controls. Exposure to ionizing radiation did not alter the amount of DNA-binding activity in A-T nuclei but led to an increase in activity in nuclei from five control cell lines. Purification of the binding activities from A-T nuclei and control cytoplasm revealed a similar pattern of activity (unpublished results). South-western blot analysis and UV-crosslinking identified a major activity at 70 kDa and two minor binding species at 31 kDa and 47 kDa. Comparison of some of the properties of the binding factor in control and A-T samples failed to reveal any differences in activity or stability.

The initial response of cells to a variety of stimuli relies on the presence of pre-existing proteins (Kingston et al 1987; Glazer et al 1989; Kramer et al 1990). These proteins may be present in the cytoplasm or as part of a complex as in the case of the glucocorticoid receptor and heat shock protein 90 (Schuh et al 1985; Lindquist 1986), bound to an inhibitor as for NF-kB (Baeuerle and Baltimore 1988), or in free-form but requiring modification prior to translocation (Yamamoto et al 1988; Dale et al 1989; Gonzalez et al 1989). In the present case, a specific DNA-binding protein appears to move from the cytoplasm to the nucleus in response to radiation damage. It is possible that this protein is a transcription factor acting like the heat shock transcription factor that enters the nucleus after heat treatment and induces the transcription of several heat shock genes (Velasquez and Lindquist 1984; Wu 1985). Candidate genes for the action of a putative transcription factor would be early response genes such as c-*jun* and gadd45 (Hallahan et al 1991; Papathanasiou et al 1991). Because we have shown that there are multiple binding sites for the protein in the human genome (Hobson et al 1991), it is possible that it plays a role other than in transcription in altering the structure of chromatin and in this way modulates the DNA replicative machinery of the cell. Since the binding activity appears to be heterogeneous, it is likely that several proteins are involved in the response. The timing of the appearance of the protein in the nucleus and its subsequent loss is compatible with a role in the inhibition/recovery of DNA synthesis post-irradiation. The constitutive presence of such an activity in unirradiated A-T cells might lead to an abnormal response after irradiation. This might be compared to loss of responsiveness of cells to hormonal treatment after a period of saturation treatment or to the de-regulation of cyclic AMP responsive element binding protein (CREB) in the presence of continuing high levels of cAMP and protein kinase A (Hagiwara et al 1992). If the factor(s) had a role in the inhibition/recovery of DNA synthesis post-irradiation, prolonged exposure, leading to loss of responsiveness, might account for the radioresistant DNA synthesis observed in this syndrome (Lavin and Schroeder 1988).

Speculation and future direction

One of the consistent anomalies observed in A-T cells is the abnormal cell cycle traverse. Exposure of A-T cells to ionizing reduction leads to an abnormally high accumulation of G1 and S phase cells in the G2/M phase of the cycle (Ford et al 1984, Bates and Lavin 1985), reduced delay in passage through mitosis of cells in the G2 phase at the time of irradiation (Scott and Zampetti-Bosseler 1982), and a reduced inhibition of movement of cells from G1 into S phase post-irradiation (Nagasawa and Little 1983; Imray et al 1983). Overall it appears that A-T cells fail to show the initial delay in progression through or exit from the various phases of the cell cycle in response to radiation damage but on completion of S phase these cells undergo a prolonged accumulation if G2/M (Beamish and Lavin - unpublished data). It is of interest that the protein kinase cdc2, together with various cyclins and other factors, control the passage of cells from G1→S, through S phase and from G2→M. Thus it is possible that the defect in A-T is related to cell cycle control.

A recent report by Rowley et al (1992) demonstrated that the *wee*1 protein kinase is required for radiation-induced mitotic delay in *Schizosaccharomyces pombe*. This delay occurs in response to DNA damage, does not involve the phosphatase (Cdc25) and is thus distinct from delay due to inhibition of DNA synthesis (Enoch and Nurse 1990). It seems likely that the *wee*1 product must be activated after irradiation to impose G2 delay. As outlined in Figure 2, this implies that an unknown phosphatase (induced/activated by radiation) dephosphorylates the *wee*1 product which in turn phosphorylates cdc2 on Tyr15, inactivates it and causes mitotic delay. Such a phosphatase might be activated by ionizing radiation as described for cells undergoing radiation-induced apoptosis (Baxter and Lavin 1992). The very pronounced G2/M phase delay observed after irradiation of A-T cells might be explained by a defect in cdc2 or in the inactivation of cdc2 by phosphorylation, implying that the defect might occur as the mammalian equivalent of *wee*1 or its activation/inactivation. Passage of cells from G1→S and through S, which is also abnormal in A-T after irradiation, could also be accounted for by an abnormality in cdc2 or the related factor, cdk2. The product of the tumour suppressor gene p53 which plays an important role in the transition from G1 to S phase could also be a candidate (Lane 1992). Cell lines lacking p53 or with dominant mutations in the gene fail to exhibit G1 arrest after irradiation and as observed with A-T cells they accumulate in G2 phase (Kastan et al 1991). Determination of the level of expression of factors involved in controlling passage of cells through the cycle, the effects of irradiation on expression, and the phosphorylation states of some of these factors in the presence and absence of irradiation, should provide information on possible abnormalities in A-T cells.

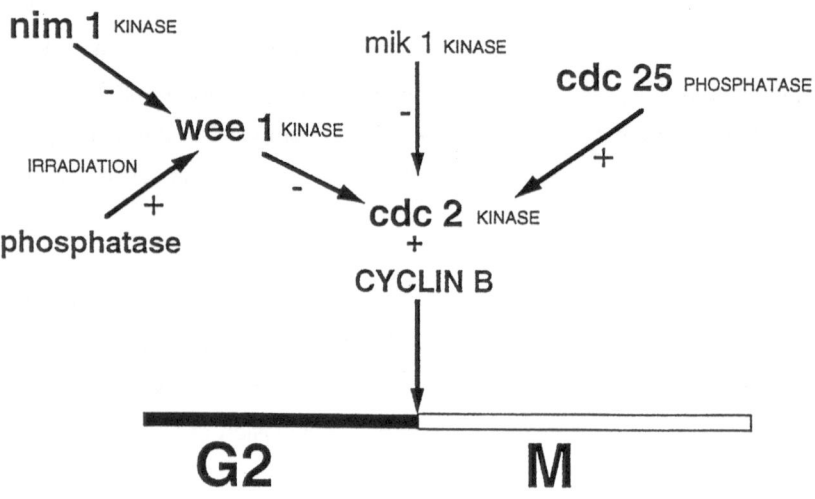

Figure 2: Radiation-induced mitotic delay   Based on Rowley et al 1992

Over the last several years the emphasis on A-T has shifted from the more phenomenonological approach to gene mapping and isolation. Attempts to isolate A-T genes using positional and complementational cloning are described elsewhere in this book. The description of five (A,C,D,E,Vi) complementation groups in this syndrome adds to the complexity. It appears likely that three of the complementation groups map to loci on the long arm of chromosome 11. The products of these genes may be part of a multimeric complex for which a defect in a single subunit may be sufficient to inactivate the molecule and produce the A-T phenotype. An example of this might be a DNA binding protein or a family of binding proteins which interacted with other proteins or families of proteins to confer specificity in the control of gene expression or in some other aspect of DNA processing in response to radiation damage. The cloning and identification of these A-T genes will no doubt clarify this picture considerably in the not too distant future.

250

References

Aggeler J and Murnane JP (1990) Enhanced expression of procollagenase in ataxia-telangiectasia and xeroderma pigmentosum fibroblasts. In Vitro Cell Dev Biol 26:915-922

Ashall F and Puck TT (1984) Cytoskeletal involvement in cAMP-induced sensitization of chromatin to nuclease digestion in transformed Chinese hamster ovary K1 cells. Proc Natl Acad Sci USA 81:5145-5149

Angel P, Poting A, Mallick U, Rahmsdorf HF, Schorpp M and Herrlich P (1986) Induction of metallothionein and other mRNA species by carcinogens and tumor promoters in primary human skin fibroblasts. Mol Cell Biol 6:1760-1766

Baeuerle PA and Baltimore D (1988) IkB: a specific inhibitor of NF-kB transcription factor. Science 242:540-546

Bates P and Lavin MF (1985) Comparison of γ-irradiation-induced accumulation of ataxia-telangiectasia and control cells in G2 phase. Mutation Res 218:165-170

Baxter GD and Lavin MF (1992) Specific protein dephosphorylation in apoptosis induced by ionizing radiation and heat shock in human lymphoid tumor lines. J Immunol 148:1949-1954

Becker Y (1986) Cancer in ataxia-telangiectasia patient: analysis of factors leading to radiation-induced and spontaneous tumors. Anticancer Res 6:1021-1032

Boder E. (1985) Ataxia-telangiectasia: An overview. In: Ataxia-telangiectasia: Genetics, Neuropathology and Immunology of a Degenerative Disease of Childhood (RA Gatti and M Swift eds) Liss, New York, pp 1-63

Boothman DA, Bonvard I and Hughes EN (1989) Identification and characterization of x-ray-induced proteins in human cells. Cancer Res 49:2871-2878

Boutin B, Wagner DK and Nelson DL (1987) Analysis of CD3 antigen expression in patients with ataxia-telangiectasia. Clin Exp Immunol 68:320-330

Carbonari M, Cherchi M, Paganelli R, Giannini G, Galli E, Gaetano C, Papetti C and Fiorilli M (1990) Relative increase of T cells expressing the gamma/delta rather than the alpha/beta receptor in ataxia-telangiectasia. New Engl J Med 322:73-76

Chen PC, Lavin MF, Kidson C and Moss D (1978) Identification of ataxia-telangiectasia heterozygotes; a cancer prone population. Nature 274:484-486

Cleaver JE (1968) Defective repair replication of DNA in xeroderma pigmentosum. Nature 218:652-656

Cleaver JE and Kraemer KH (1989) Xeroderma pigmentosum. In: The metabolic basis of inherited disease (CR Scriver, AL Beandet, WS Sly and D Vall, eds) McGraw-Hill, New York vol 2 pp 2949-2971

Cole J, Arlett CF, Green MHL, Harcourt SA, Priestley A, Henderson L, Cole H, James E and Richmond F (1988) Comparative human cellular radiosensitivity: II. The survival following gamma-irradiation of unstimulated (G₀) T-lymphocytes, T-lymphocyte lines, lymphoblastoid cell lines and fibroblasts from normal donors, from ataxia-telangiectasia patients and from ataxia-telangiectasia heterozygotes. Int J Radiat Biol 54:929-942

Cornforth MN and Bedford JS (1985) On the nature of a defect in cells from individuals with ataxia-telangiectasia. Science 227:1589-1591

Dale TC, Ali Iman AM, Kerr IM and Stark GR (1989) Rapid activation by interferon α of a latent DNA-binding protein present in the cytoplasm of untreated cells. Proc Natl Acad Sci USA 86:1203-1207

Davis MM, Gatti RA and Sparkes RS (1985) Neoplasia and chromosomal breakage in ataxia-telangiectasia: A 2:14 translocation. in: R.A. Gatti and M.Swift, (Eds.), Ataxia-telangiectasia: Genetics, Neuropathology and Immunology of a Degenerative Disease of Childhood, Liss, New York, pp. 197-203

Davies SM, Harris AL and Hickson ID (1989) Overproduction of topoisomerase II in an ataxia-telangiectasia fibroblast cell line: comparison with a topoisomerase II-overproducing hamster cell mutant. Nucleic Acids Res. 17:1337-1351

Dean SW, Sykes H and Cole J (1988) Impaired glutathione biosynthesis in cultured ataxia-telangiestasia cells. Cancer Res 48:5374-5376

Dussault JH, Letarte J, Guyda H and Laberge C (1977) Serum thyroid hormone and TSH concentrations in newborn infants with congenital absence of thyroxine-binding globulin. J Pediat 90:264-265

Edwards MJ and Taylor AMR (1981) Unusual levels of (ADP-ribose) and DNA synthesis in ataxia telangiectasia cells following γ-ray irradiation. Nature 287:745-747

Enoch T and Nurse P (1990) Mutation of fission yeast cell cycle control genes abolishes dependence of mitosis on DNA replication. Cell 60:665-673

Ford MD, Martin L and Lavin MF (1984) The effects of ionizing radiation on cell cycle progression in ataxia telangiectasia. Mutation Res 125:115-22

Foroud T, Wei S, Ziv Y, Sobel E, Lange E, Chao A, Goradia T, Huo Y, Tolun A, Chessa L, Charmley P, Sanal O, Salman N, Julier C, Concannon P, McConville C, Taylor AMR, Shiloh Y, Lange K and Gatti RA (1991) Localization of an ataxia-telangiectasia locus to a 3-cM interval on chromosome 11q23. Amer J Hum Genet 49:1263-1279

Gatti RA, Bick M, Tam CF, Medici MA, Oxelius VA, Holland M. Goldstein AL and Boder E (1982) Ataxia-telangiectasia: A multiparameter analysis of eight families. Clin Immunol Immunopathol 23:501-516

Gatti RA, Berkel I, Boder E, Braedt G, Charmley P, Concannon P, Ersoy F, Foroud T, Jaspers NGJ, Lange K, Lathrop GM, Leppert M, Nakamura Y, O'Donnell P, Paterson M, Salser W, Sanal O, Silver J, Sparkes RS, Susi E, Weeks DE, Wei S, White R, Yoder F (1988) Localization of an ataxia-telangiectasia gene to chromosome 11q22-23. Nature 336:577-580

Glazer PM, Greggio, NA, Metherall JA and Summers WC (1989) UV-induced DNA binding proteins in human cells. Proc. Natl. Acad. Sci. U.S.A. 86:1163-1167

Gonzalez GA, Yamamoto KK, Fischer WH, Karr D, Menzel P, Biggs W, Vale WW and Montminy MR (1989) A cluster of phosphorylation sites on the cAMP-regulated nuclear factor CREB predicted by its sequence. Nature 337:739-752.

Gotoff SP, Amirmokri E and Liebner EJ (1967) Ataxia telangiectasia. Neoplasia, untoward response to x-irradiation, and tuberous sclerosis. Am J Dis Child 114:617-625

Hagiwara M, Alberts A, Brindle P, Meinkoth J, Feramisco J, Deng T, Karin M, Shenolikar S and Montminy M (1992) Transcriptional attenuation following cAMP induction requires PP-1-mediated dephosphorylation of CREB. Cell

70:105-113

Hallahan DE, Sukhatme VP, Sherman ML, Virudachalam S, Kufe D and Weichselbaum RR (1991) Protein kinase C mediates x-ray inducibility of nuclear signal transducers EGR1 and JUN. Proc. Natl. Acad. Sci. U.S.A. 88:2156-2160

Hanawalt P and Painter R (1985) On the nature of a "DNA processing" defect in ataxia-telangiectasia. In: Ataxia telangiectasia, genetics, neuropathology and immunology of a degenerative disease of childhood (RA Gatti and M Swift eds) Liss, New York, pp 67-71

Hanawalt PC and Sarasin A (1986) Human genetic disease and cancer. Trends in Genetics 2:124-129

Hobson K, Singh SP and Lavin MF (1991) Use of DNA-protein interaction to isolate specific genomic DNA sequences. Analytical Biochem. 193:220-224

Houldsworth J and Lavin MF (1980) Effect of ionizing radiation on DNA synthesis in ataxia-telangiectasia cells. Nucleic Acids Res 8:3709-3720

Imray FP and Kidson C (1983) Perturbations of cell cycle progression in gamma-irradiated ataxia-telangiectasia and Huntington's disease cells detected by DNA flow cytometric-analysis. Mutation Res 112:369-382

Jamil K (1984) Decondensation of human spermatozoal chromatin by nuclear actin polymerization. Arch Androl 13:137-146

Karam LR, Calsou P, Franklin WA, Painter RB, Olsson M and Lindahl T (1990) Modification of deoxyribose-phosphate residues by extracts of ataxia telangiectasia cells. Mutation Res 236:19-26

Kastan MB, Onyekwere O, Sidransky D, Vogelstein B and Craig RW (1991) Participation of p53 protien in the cellular response to DNA damage. Cancer Res. 51:6304-6311

Kingston RE, Schuetz TJ and Larin Z (1987) Heat-inducible human factor that binds to a human hsp 70 promoter. Mol. Cell Biol. 7:1530-1534

Komatsu K, Kodama S, Okumura Y and Oshimura M (1990) Restoration of radiation resistance in ataxia-telangiectasia cells by the introduction of normal human chromosome 11. Mutation Res 235:59-63.

Kramer M, Stein B, Mai S, Kunz E, Konig H, Loferer H, Grunicke HH, Ponta H, Herrlich P and Rahmsdorf HJ (1990) Radiation-induced activation of transcription factors in mammalian cells. Radiat Environ Biophys 29:303-313

Lane DP (1992) p53, guardian of the genome. Nature 358:15-16

Lavin MF and Davidson M (1981) Repair of strand breaks in superhelical DNA of ataxia telangiectasia lymphoblastoid cells. J Cell Res 48:383-391

Lavin MF and Schroeder AL (1988) Damage resistant DNA synthesis in eukaryotes. Mutation Res 193:193-206

Lavin MF and Seymour GJ (1984) Reduced levels of fibronectin in ataxia-telangiectasia lymphoblastoid cells. Int J Cancer 33:359-363

Lechner JF, Tokiwa T, La Veck M, Benedict WF, Banks-Schlegel S, Yeager H Banerjee A and Harris C (1985) Asbestos-associated chromosomal changes in human mesothelial cells. Proc Natl Acad Sci USA 82:3884-3888

Lindquist S (1986) The heat-shock response. Annu Rev Biochem 55:1151-1191

McConville CM, Formstone CJ, Hernandez D, Thick J and Taylor AMR (1990) Fine mapping of the chromosome 11q22-23 region using PFGE, linkage and haplotype analysis; localization of the gene for ataxia-telangiectasia to a 5 cM region flanked by NCAM/DRD2 and STMY/CJ52.75, ph2.22. Nucleic

Acids Res 18:4334-4343

McKinnon PJ (1987) Ataxia-telangiectasia: an inherited disorder of ionizing-radiation sensitivity in man. Hum Genet 75:197-208

McKinnon PJ and Burgoyne LA (1985a) Evidence for the existence of an actin-derived protein in ataxia-telangiectasia lymphoblastoid cell lines. Exp Cell Res 158:413-422

McKinnon PJ and Burgoyne LA (1985b) Altered cellular morphology and microfilament array in ataxia-telangiectasia fibroblasts. Eur J Cell Biol 39:161-166

Meredith MJ and Dobson ML (1987) Impaired glutathione biosynthesis in cultured human ataxia-telangiectasia cells. Cancer Res 47:4576-4581

Mirzayans R, Smith BP and Paterson MC (1989) Hypersentitivity to cell killing and faulty repair of 1-β-D-arabino-furanosylcytosine-detectable sites in human (Ataxia-telangiectasia) fibroblasts treated with 4-nitroquinoline 1-oxide. Cancer Res 49: 5523-5529

Mohamed R, Singh SP, Kumar S and Lavin MF (1987) A defect in DNA topoisomerase II activity in ataxia-telangiectasia cells. Biochem Biophys Res Commun 149:233-238

Morgan JL, Holcomb TM and Morrissey RW (1968) Radiation reaction in ataxia telangiectasia. Am J Dis Child 116:557-558

Morris C, Mohamed R and Lavin MF (1983) DNA replication and repair in ataxia-telangiectasia cells exposed to bleomycin. Mutat Res 112:67-74

Murnane JP and Painter RB (1983) Altered protein synthesis in ataxia-telangiectasia fibroblasts. Biochemistry 22:1217-1222

Nagasawa H and Little JB (1983) Comparison of kinetics of x-ray-induced cell killing in normal, ataxia-telangiectasia and hereditary retinoblastoma fibroblasts. Mutation Res. 109, 297-308

O'Connor RD and Scott-Linthicum D (1980) Mitogen receptor redistribution defects and concomitant absence of blastogenesis in ataxia-telangiectasia T lymphocytes. Clin Immun Immunopathol 15:66-75

Oxelius V-A, Berkel AI and Hanson LA (1982) N Engl J Med 305:515-520

Ozer NK, Ciliv G, Berkel AI, Sanal O, Yegin O and Fugen E (1985) Studies on lymphocyte cell surface in ataxia-telangiectasia. Clin Exp Immunol 61:118-124

Painter RB (1982) Structural changes in chromatin as the basis for radiosensitivity in ataxia-telangiectasia. Cytogenet Cell Genet 33:139-144

Painter RB and Young BR (1980) Radiosensitivity in ataxia-telangiectasia: A new explanation. Proc Natl Acad Sci 77:7315-7317

Pandita TK and Hittleman WN (1992) Initial chromosome damage but not DNA damage is greater in ataxia telangiectasia cells. Radiation Res 130:94-103

Pandita TK and Hittleman WN (1992b) The contribution of DNA and chromosome repair deficiencies to the radiosensitivity of ataxia-telangiectasia. Radiat Res 131:214-223.

Papathanasiou MA, Kerr NCK, Robbins JH, McBride OW, Alamo I, Barrett SF, Hickson ID and Fornace AJ (1991) Induction by ionizing radiation of the gadd45 gene in cultured human cells. Mol Cell Biol 11:1009-1016

Paterson MC, Anderson AK, Smith BP, Smith PJ (1979) Enhanced radiosensitivity of cultured fibroblasts from ataxia-telangiectasia heterozygotes manifested by defective colony forming ability and reduced DNA repair replication after hypoxic-irradiation. Cancer Res 39:3225-34

Paterson MC, Smith BP, Loham PHM, Anderson AK and Fishman L (1976) Defective excision repair of gamma ray-damaged DNA in human (ataxia-telangiectasia) fibroblasts. Nature 260:444-447

Paterson MC (1991) Radiosensitivity in ataxia-telangiectasia: A new explanation involving anomalous signal transduction. AACR Special Conference on Cellular Responses to Environmental DNA Damage. Banff, Canada. December 1-6 1991

Rivat-Peran L, Buriot D, Salier J-P, Rivat C, Dumitresco S-M and Griscelli C (1981) Clin Immunol Immunopathol 20:99-105

Robbins JH (1989) No lack of complementation for unscheduled DNA synthesis between xeroderma pigmentosum complementation groups D and H. Human Genetics 84:99-100

Rowley R, Hudson J and Young PG (1992) The wee1 protein kinase is required for radiation-induced mitotic delay. Nature 356:353-355

Scheer U, Hinssen H, Franke WW and Jockusch BM (1984) Microinjection of actin-binding proteins and actin antibodies demonstrates involvement of nuclear actin in transcription of lampbrush chromosomes. Cell 39:111-122

Scott D and Zampetti-Bosseler F (1982) Cell cycle dependence of mitotic delay in X-irradiated normal and ataxia-telangiectasia fibroblasts. Int J Radiat Biol 42:679-683

Sedgwick RP and Boder E (1991) Ataxia-telangiectasia (208900; 208910; 208920). In: Hereditary Neuropthaies and Spinocerebellar Atrophies (JMB Vianney De Jong ed). Elsevier Science Publishers, Amsterdam, pp347-423

Schuh S, Yonemoto W, Brugge J, Bauer VJ, Riehl RM, Sullivan WP and Toft DO (1985) A 90,000-dalton binding protein common to both steroid receptors and the rous sarcoma virus transforming protein, pp60^{v-src}. J Biol Chem 260:14292-14296.

Shiloh Y, Tabor E and Becker Y (1982) Colony-forming ability of ataxia-telangiectasia skin fibroblasts is an indicator of their early senescence and increased demand for growth factors. Expt Cell Res 140:191-199

Shiloh Y, Tabor E and Becker Y (1985) Cells from patients with ataxia-telangiectasia are abnormally sensitive to the cytotoxic effect of a tumor promoter, phorbol-12-myristate-13-acetate. Mutat Res 149:283-286

Singh SP, Mohamed R, Salmond C and Lavin MF (1988) Reduced DNA topoisomerase II activity in ataxia-telangiectasia cells. Nucleic Acids Res 16:3919-3923

Singh SP and Lavin ML (1989) Study of DNA topoisomerase II in ataxia-telangiectasia cells. Carcinogenesis 10:1215-1218

Singh SP and Lavin MF (1990) DNA-binding protein activated by gamma radiation in human cells. Mol Cell Biol 10:5279-5285

Smith PJ (1984) Relationship between a chromatin anomaly in ataxia telangiectasia cells and enhanced sensitivity to DNA damage. Carcinogenesis 5:1345-1350

Taylor AMR, Harnden DG, Arlett CF, Harcourt AR, Lehmann AR, Stevens S and Bridges BA (1975) Ataxia-telangiectasia: a human mutation with abnormal radiation sensitivity. Nature 258:427-429

Taylor AMR (1982) Cytogenetics of ataxia-telangiectasia. In: Ataxia-telangiectasia - a Cellular and Molecular link between Cancer, Neuropathology and Immune

Deficiency (BA Bridges, DG Harnden eds) Wiley, New York, pp 53-83

Teale B, Singh S, Khanna KK, Findik D and Lavin MF (1992) Purification and characterization of a DNA-binding protein activated by ionizing radiation. J Biol Chem 267:10295-10301

Thieffry S, Arthuis M, Aicardi J and Lyon G (1961) L'ataxie-telangiectasie. Rev Neurol 105:390-405

Tsai-Pflugfelder M, Lin LF, Lin HA, Tewey KM, Whang-Peng J, Knutsen T, Huebner K, Croce CM and Wang JC (1988) Cloning and squencing of cDNA encoding human DNA topoisomerase II and locations of the gene to chromosome region 17g 21-22. Proc Natl Acad Sci USA 85:7177-7180

Vandekerckhove J (1990) Actin-binding proteins. Current Opinion in Cell Biology 2:41-50

Velasquez JM and Linquist S (1984) hsp70: Nuclear concentration during environmental stress and cytoplasmic storage during recovery. Cell 36:655-662

Vincent RA, Sheridan RB and Huang PC (1975) DNA strand breakage repair in ataxia telangiectasia fibroblast-like cells. Mutat Res 33:357-366

Waldmann TA (1982) Immunological abnormalities in ataxia-telangiectasia. In: Ataxia-telangiectasia - a Cellular and Molecular link between Cancer, Neuropathology and Immune Deficiency (BA Bridges, DG Harnden eds) Wiley, New York, pp 37-51

Wu BJ, Hunt C and Morimoto RI (1985) Structure and expression of the human gene encoding major heat shock protein hsp70. Mol Cell Biol 5:330-341

Yamamoto KK, Gonzalez GA, Biggs WH and Montminy MR (1988) Phosphorylation-induced binding and transcriptional efficacy of nuclear factor CREB. Nature 334:494-498.

RADIOBIOLOGY OF ATAXIA-TELANGIECTASIA

Robert B. Painter
Laboratory of Radiobiology and Environmental Health
Box 0750
University of California, San Francisco
San Francisco, CA 94143-0750

INTRODUCTION

The discovery that ataxia-telangiectasia (A-T) patients (Morgan et al., 1968; Gotoff et al., 1967; Cunliffe et al., 1975), as well as cells from these patients (Taylor et al., 1975), are hypersensitive to ionizing radiation (Fig. 1) has sparked an outpouring of research aimed at determining the basis of this radiosensitivity and its relationship to the pathology of the disease.   The increased susceptibility of A-T cells to killing by ionizing radiation can largely be correlated with the increased frequency of radiation-induced chromosomal aberrations (Bender et al., 1985, 1988; Higurachi and Conen, 1973; Nagasawa et al., 1985; Natarajan and Meyers, 1979; Taylor, 1982; Zampetti-Bosseler and Scott, 1981);   however, the molecular basis of this extraordinary radiosensitivity is still not understood.   Many chromatid-type aberrations are observed after irradiation of A-T cells in the G_1 phase of the cell cycle (Bender et al., 1985; Natarajan and Meyers, 1979; Taylor et al., 1976; Taylor, 1978), something almost never seen in normal cells or in cells from patients with other genetic diseases. This suggests that some kind of damage that is always repaired in normal cells before they move into S phase is not repaired in A-T cells.   Unfortunately, this is a clue that no one has yet been able to exploit.

NATO ASI Series, Vol. H 77
Ataxia-Telangiectasia
Edited by R. A. Gatti and R. B. Painter
© Springer-Verlag Berlin Heidelberg 1993

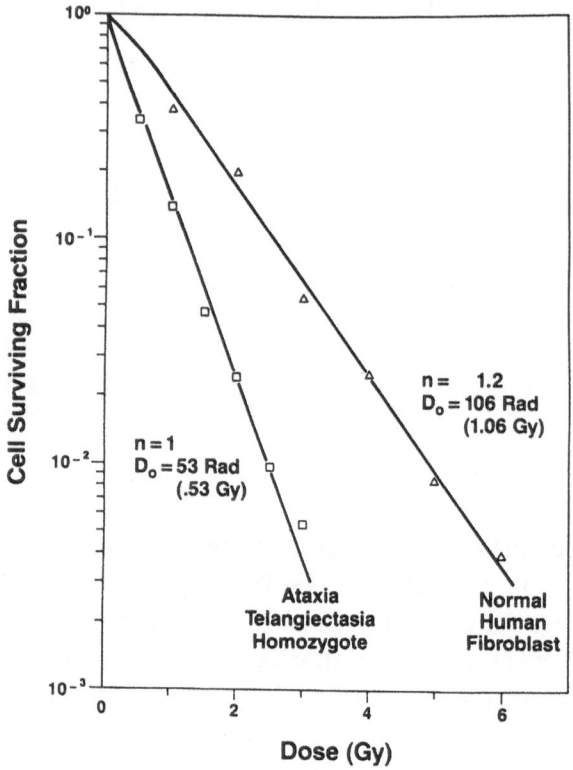

Fig. 1   Dose-response curves for normal human fibroblasts and for cells from a patient with Ataxia-telangiectasia (A-T). Note that human cells tend to have a smaller shoulder than cells of rodent origin. The A-T cells are much more sensitive to x-rays with D_0 of about 50 rads (0.5 Gy) compared with 120 rads (1.2 Gy) for the normal fibroblasts. From Hall (1973) with permission.

DNA REPAIR IN A-T

In general, the most likely possibility for hypersensitivity to a DNA-damaging agent is a defect in DNA repair. The outstanding example of this is the defective repair of ultraviolet light-induced DNA damage exhibited by patients with the autosomal recessive disease xeroderma pigmentosum (Cleaver, 1968). This syndrome has several complementation groups; some are more sensitive to UV light than others, and the sensitivity is, to a first approximation, correlated with the extent of the defect in DNA repair. For A-T, however, the situation is more complicated. First, there is at best only a very subtle defect in DNA repair in A-T cells; a recent report indicates that A-T cells in the G_1 and G_2 phases of the cell cycle repair DNA double-strand breaks to a slightly lesser extent than do normal cells (Pandita and Hittelman, 1992). All previous reports indicated that the repair of DNA single- and double-strand breaks and of DNA base damage was normal in A-T cells. Second, although there are at least five complementation groups in A-T (Jaspers et al., 1988), they all have about the same average radiosensitivity. These attributes of A-T cells suggest that the basis of their hypersensitivity to ionizing radiation lies in the failure of some function other than DNA repair.

RADIORESISTANT DNA SYNTHESIS IN A-T CELLS

There is a distinctive abnormality of DNA metabolism in A-T cells: the paradoxical phenomenon called radioresistant DNA synthesis (RDS). Despite the increased sensitivity of A-T cells for killing by ionizing radiation, DNA synthesis in A-T cells is more resistant to ionizing radiation than that in normal cells (Houldsworth and Lavin, 1980; Painter and Young, 1980). In normal cells, ionizing radiation depresses the rate of DNA synthesis so that when rate is plotted against dose a two-component curve results, with a steep initial slope followed by a shallower slope at doses greater than about 5 cGy ; in contrast, the plot of DNA synthesis rate against dose for A-T cells has no initial steep component and is a single-component curve whose slope is virtually identical to the shallow component observed for normal cells (Fig. 2). For an understanding of the basis of these curves, a discussion of mammalian DNA synthesis is necessary.

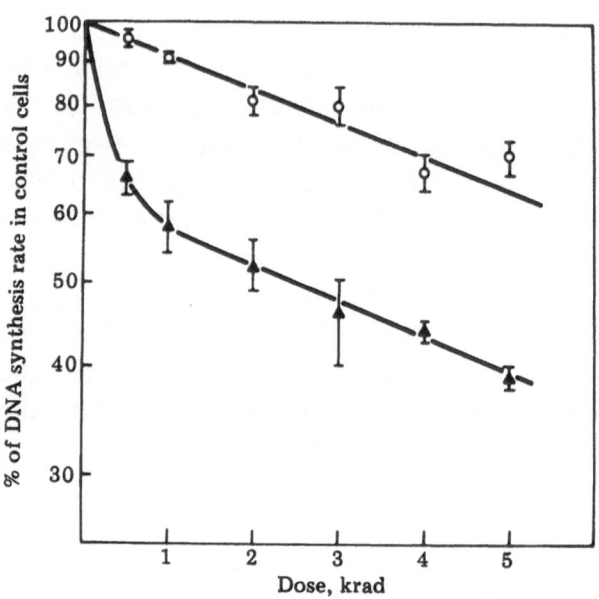

Fig. 2 Rate of DNA synthesis as a function of ionizing radiation dose in A-T (O) and normal (Δ) human fibroblasts. (From Painter and Young, 1980).

All diploid mammalian cells contain about 6 picograms of nuclear DNA, or about 6 billion base pairs. The rate of fork displacement along each DNA molecule during DNA replication is about 500 base pairs per minute. Since the average time required for a mammalian cell to replicate its DNA (the length of S phase) is about 6 hours, it is obvious that very many molecules must be replicated simultaneously. Indeed, there are about ten thousand DNA molecules in the process of replication at any one time during the mammalian S phase. Replication is initiated at so-called origins and proceeds bidirectionally. These initiations occur in groups, or clusters, of adjacent "replicons," and replication terminates when the growing points from adjacent replicons merge. There is an average of about 25 replicons per cluster. Control of initiation of replicon clusters is semi-stringent, and the molecular mechanisms for this control are largely unknown.

Ionizing radiation inhibits mammalian cell DNA replication in two ways: it blocks chain elongation ahead of DNA growing points that had initiated replication before irradiation, and it blocks the initiation of replicon clusters scheduled to initiate after irradiation. Because the latter effect requires only one "hit" in a cluster of many replicons, the target size is large and the dose of radiation required to cause the effect is relatively small. This then is observed as the initial steep component of the curve for inhibition of DNA synthesis by radiation. In contrast, for chain elongation to be blocked in DNA already undergoing replication, the effective ionization must occur close to the advancing replication fork; therefore, the target size is small, and the dose required for the effect is relatively high. The effect of ionizing radiation on chain elongation is thus reflected as the high-dose, shallow-slope region of the curve for radiation-induced inhibition of DNA synthesis (Makino and Okada, 1975; Walters and Hildebrand, 1975; Painter and Young, 1976).

The curve for inhibition of DNA synthesis by ionizing radiation in A-T cells (i.e., RDS) shows only a single component that is parallel to the shallow component observed for inhibition in normal cells. Thus, it would appear that initiation in A-T cells is not inhibited at all by ionizing radiation and that chain elongation is inhibited to the same extent as in normal cells. Surprisingly, however, experiments using both velocity sedimentation techniques (Painter, 1983) and fiber autoradiography (Ockey, 1983) have shown just the opposite: DNA chain elongation is almost completely resistant to ionizing radiation in A-T cells, and the inhibition of DNA synthesis is due solely to inhibition of replicon initiation. These results imply that in A-T cells radiation blocks initiation of individual replicons rather than clusters of replicons (Fig. 3). Thus, it appears that an effector molecule, which in normal cells is responsible for delaying the initiation of whole clusters of replicons and for blocking chain elongation at lesions near the growing forks, is defective in A-T cells. The nature of this effector is unknown; it is not poly(ADP-ribose) (James and Lehmann, 1982; Painter, 1985). Identification of this effector would be important not only for understanding RDS but also for establishing the relationship of RDS to the pathology of A-T.

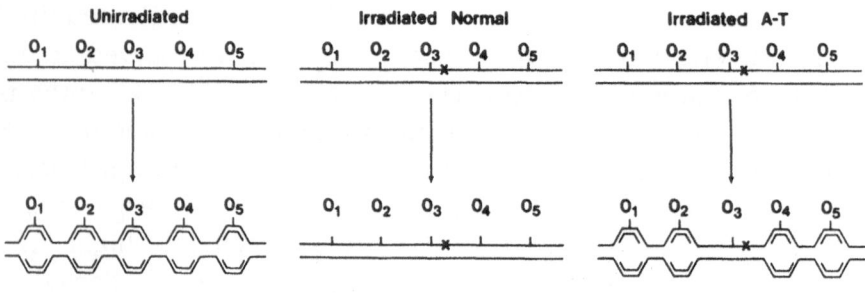

Fig. 3 Diagram of the difference between the effects of ionizing radiation on DNA replicon initiation in normal cells and in A-T cells. In unirradiated cells of either type, initiation occurs synchronously in a cluster of five replicons at their origins (O1-O5). In irradiated normal cells a lesion (X) blocks the initiation of all five replicons, whereas in irradiated A-T cells initiation is blocked only in the lesion containing the lesion. (From R.B. Painter, International Journal of Radiation Biology 49,771-781, 1986).

It has been suggested that the failure of A-T cells to shut down DNA synthesis after irradiation to the same extent as in normal cells permits replication of damaged DNA and is the cause of at least some of the hypersensitivity to ionizing radiation (Painter and Young, 1980). However, experiments in which extended times were allowed for repair of lesions in A-T cells showed that delaying the onset of S phase by many hours did not increase survival (Cox et al., 1981; Smith and Paterson, 1983). Moreover, experimentally derived strains of A-T cells, produced by transfection with DNA from normal human cells, showed increased survival after irradiation but retained RDS (Lehmann et al., 1989; Kapp and Painter, 1989). It does not seem likely, therefore, that enhanced replication of radiation-induced lesions is the cause of radiosensitivity of A-T cells.

RADIOSENSITIVTY OF A-T HETEROZYGOTES

The consensus of opinion is that many but not all A-T heterozygotes (A-T hets) are slightly hypersensitive to ionizing radiation. When survival curves from cells derived from A-T hets are compared with a spectrum of survival curves from normal cells, the cells from A-T hets generally overlap with the more sensitive normal cells. Thus, the once-attractive possibility of using radiosensitivity to identify A-T hets seems to be invalid. (A-T hets also do not exhibit RDS.) However, the slight radiosensitivity of A-T hets does have importance for public health. Swift et al. (1991) claim that the higher incidence of breast cancer in A-T hets (Swift et al., 1986, 1991) is caused by radiation exposure, i.e., A-T hets are extremely prone to radiation-induced breast cancer. Although this claim was made on the basis of scanty epidemiological evidence and there is no radiobiological precedent for such an effect, the possibility that A-T hets are prone to radiation-induced breast cancers should be kept in mind, at least until more data are compiled.

OTHER RADIATION EFFECTS IN A-T CELLS

When A-T cells in G_2 phase are exposed to ionizing radiation, the dose-dependent mitotic delay is less than that observed in normal human cells (Zampetti-Bosseler and Scott, 1981; Scott and Zampetti-Bosseler, 1982). It is probable that this reduced delay permits cells to enter into mitosis before repair is complete, thereby increasing the frequency of chromosomal aberrations and enhancing cell killing. Again, a defective effector is suspect; it might be the same as the one that causes RDS. The opposite effect occurs for cells irradiated in S phase. When these cells reach G_2 they accumulate in this phase for extended periods of time (Ford et al., 1984). This effect presumably is caused by misrepair (or misreplication) of molecules in S, and these abnormal molecules somehow block the cells that harbor them from entering mitosis. This phenomenon is especially difficult to understand in the context of the A-T cell, in which other responses to radiation are speeded up relative to those in normal cells (e.g., RDS, decreased mitotic delay).

A-T cells do not repair sublethal damage (i.e., there is no recovery between split doses of radiation) (Cox et al., 1981), and they do not demonstrate liquid holding repair (i.e., retention of cells in G_1 phase for extended times does not improve survival) (Smith and Paterson, 1983). In contrast to early unrefereed reports for diploid A-T fibroblasts, which suggested that A-T cells are hypomutable, gamma-irradiated shuttle vectors show the same frequency of ionizing radiation-induced mutations in A-T lymphocytes as in normal lymphocytes, and the mutation spectrum of these irradiated plasmids is the same in A-T and normal lymphocytes (Sikpi et al., 1992).

CONCLUSIONS

A-T cells show remarkable differences from normal cells in several radiobiological endpoints. They are hypersensitive for radiation-induced chromosomal aberrations and cell killing. In contrast, DNA synthesis and G_2 delay are more resistant to radiation in A-T cells than in normal cells. No DNA repair defect has been found in A-T cells that is sufficient to explain their radiosensitivity. With the cloning of one of the genes nearly accomplished (Kapp et al., 1992), it should be possible in the near future to determine the abnormal function that is responsible for these radiobiological anomalies and to establish the relationship of this abnormality to the pathology associated with the A-T syndrome.

REFERENCES

Bender MA, Rary JM, Kale RP (1985) G_0 chromosomal sensitivity in ataxia telangiectasia lymphocytes. Mutat Res 150:277-282

Bender MA, Viola MV, Fiore J, Thompson MH, and Leonard RC (1988) Normal G_2 chromosomal radiosensitivity and cell survival in the cancer family syndrome. Cancer Res 48:2579-2584

Cleaver JE (1968) Defective repair replication of DNA in xeroderma pigmentosum. Nature 218: 652-656

Cox R, Masson WK, Weichselbaum RR, Nove J, Little JB (1981) The repair of potentially lethal damage in ataxia telangiectasia fibroblasts. Int J Radiat Biol 39:357-365

Cunliffe PN, Mann JR, Cameron AH, Roberts KD, and Ward HWC (1975) Radiosensitivity in ataxia telangiectasia. Br J Radiol 48:374-376

Ford MD, Martin L, Lavin MF (1984) The effects of ionizing radiation on cell cycle progression in ataxia telangiectasia. Mutat Res 125:115-124

Gotoff P, Amirmokri E, and Liebner EJ (1967) Ataxia telangiectasia. Neoplasia, untoward response to x-irradiation, and tuberous sclerosis. Am J Dis Child 114:617-625

Hall EJ (1973) Radiobiology for the radiologist. Harper & Row, Hagerstown, Maryland

Higurachi M, Conen PE (1973) In vitro chromosomal radiosensitivity in "chromosomal breakage syndromes." Cancer 32:380-383

Houldsworth J, Lavin MF (1980) Effect of ionizing radiation on DNA synthesis in ataxia telangiectasia cells. Nucl Acids Res 8: 3709-3720

James MR, Lehmann AR (1982) Role of adenosine poly (adenosine diphosphate ribose) in deoxyribonucleic acid repair in human fibroblasts. Biochemistry 21: 4007-4013

Jaspers NGJ, Gatti RA, Baan C, Linssen PC, Bootsma D (1988) Genetic complementation analysis of ataxia telangiectasia and the Nijmegen breakage syndrome: a survey of 50 patients. Cytogenet Cell Genet 49:259-263

Kapp LN, Painter RB (1989) Stable radioresistance in ataxia-telangiectasia cells containing DNA from normal human cells. Int J Radiat Biol 56:667-675

Kapp LN, Painter RB, Yu L-C, van Loon N, Richard CW, III, James MR, Cox DR, Murnane JP (1992) Cloning of a candidate gene for ataxia-telangiectasia group D. Am J Hum Genet 51:45-54

Lehmann AR, Jaspers NGJ, Gatti RA (1989) Fourth International Workshop on Ataxia-Telangiectasia (meeting report). Cancer Res 49:6162-6163

Makino F, Okada S (1975) Effects of ionizing radiations on DNA replication in cultured mammalian cells. Radiat Res 62: 37-51

Morgan JL, Holcomb TM, Morrissey RW (1968) Radiation reaction in ataxia-telangiectasia. Am J Dis Child 116:557-558

Nagasawa H, Latt SA, Lalande ME, and Little JB (1985) Effects of X-irradiation on cell cycle progression, induction of chromosomal aberrations and cell killing in ataxia telangiectasia (A-T) fibroblasts. Mutat Res 148:71-82

Natarajan A-T, Meyers M (1979) Chromosome radiosensitivity of ataxia telangiectasia cells at different cell stages. Hum Genet 52:127-132

Ockey CH (1983) Differences in replicon behavior between X-irradiation-sensitive mouse lymphoma cells and A-T fibroblasts using fiber autoradiography. Radiat Res 94: 427-438

Painter RB (1983) Are lesions induced by ionizing radiation direct blocks to DNA chain elongation? Radiat Res 95: 421-426

Painter RB (1985) 3-Aminobenzamide does not affect radiation-induced inhibition of DNA synthesis in human cells. Mutat Res 143: 113-115

Painter RB (1986) Inhibition of mammalian cell DNA synthesis by ionizing radiation. Int J Radiat Biol 49:771-781

Painter RB, Young BR (1976) Formation of nascent DNA molecules during inhibition of replicon initiation in mammalian cells. Biochim Biophys Acta 418: 146-153

Painter RB, Young BR (1980) Radiosensitivity in ataxia-telangiectasia: a new explanation. Proc Natl Acad Sci USA 77: 7315-7317

Pandita TK, Hittelman WN (1992) The contribution of DNA and chromosome repair deficiencies to the radiosensitivity of ataxia-telangiectasia. Radiation Res 131, in press

Scott D, Zampetti-Bosseler F (1982) Cell cycle dependence of mitotic delay in x-irradiated normal and ataxia-telangiectasis fibroblasts. Int J Radiat Biol 42: 679-683

Sikpi MO, Freedman ML, Dry SM, Lurie AG (1992) Mutation spectrum in γ-irradiated shuttle vector replicated in ataxia-telangiectasia lymphoblasts. Radiat Res 130: 331-339

Smith PJ, Paterson MC (1983) Effect of aphidicolin on *de novo* DNA synthesis, DNA repair and cytoxicity in γ-irradiated human fibroblasts: implications for the enhanced radiosensitivity in ataxia telangiectasia. Biochim Biophys Acta 739:17-26

Swift M, Morrell D, Chamberlain AR, Skolnick MH, Bishop DT (1986) The incidence and gene frequency of ataxia-telangiectasia in the United States. Am J Hum Genet 39:573-583

Swift M, Morrell D, Massey RB, Chase CL (1991) Incidence of cancer in 161 families affected by ataxia-telangiectasia. N Engl J Med 325: 1831-1836

Taylor AMR (1978) Unrepaired DNA stand breaks in irradiated ataxia telangiectasia lymphocytes suggested from cytogenetic observations. Mutat Res 50:407-418

Taylor AMR (1982) Cytogenetics of ataxia telangiectasia. In BA Bridges and DG Harnden (eds). Ataxia telangiectasia - a cellular and molecular link between cancer, neuropathology and immune deficiency. pp 53-82. Chichester: Wiley

Taylor AMR, Harnden DG, Arlett CF, Harcourt SA, Lehmann AR, Stevens S, and Bridges BA (1975) Ataxia-telangiectasia: a human mutation with abnormal radiation sensitivity. Nature 258:427-429

Taylor AMR, Metcalfe JA, Oxford JM, and Harnden DG (1976) Is chromatid-type damage in ataxia telangiectasia after irradiation at G0 a consequence of defective repair. Nature 260:441-443

Walters RA, Hildebrand CE (1975) Evidence that X-irradiation inhibits replicon initiation in Chinese hamster cells. Biochem Biophys Commun 65: 265-271

Zampetti-Bosseler F, Scott D (1981) Cell death, chromosome damage and mitotic delay in normal human, ataxia telangiectasia and retinoblastoma fibroblasts after X-irradiation. Int J Radiat Biol 49:485-494

Treatment of Ataxia-Telangiectasia

Susan L. Perlman, M.D.
Department of Neurology
University of California at Los Angeles
Los Angeles, CA 90024-6975

The greatest areas of concern are pulmonary disease and malignancy. Recurrent sinopulmonary infections must be recognized and treated aggressively to lower the risk of developing chronic bronchiectasis. When chronic bronchiectatic changes are present, care must be taken with pulmonary toilet to remove secretions and protect the oxygenating capability of the lungs. Periodic pulmonary function studies can help monitor this, and assistance from respiratory therapists and pulmonary physicians is invaluable. Various immunotherapies have been tried to build up the patient's resistance to infection. The most reliable remains the use of intravenous gamma globulin (0.6 - 0.8 ml perkg) IV q 3-4 weeks (when immunoglobulin levels are less than 200 mg per 100 ml). Increasing bulbar dysfunction in the later stages of disease predisposes to aspiration pneumonia. This may be helped by anticholinergic drugs to dry up secretions or by fluoxitine 10 - 20 mg q AM.

There is a 10 - 40% risk of malignancy in patients with A-T. This is primarily due to lymphomas, the leukemias, basal cell carcinoma, and gynecologic, thyroid, liver, kidney, and brain neoplasms. The patient's physical and neurologic status should be monitored regularly to assure the earliest possible diagnosis of these complications. Preferred treatments depend on tumor type and may include surgery, reduced-dose radiotherapy (less than 1200-2000 RADS), or chemotherapy (avoiding radiomimetic or neurotoxic agents). A-T carriers (heterozygotes) may make up 1-3% of the general population and are also hypersensitive to ionizing radiation and radiomimetic agents. Female carriers of the A-T gene appear to be at increased risk of developing breast cancer (Swift et al. 1987, 1991).

Increased photosensitivity of skin in A-T patients may lead to oculocutaneous telangiectases, progeric skin changes, and basal cell carcinoma. Dermatologic health should be monitored and avoidance of sun exposure and use of sun blocking agents recommended.

Insulin-resistant diabetes mellitus is also seen (as it is seen in other inherited spinocerebellar degenerations, e.g. Friedreich's ataxia). It is easily screened for in blood (blood sugars, glycosylated hemoglobin levels, and insulin levels). Other endocrine abnormalities are also noted (hypogonadism, thyroid changes, and adrenal abnormalities).

Orthopedic and rehabilitation needs must be monitored. All patients with progressive neuromuscular disease benefit from some form of daily home or therapist-assisted exercise program, to include strengthening, stretching, coordination-related activities and conditioning (Perlman et al 1986). Nonambulatory patients may experience orthopedic complications relating to postural habits that can lead to severe osteoporosis, scoliosis, and foot deformities.

Psychological needs of the patient and family must be addressed at each visit. Questions about diagnosis, prognosis, treatment availability, and ongoing research should be explored. Frequently misunderstandings come to light regarding the genetic risk to other family members. Risks for carrying the A-T gene should be explained. The better a clinician understands the knowledge, beliefs, and desires of the patient and family, the better relationship he/she will have with them. Emotional issues may include adjustment problems of patient and family (denial, depression, anger) which could require professional counseling for resolution. Support groups for patient and family can also be helpful (e.g.. National Ataxia Foundation, Wayzata, MN, (612) 473-7666 and the AT Medical Research Foundation, Los Angeles, CA (310) 476-1218.)

The long term management of diseases like AT is often facilitated by a case manager, to coordinate needs of the patient, family and health care team.

Medications for ataxia and tremor

Several medicines of different neurochemical specificity have been used to treat the symptoms of cerebellar disease (ataxia, tremor, dizziness) (Table 1).

Table 1. Medications For Ataxia

AVAILABLE

	Dose	Effect
AMANTIDINE (SYMMETREL)	100 mg bid	dopaminergic
VALPROIC ACID (DEPAKOTE)	250-500 mg bid-tid	GABAergic
BACLOFEN (LIORESAL)	up to 20 mg qid	GABAergic
ACETAZOLAMIDE (DIAMOX)	250 mg bid-qid (for paroxysmal ataxia)	carbonic anhydrase inhibitor

EXPERIMENTAL/UNPROVEN

PHYSOSTIGMINE (ESERINE)	1-4 mg q 2 hours (ave 6-24 mg/d)	cholinergic
L-5-OH - TRYPTOPHAN	5 mg/kg/d	serotonergic
AMPHETAMINES		CNS stimulants sympathomimetic
D - TOCOPHERYL (VITAMIN E)	1000-1600 mg/d	anti-oxidant

Amantidine is reported to improve balance, coordination, and energy levels in Friedreich's ataxia (Peterson PL et al 1988). Side effects include blurred vision, dry mouth, urinary retention, constipation, and fluid retention with peripheral edema.

Valproic acid (VPA) and baclofen are both ostensibly GABAergic. VPA may work best for trunkal instability and tremor. Baclofen is reported to be useful for eye movement incoordination and nystagmus (Yee, RD et al 1982) Both drugs can cause significant nausea and drowsiness/or a paradoxical increase in ataxia.

Acetazolamide is used primarily for episodic ataxia (Baloh, RW et al 1991)

Experimental drugs and unproven therapies may provide future options.

When tremor is the primary problem, a wider range of drug choices is available (Table 2).

Table 2. Medications for Tremor

ESSENTIAL TREMOR / POSTURAL TREMOR

<u>Dose</u>

PROPRANOLOL (INDERAL) up to 240 mg/d in divided doses or time-released

OTHER BETA BLOCKERS (NADOLOL PINDOLOL METOPROLOL, ATENOLOL/CORGARD, VISKEN, LOPRESSOR, TENORMIN)

PRIMIDONE (MYSOLINE) up to 250 mg dd (often less)

METHAZOLAMIDE(NEPTAZINE) 50 mg dd

LOW DOSE BENZODIAZEPINES FOR ANXIOLYTIC EFFECTS
 (e.g., diazepam, clonazepam, alprazolam)

CEREBELLAR TREMOR/MYOCLONUS

CLONAZEPAM (KLONOPIN) up to 2 mg tid (often less)

VALPROIC ACID (DEPAKOTE) 250 - 500 mg bid-tid

L-5-OH-TRYPTOPHAN (EXPERIMENTAL) 5 mg/kg/d

CARBAMAZEPINE (TEGRETOL) average 200 mg tid

For static postural tremor, low dose beta blockers are often quite effective, but may cause serious cardiac side effects (hypotension, arrhythmias, syncope) or depression. Primidone is metabolized to phenobarbitol and may be too sedating, as may the benzodiazepines.

Action tremor or myoclonus often responds well to low doses of clonazepam or valproic acid, although a paradoxical increase in ataxia has been seen. Drowsiness continues to complicate the use of clonazepam and dosing may be restricted to bedtime only (2 mg maximum). Carbamazepine is reported to help cerebellar tremor as well, but we are less impressed with its usefulness in view of its many potential side effects (nausea, drowsiness, ataxia, bone marrow suppression, liver dysfunction).

When complaints of dizziness are present, many drug strategies are available, but side effects must be weighed carefully (Baloh, RW 1984) (Table 3).

Table 3. Medications for Dizziness

Class	Drug	Dosage	Sedation	Antiemetic	Dryness Mucous Membranes	Extra Pyramidal Symptoms
Anticholinergic	Scopolamine	0.6 mg orally q 4-6 h. 0.5 mg transdermally q.3 days	+	+	+ + +	–
	Atropine	0.4 mg orally or intramuscularly q.4-6 h.	–	+	+ + +	–
Monoaminergic	Amphetamine	5 or 10 mg orally q.4-6 h.	–	+	+	+
	Ephedrine	25 mg orally q.4-6 h.	–	+	+	–
Antihistamine	Meclizine	25 mg orally q.4-6 h.	+	+	+	–
	Cyclizine	60 mg orally or intramuscularly q.4-6 h. or 10C mg suppository q.8 h.	+	+	+ +	–
	Dimenhydrinate	50 mg orally or intramuscularly q. 4-6 h. or 100 mg suppository q.8 h.	+	+	+	–
	Promelhazine	25 or 50 mg orally or intramuscularly or suppository q.6 h.	+ +	+	+ +	+
Phenothiazine	Prochlorperazine	5 or 10 mg orally or intramuscularly q.6 h. or 25 mg suppository q.12 h.	+	+ + +	+	+ + +
	Chlorpromazine	25 mg orally or intramuscularly q.6 h.	+ + +	+ +	+	+ + +
Benzodiazepine	Diazepam	5 or 10 mg orally, intramuscularly or intravenously q.4-6 h.	+ + +	+	–	–
Butyrophenone	Haloperidol	1.0 or 2.0 mg orally or intramuscularly q.8-12 h.	+ + +	+ +	+	+ +
	Droperidol	2.5 or 5 mg intramuscularly q.12 h.	+ + +	+ +	+	+ +

Medication for basal ganglia symptoms

Dystonia may complicate the later stages of A-T. Dopaminergic, anticholinergic, dopamine depleting and GABAergic medications can be tested for efficacy. Some dystonic syndromes respond well to low dose DOPA therapy (Sinemet 25/100 tid) or anticholinergic drugs (trihexyphenidyl 2 mg tid or more), but side effects may be limiting (Table 4).

Table 4. Medications For Basal Ganglia Symptoms

TREMOR, RIGIDITY, BRADYKINESIA

	Dose
L-DOPA/CARBIDOPA (SINEMET) 100/25	1-3 TABLETS TID (now available as time-released)
AMANTIDINE (SYMMETREL) (dopamine releaser)	100 mg bid
SELEGILINE (ELDEPRYL) (MAB-B inhibiter)	5 mg bid
DOPAMINE AGONISTS -	
BROMOCRIPTINE (PARLODEL)	10-40 mg/d in divided doses
PERGOLIDE (PERMAX)	1 mg tid
LISURIDE (Not available in U.S.A.)	
ANTICHOLINERGIC, ANTIHISTAMINIC DRUGS AS ADJUNCTIVE AGENTS	

CHOREOATHETOSIS

HALOPERIDOL (HALDOL) (rather than phenothiazines)	05 - 5 mg bid-tid
BACLOFEN (LIORESAL)	up to 20 mg qid
ISONIAZID (INH)	10 - 20 mg/kg/d
GABA aminotransferase inhibitor	with 100 mg pyridoxine/d
TETRABENAZINE (not available in U.S.A.) dopamine depleter	200 mg /d

Treatment of fatigue and muscle cramps or twitching

Fatigue is a common complaint in many neuromuscular conditions, especially (but not solely) when there is a peripheral nerve component to the disease. A daily exercise program can do much to boost energy levels. Several medications have also proven helpful (Table 5).

Table 5. Medications for Fatigue

	Dose
PYRIDOSTIGMINE (MESTINON)	up to 180 mg bid in divided dose or time-released
AMANTIDINE (SYMMETREL)	100 mg bid
SELEGILINE (ELDEPRYL)	5 mg bid
PEMOLiNE (CYLERT)	18.95 - 75 mg of a.m.
EPHEDRINE	25 mg bid-qid

Pyridostigmine use may be limited by stomach cramps and diarrhea. Amantidine may be constipating. Muscle cramps respond well to stretching, calcium/potassium supplements, or a variety of medications (quinine, phenytoin, baclofen, clonazepam). As always, benefits must be weighed against potential adverse effects.

Summary

Many treatment options are available for managing the whole patient with A-T (Table 6). Effective treatment requires a caring and committed team effort.

Table 6. Treatment Options

SYMPTOMATIC MEDICATION FOR

    ATAXIA
    DIZZINESS
    TREMOR
    SPASTICITY
    BASAL GANGLIA SYMPTOMS
    BULBAR DYSFUNCTION
    FATIGUE
PHYSICAL THERAPY/OCCUPATIONAL THERAPY
ORTHOTICS FOR BRACING AND EQUIPMENT
SPEECH THERAPY
NUTRITIONAL COUNSELING
GENETICS COUNSELLING
PSYCHOSOCIAL INTERVENTION
SUPPORT GROUPS
LEGAL AID
NEURO-OPHTHALMOLOGY
SLEEP DISORDERS CLINIC
GASTROENTEROLOGY
NEURO-UROLOGY
CARDIOLOGY
ORTHOPEDICS
INTERNAL MEDICINE/TB TESTING, FLU SHOT
FDA REFERRAL FOR NEW DRUGS

References

Baloh, RW (1984) The Essentials of Neurotology. FA Davis Company, Philadelphia

Baloh, RW; Winder, A (1991) Acetazolamide - Responsive Vestobulocerebellar Syndrome, clinical and oculographic features. Neur 41:429-33

Perlman, SL; Kern, R (1986) Intensive Physical Therapy for Chronic Progressive Neuromuscular Disease. Muscle and Nerve 9:257 (#55)

Peterson, PL; Saad, J; Nigro, MA (1988) The Treatment of Friedreich's Ataxia
with Amantidine Hydrochloride. Neur 38:1478-80

Swift, M; Reitnauer, PJ; Morrell, D; Chase, CL (1987) Breast and other Cancers in Families with Ataxia-Telangiectasia. N Engl J Med 316:1289-94

Swift, M; Morrell, D; Massey, RB; Chase, CL (1991) Incidence of Cancer in
161 Families Affected by Ataxia-Telangiectasia, N Engl J Med 325:183136

Yee, RD; Baloh, RW; Honrubia, V (1982) Effect of Baclofen on Congenital
Nystagmus. Functional Basis of Ocular Motility Disorders Pergamon
Press

INDEX

acetazolamide, 270
amantidine, 270-271, 274-275
amygdala, 176
alphafetoprotein, 184-187, 195, 205
Alu sequences, 80-81
antigen receptor, 147
ataxia, treatment of, 270-271
A-T$_{Fresno}$, 49-50, 224
AT-like disorders, 49
biochemical defects, 235-249
brain, DNA recombination, 175-179
breast cancer, 113, 168
    BRCA1 gene, 127-132
    combined relative risk estimates, 143
    families, 127-128
    ovarian cancer family, 127
    risk, 22, 132-134, 137-140, 168
caffeine, 165
cancer. *See* malignancy
candidate genes
    ATDC, 14-17
    complementing cDNAs, 54
capping in A-T cells, 239-240
carcinogenesis, 164-168, 170
cardiac defects, 195-196
carrier detection, 101-116
    See also heterozygotes
CD3, increased expression, 239
cell cycle, 103-105, 163, 166, 247-248
    DNA damage, 163
    G1 arrest, 169
    G1 sensitivity, 243, 248
    G2 sensitivity, 219, 243, 248, 264
    RAD9, 168
    S-phase, 169, 264
    See also G2 assay
cell lines, 65, 118, 195
    Group A, 123
cell phase. *See* cell cycle
cell survival, 108
cellular abnormalities, 237
cerebellum, 176
cerebral cortex, 176
checkpoints. *See* cell cycle
chromosomal anomalies, 103, 169, 217-218, 242
chromosome
    damage, radiation-induced, 101, 243
    fragility. *See* chromosomal anomalies
    rearrangement, 155
    transfer, 159
classification. *See* variants

cloning
    complementation, 54-63, 64-73
    cosmids, 26-27
    EBV vector, 54, 60, 66
    Group D, 13, 17-19
clubbing, 201-203
coding joint, 149-150
complementation analysis, 65, 158, 167, 259
    Group A, 119, 123
consanguinity, 184-186, 191-192, 205
Costa Rica, 199-205
CpG density, 147
cytogenetics. *See* chromosome anomalies
cytoskeletal abnormalities
diabetes, 195, 270
dizziness, treatment of, 272-273
DNA
    chain elongation, 261
    double strand breaks, 155
    hairpins, 151
    repair, 258-259, 264-265
    replication, 144, 260-262
epidemiology
    Costa Rica, 199-206
    Italy, 191-197
    Turkey, 183-189
excision repair genes
    XRCC 2, 160
    XRCC 4, 160
families, A-T, 23, 184-186
fatigue, treatment of, 275
FISH. *See* fluorescent in situ hybridiation
fluorescent in situ hybridiation, 25, 29, 59, 159
frequency. *See* gene frequency or heterozygosity frequency
fusion, somatic cell, 158
    See also compelemntation analysis
G1 arrest, 169
G2 assay, 101-116, 103, 105, 219, 264
GADD45, 167
galactosidase, beta, 176-178
gamma irradiation, low dose rate, 102, 103, 117
gastic carcinoma, 193, 201
    See also malignancy
gene frequency, 22, 200
gene induction, 245
genetic heterogeneity, 41-45, 50, 210-227
genetic map, 17, 26, 28, 37, 159
genome stability, 148, 168
glia, 178
glutathione synthesis, 238
haplotype analysis, 39, 133
heterogeneity. *See* genetic heterogeneity
heterozygotes, 101-116, 263, 270
heterozygosity frequency, 22

hippocampus, 176
historical, 1-2, 39
Hodgkin disease. *See* malignancy
immune rearrangement, 155
immunodeficiency, 186-187, 203-204, 217, 241
    with hyperIgM, 184, 185, 195
    IgA deficiency, 205
    IgG2 deficiency, 205
immunoglobulin gene superfamily, 175
incidence. *See* frequency
initiation, 262
insertions. *See* chromosomal anomalies
Italy, 191-197
lacZ gene, 175-178
leukemia. *See* malignancy
libraries
    genomic, human, 8
    cDNA, 56, 66
linkage analyses, 22-25, 29, 31, 36, 50, 127-135, 185-187
localization of A-T gene(s)
    chromosome 11, 13, 16-17, 30, 127-135, 185-187, 212-
        213
    not chromosome 11, 91, 213
location scores, 30, 40
  See also localization
lod scores, 29, 39, 129-132
  See also localization and genetic map
lymphoblastoid cell lines. *See* cell lines
lymphocytes, 101, 147, 175-176
lymphoma, 168
    See also malignancy
malignancy, 1, 186-187, 193, 195-6, 201, 269
mammography, 137-140
map. *See* genetic map
maximum likelihood procedure, 43
membrane proteins/receptors, 239
mental retardation, 184-186
methylation, CpG, 145, 147-150
microcell hybrids, 76
microcephaly, 186-187
microfilaments in A-T, 239-240
Monte Carlo method, 40
mortality, 201
mutants
    AT-like, 90
    rodent, 86-96
NBS. *See* Nijmegen Breakage Syndrome
neocarzinostatin sensitivity, 67
neoplasm. *See* malignancy
Nijmegen Breakage Syndrome, 48, 158, 223-225
nucleocytomegaly, 1
oculomotor signs, 196, 216
orthopedic/rehabilitation, treatment, 270
p53, 124, 127, 164-168

PCR. *See* polymerase chain reaction
PKC. *See* protein kinase C
polymerase,
    DNA, 120
    chain reaction, 77
polymorphisms, genetic, 24, 26
    microsatellite markers, 129, 131-132
poly(ADP-ribose), 165
post-irradiation DNA synthesis, 157
protein activation, 245
protein kinase C, 124
psychological needs, 270
pulmonary disease, chronic, 201
radiation hybrid, 160
radiation sensitivity, 1, 261, 263-264
radiobiology of A-T, 257-265
radioresistant DNA synthesis, 89, 246, 259-263
    normal in A-T, 195-196, 219-223
radiosensitivity, 76, 79, 169, 242
    to Ara-C, 119
    G0 cells, 104
    G2 cells, 103, 105
radiotherapy, normal tissue response, 102
RDS. *See* radioresistant DNA snythesis
recombination, 144
    DNA, in brain, 175-179
    fraction. *See* lod scores
    mitotic, 57
    site specificity, 175-176
    V(D)J, 143-151, 155
repair
    AraC-detectable sites, 122
    of single strand breaks, 244
replication, 144
replicons, 261
    initiation, 262
reporter gene, 175-176
rescue, cDNA, 59
RFLP. *See* polymorphisms
rigidity, treatment of, 274
risk
    cancer, 133-134
    X-ray sensitivity, 137-140, 102, 263
    sun exposure, 269
    See also breast cancer risk
SCID
    cells, 155-161
    mouse, 149
sensitivity
    caffeine, 175
    G2, 219
    neocarzinostatin, 67
    streptonigrin, 56
    X-ray, 60, 67

signal joint, 149-150
signal sequences, 175, 178
signal transduction, 124
    pathway, 167
somatic cell hybridization
stomach cancer. *See* gastric carcinoma
strand breaks, 120
streptonigrin, 56
sun exposure, 269
suppression, secondary, 61
SV40, 169
telangiectasia, 202
    without ataxia, 48, 50, 186, 188, 217-219
topoisomerase, 244
transcription, 144
transfection, 8, 56, 66
    synchrony, 9
transformation, secondary, 59
    primary, 58
    secondary, 59
transgenic mice, 176-178
translocation, 143
    See also chromosomal anomalies
treatment, 269-276
tremor, treatment of, 270-271, 274
Turkey, 183-189
twitching, 275
variants, 45-49, 183-188, 191-197, 199-205, 209-227
    clinical, 47, 183
    laboratory, 47, 184-187, 195
    normal RDS, 195-196, 219-223
X-ray risk, 137-140

NATO ASI Series H

Vol. 1: Biology and Molecular Biology of Plant-Pathogen Interactions.
Edited by J.A. Bailey. 415 pages. 1986.

Vol. 2: Glial-Neuronal Communication in Development and Regeneration.
Edited by H.H. Althaus and W. Seifert. 865 pages. 1987.

Vol. 3: Nicotinic Acetylcholine Receptor: Structure and Function.
Edited by A. Maelicke. 489 pages. 1986.

Vol. 4: Recognition in Microbe-Plant Symbiotic and Pathogenic Interactions.
Edited by B. Lugtenberg. 449 pages. 1986.

Vol. 5: Mesenchymal-Epithelial Interactions in Neural Development.
Edited by J. R. Wolff, J. Sievers, and M. Berry. 428 pages. 1987.

Vol. 6: Molecular Mechanisms of Desensitization to Signal Molecules.
Edited by T M. Konijn, P J. M. Van Haastert, H. Van der Starre,
H. Van der Wel, and M.D. Houslay. 336 pages. 1987.

Vol. 7: Gangliosides and Modulation of Neuronal Functions.
Edited by H. Rahmann. 647 pages. 1987.

Vol. 8: Molecular and Cellular Aspects of Erythropoietin and Erythropoiesis.
Edited by I.N. Rich. 460 pages. 1987.

Vol. 9: Modification of Cell to Cell Signals During Normal and Pathological Aging.
Edited by S. Govoni and F Battaini. 297 pages. 1987.

Vol. 10: Plant Hormone Receptors. Edited by D. Klämbt. 319 pages. 1987.

Vol. 11: Host-Parasite Cellular and Molecular Interactions in Protozoal Infections.
Edited by K.-P. Chang and D. Snary. 425 pages. 1987.

Vol. 12: The Cell Surface in Signal Transduction.
Edited by E. Wagner, H. Greppin, and B. Millet. 243 pages. 1987.

Vol. 13: Toxicology of Pesticides: Experimental, Clinical and Regulatory
Perspectives. Edited by L.G. Costa, C.L. Galli, and S.D. Murphy.
320 pages. 1987.

Vol. 14: Genetics of Translation. New Approaches.
Edited by M.F. Tuite, M. Picard, and M. Bolotin-Fukuhara. 524 pages. 1988.

Vol. 15: Photosensitisation. Molecular, Cellular and Medical Aspects.
Edited by G. Moreno, R. H. Pottier, and T. G. Truscott. 521 pages. 1988.

Vol. 16: Membrane Biogenesis. Edited by J.A.F Op den Kamp. 477 pages. 1988.

Vol. 17: Cell to Cell Signals in Plant, Animal and Microbial Symbiosis.
Edited by S. Scannerini, D. Smith, P. Bonfante-Fasolo, and V. Gianinazzi-
Pearson. 414 pages. 1988.

Vol. 18: Plant Cell Biotechnology.
Edited by M.S.S. Pais, F. Mavituna, and J. M. Novais. 500 pages. 1988.

Vol. 19: Modulation of Synaptic Transmission and Plasticity in Nervous Systems.
Edited by G. Hertting and H.-C. Spatz. 457 pages. 1988.

Vol. 20: Amino Acid Availability and Brain Function in Health and Disease.
Edited by G. Huether. 487 pages. 1988.

NATO ASI Series H

Vol. 21: Cellular and Molecular Basis of Synaptic Transmission.
Edited by H. Zimmermann. 547 pages. 1988.

Vol. 22: Neural Development and Regeneration. Cellular and Molecular Aspects.
Edited by A. Gorio, J. R. Perez-Polo, J. de Vellis, and B. Haber. 711 pages.
1988.

Vol. 23: The Semiotics of Cellular Communication in the Immune System.
Edited by E.E. Sercarz, F. Celada, N.A. Mitchison, and T. Tada. 326 pages.
1988.

Vol. 24: Bacteria, Complement and the Phagocytic Cell.
Edited by F. C. Cabello und C. Pruzzo. 372 pages. 1988.

Vol. 25: Nicotinic Acetylcholine Receptors in the Nervous System.
Edited by F. Clementi, C. Gotti, and E. Sher. 424 pages. 1988.

Vol. 26: Cell to Cell Signals in Mammalian Development.
Edited by S.W de Laat, J.G. Bluemink, and C.L. Mummery. 322 pages.
1989.

Vol. 27: Phytotoxins and Plant Pathogenesis.
Edited by A. Graniti, R. D. Durbin, and A. Ballio. 508 pages. 1989.

Vol. 28: Vascular Wilt Diseases of Plants. Basic Studies and Control.
Edited by E. C. Tjamos and C. H. Beckman. 590 pages. 1989.

Vol. 29: Receptors, Membrane Transport and Signal Transduction.
Edited by A. E. Evangelopoulos, J. P. Changeux, L. Packer, T. G.
Sotiroudis, and K.W.A. Wirtz. 387 pages. 1989.

Vol. 30: Effects of Mineral Dusts on Cells.
Edited by B.T. Mossman and R.O. Begin. 470 pages. 1989.

Vol. 31: Neurobiology of the Inner Retina.
Edited by R. Weiler and N.N. Osborne. 529 pages. 1989.

Vol. 32: Molecular Biology of Neuroreceptors and Ion Channels.
Edited by A. Maelicke. 675 pages. 1989.

Vol. 33: Regulatory Mechanisms of Neuron to Vessel Communication in Brain.
Edited by F. Battaini, S. Govoni, M.S. Magnoni, and M. Trabucchi.
416 pages. 1989.

Vol. 34: Vectors asTools for the Study of Normal and Abnormal Growth and
Differentiation.
Edited by H. Lother, R. Dernick, and W. Ostertag. 477 pages. 1989.

Vol. 35: Cell Separation in Plants: Physiology, Biochemistry and Molecular
Biology. Edited by D. J. Osborne and M. B. Jackson. 449 pages. 1989.

Vol. 36: Signal Molecules in Plants and Plant-Microbe Interactions.
Edited by B.J.J. Lugtenberg. 425 pages. 1989.

Vol. 37: Tin-Based Antitumour Drugs. Edited by M. Gielen. 226 pages. 1990.

NATO ASI Series H

Vol. 38: The Molecular Biology of Autoimmune Disease.
Edited by A.G. Demaine, J-P. Banga, and A.M. McGregor. 404 pages.
1990.

Vol. 39: Chemosensory Information Processing.
Edited by D. Schild. 403 pages. 1990.

Vol. 40: Dynamics and Biogenesis of Membranes.
Edited by J. A. F. Op den Kamp. 367 pages. 1990.

Vol. 41: Recognition and Response in Plant-Virus Interactions.
Edited by R. S. S. Fraser. 467 pages. 1990.

Vol. 42: Biomechanics of Active Movement and Deformation of Cells.
Edited by N. Akkas. 524 pages. 1990.

Vol. 43: Cellular and Molecular Biology of Myelination.
Edited by G. Jeserich, H. H. Althaus, and T. V. Waehneldt. 565 pages.
1990.

Vol. 44: Activation and Desensitization of Transducing Pathways.
Edited by T. M. Konijn, M. D. Houslay, and P. J. M. Van Haastert.
336 pages. 1990.

Vol. 45: Mechanism of Fertilization: Plants to Humans.
Edited by B. Dale. 710 pages. 1990.

Vol .46: Parallels in Cell to Cell Junctions in Plants and Animals.
Edited by A. W Robards, W. J . Lucas, J . D. Pitts, H . J . Jongsma,
and D. C. Spray. 296 pages. 1990.

Vol. 47: Signal Perception and Transduction in Higher Plants.
Edited by R. Ranjeva and A. M. Boudet. 357 pages. 1990.

Vol. 48: Calcium Transport and Intracellular Calcium Homeostasis.
Edited by D. Pansu and F. Bronner. 456 pages. 1990.

Vol. 49: Post-Transcriptional Control of Gene Expression.
Edited by J. E. G. McCarthy and M. F. Tuite. 671 pages. 1990.

Vol. 50: Phytochrome Properties and Biological Action.
Edited by B. Thomas and C. B. Johnson. 337 pages. 1991.

Vol. 51: Cell to Cell Signals in Plants and Animals.
Edited by V. Neuhoff and J. Friend. 404 pages. 1991.

Vol. 52: Biological Signal Transduction.
Edited by E. M . Ross and K . W. A. Wirtz. 560 pages. 1991.

Vol. 53: Fungal Cell Wall and Immune Response.
Edited by J. P. Latge and D. Boucias. 472 pages. 1991.

Vol. 54: The Early Effects of Radiation on DNA.
Edited by E. M. Fielden and P. O'Neill. 448 pages. 1991.

Vol. 55: The Translational Apparatus of Photosynthetic Organelles.
Edited by R. Mache, E. Stutz, and A. R. Subramanian. 260 pages. 1991.

NATO ASI Series H

Vol. 56: Cellular Regulation by Protein Phosphorylation.
Edited by L. M. G. Heilmeyer, Jr. 520 pages. 1991.

Vol. 57: Molecular Techniques in Taxonomy.
Edited by G . M . Hewitt, A. W. B. Johnston, and J. P. W. Young .
420 pages. 1991.

Vol. 58: Neurocytochemical Methods.
Edited by A. Calas and D. Eugene. 352 pages. 1991.

Vol. 59: Molecular Evolution of the Major Histocompatibility Complex.
Edited by J. Klein and D. Klein. 522 pages. 1991.

Vol. 60: Intracellular Regulation of Ion Channels.
Edited by M. Morad and Z. Agus. 261 pages. 1992.

Vol. 61: Prader-Willi Syndrome and Other Chromosome 15q Deletion Disorders.
Edited by S. B. Cassidy. 277 pages. 1992.

Vol. 62: Endocytosis. From Cell Biology to Health, Disease and Therapie.
Edited by P. J. Courtoy. 547 pages. 1992.

Vol. 63: Dynamics of Membrane Assembly.
Edited by J. A. F. Op den Kamp. 402 pages. 1992.

Vol. 64: Mechanics of Swelling. From Clays to Living Cells and Tissues.
Edited by T. K. Karalis. 802 pages. 1992.

Vol. 65: Bacteriocins, Microcins and Lantibiotics.
Edited by R. James, C. Lazdunski, and F. Pattus. 530 pages. 1992.

Vol. 66: Theoretical and Experimental Insights into Immunology.
Edited by A. S. Perelson and G. Weisbuch. 497 pages. 1992.

Vol. 67: Flow Cytometry. New Developments.
Edited by A. Jacquemin-Sablon. 1993.

Vol. 68: Biomarkers. Research and Application in the Assessment of
Environmental Health. Edited by D. B. Peakall and L. R. Shugart.
138 pages. 1993.

Vol. 69: Molecular Biology and its Application to Medical Mycology.
Edited by B. Maresca, G. S. Kobayashi, and H. Yamaguchi. 271 pages.
1993.

Vol. 70: Phospholipids and Signal Transmission.
Edited by R. Massarelli, L. A. Horrocks, J. N. Kanfer, and K. Löffelholz.
448 pages. 1993.

Vol. 71: Protein Synthesis and Targeting in Yeast.
Edited by A. J. P. Brown, M. F. Tuite, and J. E. G. McCarthy. 425 pages.
1993.

Vol. 72: Chromosome Segregation and Aneuploidy.
Edited by B. K. Vig. 425 pages. 1993.

NATO ASI Series H

Vol. 73: Human Apolipoprotein Mutants III. In Diagnosis and Treatment.
Edited by C. R. Sirtori, G. Franceschini, B. H. Brewer Jr. 302 pages. 1993.

Vol. 74: Molecular Mechanisms of Membrane Traffic.
Edited by D. J. Morré, K. E. Howell, and J. J. M. Bergeron. 429 pages.
1993.

Vol. 75: Cancer Therapy. Differentiation, Immunomodulation and Angiogenesis.
Edited by N. D'Alessandro, E. Mihich, L. Rausa, H. Tapiero, and T. R.Tritton.
299 pages. 1993.

Vol. 76: Tyrosine Phosphorylation/Dephosphorylation and Downstream Signalling.
Edited by L. M. G. Heilmeyer Jr. 388 pages. 1993.

Vol. 77: Ataxia-Telangiectasia. Edited by R. A. Gatti, R. B. Painter. 306 pages. 1993.